Population Dynamics of Rabies in Wildlife

Contributors

P. J. Bacon

Frank G. Ball

L. H. Broekhoven

Andrew B. Carey

C. O. R. Everard

J. D. Everard

C. Kaplan

Kari Kuulasmaa

David W. Macdonald

B. G. Mansourian

Denis Mollison

A. Jane Ross

P. Saengcharoenrat

B. McA. Sayers

A. D. M. Smith

R. R. Tinline

Dennis R. Voigt

Population Dynamics of Rabies in Wildlife

Edited by

PHILIP J. BACON

Institute of Terrestrial Ecology
Merlewood Research Station
Grange-over-Sands, Cumbria, England

1985

ACADEMIC PRESS

Harcourt Brace Jovanovich, Publishers

London Orlando San Diego New York Austin
Montreal Sydney Tokyo Toronto

ACADEMIC PRESS INC. (LONDON) LTD.
24–28 Oval Road
LONDON NW1 7DX

United States Edition published by
ACADEMIC PRESS, INC.
Orlando, Florida 32887

British Library Cataloguing in Publication Data

Population dynamics of rabies in wildlife.
  1. Rabies—Mathematical models 2. Animals
  as carriers of disease—Mathematical models
  I. Bacon, Philip J.
  614.5'63   RC148

Library of Congress Cataloging in Publication Data
Main entry under title:

Population dynamics of rabies in wildlife.

  Includes index.
  1. Rabies. 2. Rabies—Prevention. 3. Wildlife
diseases. 4. Vector control. 5. Veterinary epidemiology.
6. Rabies—Mathematical models. 7. Rabies—Prevention—
Mathematical models. 8. Wildlife diseases—Mathematical
models. 9. Vector control—Mathematical models.
10. Veterinary epidemiology—Mathematical models.
I. Bacon, Philip J.
SF797.P66 1985   636.089'4563   84-28216
ISBN 0-12-071350-0 (alk. paper)
ISBN 0-12-071351-9 (paperback)

PRINTED IN THE UNITED STATES OF AMERICA

85 86 87 88   9 8 7 6 5 4 3 2 1

Dedicated to the memory of Dr. Franz Steck, one of the pioneers of the successful Swiss campaign for the oral immunisation of wild foxes against rabies, who was tragically killed in a helicopter accident during the early field trial years of the project.

Contents

3   Mongoose Rabies in Grenada

C. O. R. Everard and J. D. Everard

4   The Biological Basis of Rabies Models

David W. Macdonald and Dennis R. Voigt

5   A Systems Analysis of Wildlife Rabies Epizootics

P. J. Bacon

6 A Continuous Time Deterministic Model of Temporal Rabies

A. D. M. Smith

7 Discrete Time Temporal Models of Rabies

P. J. Bacon

8 Spatial Models for the Spread and Control of Rabies Incorporating Group Size

Frank G. Ball

9 Sensitivity Analysis of Simple Endemic Models

Denis Mollison

10 Pattern Analysis of the Case Occurrences of Fox Rabies in Europe

B. McA. Sayers, A. Jane Ross, P. Saengcharoenrat and B. G. Mansourian

Contributors

Numbers in parentheses indicate the pages on which the authors' contributions begin.

P. J. Bacon (109, 147), Institute of Terrestrial Ecology, Merlewood Research Station, Grange-over-Sands, Cumbria LA11 6JU, England

Frank G. Ball[1] (197, 255), Department of Biomathematics, University of Oxford, Oxford OX1 3UB, England

L. H. Broekhoven (311), Department of Mathematics and Statistics, Queen's University, Kingston, Ontario, Canada K7L 3N6

Andrew B. Carey (23), Forest Service, United States Department of Agriculture, Olympia, Washington, U.S.A. 98502

C. O. R. Everard (43), Leptospirosis Laboratory, Medical Research Council, The Pine, St Michael, Barbados

J. D. Everard (43), Leptospirosis Laboratory, Medical Research Council, The Pine, St Michael, Barbados

C. Kaplan (1), Department of Microbiology, University of Reading, Reading RG1 5AQ, England

Kari Kuulasmaa[2] (291), Department of Actuarial Mathematics and Statistics, Heriot-Watt University, Riccarton, Edinburgh EH14 4AS, Scotland

David W. Macdonald (71), Department of Zoology, University of Oxford, Oxford OX1 3PS, England

B. G. Mansourian (235), World Health Organization, Geneva 1211, Switzerland

Denis Mollison (223, 291), Department of Actuarial Mathematics and Statistics, Heriot-Watt University, Riccarton, Edinburgh EH14 4AS, Scotland

A. Jane Ross (235), Department of Electrical Engineering, Imperial College, London SW7 2BT, England

[1]Present address: Department of Mathematics, University of Nottingham, University Park, Nottingham NG7 2RD, England.

[2]Present address: National Public Health Institute, Mannerheimintie 166, SF-00280 Helsinki, Finland.

P. Saengcharoenrat (235), Department of Electrical Engineering, Imperial College, London SW7 2BT, England

B. McA. Sayers (235), Department of Electrical Engineering, Imperial College, London SW7 2BT, England

A. D. M. Smith[3] (131), Centre for Environmental Technology, Imperial College, London SW7 2BT, England

R. R. Tinline (311), Department of Geography, Queen's University, Kingston, Ontario, Canada K7L 3N6

Dennis R. Voigt (71, 311), Wildlife Branch, Ontario Ministry of Natural Resources, Maple, Ontario, Canada L0J 1E0

[3]Present address: Department of Zoology, University of Adelaide, Adelaide, South Australia, Australia 5001.

Preface

Rabies has been known and feared as a killer disease for over 2000 years. Its association with 'mad dogs' has also been understood since then, although it was not until the early nineteenth century that it was shown that the disease was passed from one animal to another and did not arise, spontaneously, during inclement weather. By the end of the nineteenth century a vaccine had been developed, but it often had serious side effects and was painful to receive. During the last few decades great strides have been made in vaccine development so that, in the developed nations, the disease has lost much of its aura. However, its associations with the stigma of madness (the faithful pet that turns on its owner), the horrifying symptoms in man and the inevitability of death once symptoms appear maintain the awesome image of the disease. In developing countries the disease is still a very serious problem. It is estimated to cause at least 15,000 human deaths annually, and the economic losses of cattle in Latin America alone cost around U.S. $250,000,000 directly and U.S. $250,000,000,000 indirectly a year. In the poorer developing nations, the lack of diagnosis and high costs of the effective vaccines prevent treatment in man, whereas, in the richer nations, vaccination of domestic animals, especially dogs, cats and livestock, has reduced the disease to a minor problem, predominantly in wild animals. Even so, the fear of rabies is so great that about 99% of all 'post-exposure' treatments are probably unnecessary, and this, plus the losses of cattle (or cost of immunising them), makes the disease expensive even to developed countries.

During the last hundred years or so the role that wildlife plays in rabies outbreaks has become clear, and the qualitative observations indicating that the disease did not spread in areas where its wild hosts were rare led to the expectation that killing the hosts would eliminate the disease. In practice this qualitative expectation has not been realised, and it is now widely accepted that attempts to control rabies on a wide scale by killing the wild host populations have generally proved both costly and ineffective (although there has been some success in containing local outbreaks and rigorous quarantine has been most effective for protecting isolated 'islands'). These failures arise because the control measures are not able to reduce the host populations to a low enough level for a sufficiently long period for the disease to die out, but the detailed circumstances allowing the disease to persist are not clearly understood. The failure of such qualitative control policies led to the development of quantitative attempts to assess chances of disease spread and persistence. The aim of this book is to show how biologists, veterinarians and mathematicians have collaborated to elucidate the mechanisms underlying rabies epidemics, with a view to formulating better control measures.

The book was envisaged as a case study of the practical application of mathematics to biology. As such it aims both to explain the mathematics in simple terms that non-mathematical biologists can follow (albeit with some effort) and also to give enough biological and ecological background information so that mathematicians with no knowledge of these subjects will be able to appreciate adequately the assumptions underlying the mathematical approximations that are used. Accordingly, the first chapter gives the medical, virological and epidemiological information needed to set the scene of rabies as a world health hazard and the various mechanisms by which it spreads. The next three chapters deal with the ecologies of various communities of hosts: the multi-species host complex in the United States; the single mongoose host on Grenada; and a contrast between the 'fox' rabies epizootics in Canada and Europe, relating these to the different environments. The fifth chapter attempts to digest some of the previous information into general concepts that can be of use when considering mathematical models of the processes and indicates some of the practical difficulties likely to be encountered. The remaining chapters describe a variety of different models (concise explicit *simplified* descriptions) of rabies. Chapters 6 and 7 consider only epizootics in time, ignoring spatial and stochastic factors, but showing how the main aspects of the disease will affect the nature of its outbreaks. As a contrast, Chapter 8 concentrates on aspects ignored by the previous models and produces a system based on social groupings of hosts, stochastic infections and spatial spread. Chapter 9 investigates the structures of simple models and shows clearly how some predictions of a model are robust, depending on accurately known parameters, whereas others may be highly sensitive to qualitative assumptions incorporated into the models' 'faute de mieux'. Chapters 10 and 11 provide yet another change of tack and describe the fitting of analytical statistical models to data on rabies spread in Europe. These analyses elucidate the underlying patterns and thereby attempt to uncover factors affecting the course of the outbreaks. Chapter 12 considers spatial epidemics with respect of mathematical approaches especially developed for such studies and indicates alternative routes, whereby rather similar effects can be produced. Finally, Chapter 13 presents a most interesting 'hybrid' model that is based both on 'rules' of host social behaviours and mathematical descriptions of disease and on host population processes.

This book does not intend to give 'definitive answers', far less to present 'ultimate' models of how rabies spreads and persists in the real world. It is hoped, however, that readers of the book will come to appreciate how such understanding can be achieved and will be better able to assess the strengths and weaknesses of these, and similar, models. If it achieves this, the book will have served its main purpose; if it should also contribute, in some small way, to the practical control of wildlife rabies, this will be a bonus, but a very welcome one.

Cumbria   *Philip J. Bacon*
September 1985

Rabies: A Worldwide Disease

1

C. Kaplan
Department of Microbiology,
University of Reading,
Reading, England

I. Introduction

Since the end of the Second World War, there has undoubtedly been a secular increase in the incidence of rabies, which cannot be ascribed entirely either to improvements in diagnostic methods or to increased scientific interest in the disease. This increased incidence has been most notable in Europe, where, as in North America, cases are reported and registered more efficiently than in many other parts of the world. With the exception of areas such as Europe, North America and parts of Africa and Asia Minor, the lack of adequate statistics—especially in developing countries—means that the true worldwide incidence of the disease can only be guessed at. Even in those countries with good statistical services for both human and animal health, the incidence of rabies in wildlife must be estimated from the cases recognized among wildlife—certainly fewer than the (unknown) numbers actually occurring in populations of an unknown size. There are many problems to be resolved in the quantitative study of rabies.

The disease has been recognized for more than 2000 years. The Greek physician, Hippocrates, described the condition as it occurs in man, and it was clearly understood in his period that clinical symptoms in human beings were related to previous attacks by mad dogs. It was widely believed for many years (and as late as the third quarter of the nineteenth century) that rabies could occur spontaneously in dogs as a result of, for example, weather conditions. The 'dog days' of summer were felt to contribute to the causation of rabies in some unspecified way. Zincke, in 1804, passed the disease from a rabid dog to a healthy one by contaminating superficial skin incisions in the healthy animal with saliva from the diseased beast. Other observations were made during the nineteenth century on the infectious nature of rabies, especially by Rey and other members of the veterinary school at Lyons from about 1840 onwards.

Louis Pasteur (Pasteur *et al.*, 1882) showed that many of the reputed demonstrations of an infectious agent in the saliva of rabid animals were fallacious but that, nevertheless, an agent was present in such saliva that could transmit the disease. The results of his investigations suggested very strongly that the brain and spinal cord were closely involved in the development of the disease. He showed that the disease could be induced by inoculating material from the brains of rabid dogs into the brains of healthy dogs, and pointed out the advantages in using this method for experiments. Infection of healthy animals was far more certain than after inoculation with saliva, and the incubation period was reduced to 1 or 2 weeks. Pasteur used dried spinal cords of infected rabbits to prepare a vaccine for the treatment of victims of dog bites after the attack but before the appearance of symptoms.

Pasteur called the virus that he isolated from rabid dogs *le virus des rues* (street virus). He infected a rabbit by inoculating this virus directly into the brain (intracerebral inoculation). The infection was then passed successively from rabbit to rabbit by intracerebral inoculation of brain material. During this process (known as *passage*), the incubation period, originally predictable only within very wide limits, became shorter and eventually established itself at 8 or 9 days. Because of this relatively fixed incubation period Pasteur called his adapted strain *virus fixe* (fixed virus). These terms are still used to distinguish between strains freshly isolated from clinical cases of rabies in animals and strains adapted to replication in the brains of experimental animals. Fixed viruses are highly neurotropic (see Section II), a fact that has important implications for the interpretation of the results of certain types of experimental infection.

II. The Virus

A. RABIES VIRUS

Rabies virus is the prototype of the Lyssavirus subgroup of the very large group of Rhabdoviruses, the name of which is derived from the Greek word *rhabdos,* a rod. The viruses of this group are cylindrical with one end flattened and the other rounded or conical, making them what has been described as 'bullet shaped'. On average, the virus particles or virions of rabies are 180 nm long by 75 nm wide, plus the size (about 8 nm) of the numerous fine projections from the surface of the virion. The projections are not present at the flattened end of the virion (Sokol *et al.,* 1968). The published measurements of rabies virions refer to strains of fixed virus.

Purified preparations of rabies virus have been subjected to morphological, biochemical and immunological analysis. Hamparian *et al.* (1963) and Kissling and Reeve (1963) showed that it contained ribonucleic acid (RNA). The projections or 'spikes' consist of glycoprotein. When separated and purified glycoprotein is injected into experimental animals, it stimulates the production of antibody able to neutralize the infectivity of rabies virus (Crick and Brown, 1970). Other structural components of the virus are also antigenic, but appear to have no direct involvement in the stimulation of virus neutralizing or protective antibody.

During the replication in the central nervous systems, the pathological appearances that rabies virus induces are, with one exception, not specific. The exception is 'the *Negri body*' described in 1903 by Negri. The Negri body is an eosinophilic (red-staining) inclusion found in neurones of subjects infected with street virus. The presence of Negri bodies is not invariable, but when present (in about 85% in cases) they make the diagnosis of rabies certain. Negri thought that his inclusions were protozoan parasites—the cause of rabies. In this he was wrong, but the nature of the Negri body remained elusive until Miyamoto and Matsumoto (1965) showed clearly that the Negri body seen by light microscopy was identical with the amorphous matrix (visible by electron microscopy) that is present in the brains of animals infected with street virus. The matrix consists of material that condenses at its edge and is assembled into virions (virus particles), which leave the infected cell by budding from the cell membrane (see Fig. 1).

B. RABIES-RELATED VIRUSES

The members of the Rhabdovirus group that infect animals have been divided on morphological and morphogenetic grounds into the vesicular stomatitis and Rabies subgroups. The rabies subgroup contains four viruses which are morphologically similar and serologically related and two which are morphologically distinguishable but are serologically related. The viruses that are serologically

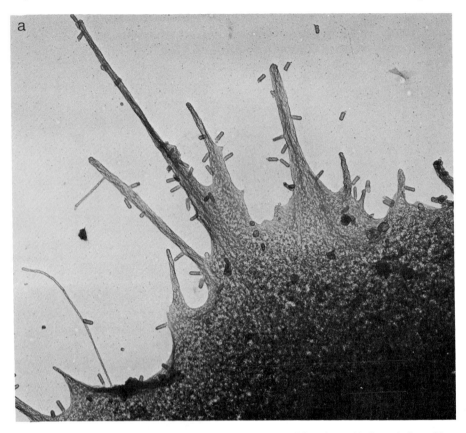

Fig. 1. Virus particles budding from an infected nerve cell in culture. (a) General view. (b) Highly magnified, showing typical bullet-shaped virions. (Reproduced by kind permission of Dr. Yuzo Iwasaki.)

related to rabies virus are Mokola (Shope *et al.*, 1970), Lagos bat (Boulger and Porterfield, 1958) and Duvenhage (Meredith *et al.*, 1971).

Nigerian horse virus, isolated by Porterfield *et al.* (1958) from a horse with 'staggers' is probably also related serologically to rabies virus (Dr. G. S. Turner, personal communication). The serologically unrelated viruses, Obodhiang (Schmidt *et al.*, 1965) and Kotonkan (Kemp *et al.*, 1970), were isolated from midges and mosquitoes, respectively, and fortunately they do not cause neurological disease. In Africa, there is thus a group of viruses more or less closely related to rabies virus antigenically, several of which cause neurological symptoms in infected animals and in human beings. At least one of this group, Duvenhage virus, has caused a clinical syndrome in man that is indistinguishable from rabies.

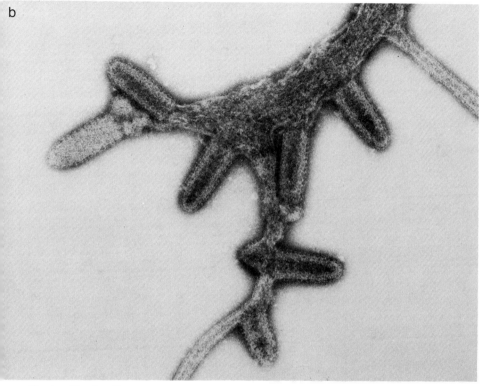

b

Fig. 1. (*Continued.*)

C. OULOU FATO

Oulou fato, which has been described as a non-fatal disease of dogs in West Africa caused either by a rabies virus of reduced virulence or by a rabies-related virus, has been shown by Remlinger (1933) to be a form of dumb rabies caused by a virus indistinguishable from the classical rabies virus. Dogs with this disease are quite capable of transmitting fatal rabies to other animals and man by their bites.

III. Pathogenesis of the Infection

For a long time after the unequivocal demonstration of the infectious nature of rabies, the mechanism by which the agent caused the symptoms and signs of the disease (the pathogenesis) was not understood. Although the general picture of the pathogenesis of rabies is now clear (Murphy *et al.*, 1973), the nature of the damage (or lesion) in neurones, which causes the behavioural changes so important in the disease, has not been elucidated. Rabies is caused by the rabies virus invading and multiplying in the central nervous system of the victim. All warm-blooded animals are susceptible, and it is widely accepted that once an infected animal develops the clinical symptoms of rabies it will inevitably die. (This is not to say, however, that every infected animal necessarily develops symptoms; for further discussion of this, see below.) In general, animals with rabies show one of the two main forms of the disease. The excited or *furious form* is regarded by many as typical of the infection, but a significant proportion of diseased animals suffers from the paralytic or *dumb form* of the disease. Animals with dumb rabies are infectious and able to transmit fatal infections. Even in the furious form, however, paralysis supervenes sooner or later and the animal (or human patient) dies from respiratory failure or from the paralysis of some other vital function.

In the infectious animal, the virus is excreted in the saliva and frequently in the urine. Salivary virus is by far the more important in the spread of the disease, but urine may play a part in some special situations. The animal with the furious form of the disease attacks other animals, man and even inanimate objects without provocation. An important feature of rabies is that animals normally wary of contact with man, e.g. foxes, lose their fear and approach and even enter human habitations and farm buildings. Crepuscular and nocturnal animals may exhibit considerable activity during daylight. Behaviour generally becomes very abnormal. The bite of such an infected and abnormally behaving animal can cause considerable tissue damage with consequent risk of relatively large areas of tissue being exposed to rabies virus in the saliva.

The primary site of virus replication in the newly infected animal is muscle. The virus enters nerve endings from infected muscle cells. When it is within a nerve, the virus ascends in the axoplasm, probably being carried passively by the movement of the fluids. Judging from immunohistological studies, the amount of virus is amplified at staging posts on its journey to the central nervous system by replication in, e.g. the neuronal cells of posterior root ganglia of the spinal cord. When it reaches the central nervous system, the virus is further amplified by stepwise multiplication in neurones of the spinal cord before passing to the next nerve fibre in the chain carrying it to the brain.

In the brain, the virus is generalized, infecting cells throughout the brain, but clinical signs of disease do not appear until the virus has been through several cycles of replication. Particularly important in the development of the disease picture is the involvement of cells in vital centres in the brain stem and also the cells of the limbic system. The limbic system, comprising interconnected collections of neurones known as nuclei, lies in the older part of the forebrain and is closely associated with the expression of emotion. The furiously rabid animal expresses rage by attacking and biting freely. Saliva and virus are deposited in the wounds it has made, thus starting the cycle of infection and disease again.

Because of the large number of neurones available in the brain, the virus undergoes considerable multiplication. It enters efferent nerves of all types—sensory, motor and autonomic or involuntary—and moves outwards from the brain to virtually all organs and tissues of the body, including, of course, the salivary glands where further multiplication occurs in infected glandular cells. The greatest concentration of virus is found in those organs with the richest nerve supply. This information has been exploited by the development of diagnostic tests, which can be made during the course of the disease by, e.g. immunofluorescent examination of histological sections of skin biopsy samples for the presence of rabies antigen (Smith et al., 1972).

The *incubation period* between the infecting bite and the appearance of symptoms is variable and may be very long. In dogs, it is generally between 2 and 6 weeks, but there are reliably documented cases of periods of more than 6 months. In man, an incubation period between 6 weeks and 3 months is common, but some authentic incubations of more than 1 year have been recorded. In man and animals, the incubation period and, indeed, the outcome of the attack in terms of development of clinical disease is related to the part of the body affected by the attacking animal and by the amount of virus deposited in the wound. Wounds of head, neck and upper or forelimbs tend to be followed by shorter incubation periods than wounds of the lower trunk or posterior part of the body and the lower or hind limbs. The increased incubation periods associated with infection of lower or hind limb wounds may be related to the rate at which the virus progesses in nerves and the distance from the entry wound to the central nervous system. Experiments in several species of animal with fixed viruses indicate a rate in nerves of about 3 mm per hour. The street virus, however, has a slower and more variable rate of progression (Baer et al., 1968). Experiments have also shown that while fixed virus moves from the inoculation site within a few hours, the street virus may remain there for many days after the initiation of infection. This difference may be related to the *neurotropism of fixed viruses,* as compared to the much wider range of cell types in which the street virus will grow. The neurotropism of fixed viruses can be demonstrated by assaying, e.g. a preparation of a vaccine strain by the intracerebral and intramuscular routes of inoculation in two groups of similar mice. The assay determines the dose of virus which kills one-half of an adequate number of test animals. This is the 50% lethal dose, or LD_{50}. By the intramuscular route, the LD_{50} will be up to 1000 times greater than by the intracerebral route.

Infection, i.e. the entry of viruses into the body of a susceptible animal, is not invariably followed by the appearance of clinical disease. Some infections in some animals may be *inapparent.* Andral and Serié (1957) found antibodies to rabies in stray dogs caught in Addis Ababa. Tierkel (1959) reported the presence of rabies antibodies in 12/24 apparently healthy foxes captured in an area where rabies was enzootic. Unfortunately, neither Andral and Serié nor Tierkel had facilities to hold their animals in quarantine for long enough to see whether or not they would develop clinical rabies.

Raccoons captured in the wild developed antibodies in captivity without developing clinical signs of rabies (McLean, 1972). This suggests that infection without subsequent disease may occur in nature. Veeraraghavan and others (1967) reported the case of a dog that bit a man and gave him rabies without the dog having shown any symptoms itself. The dog was kept in quarantine at the Pasteur Institute of South India for 37 months and 23 days. During the first 32 months, 913 samples of saliva were examined, and rabies virus was isolated 14 times. Subsequently, 131 samples of saliva were examined by animal inoculation and immunofluorescence; 14 were positive by immunofluorescence but none by animal inoculation. This suggests the presence of rabies virus antigens but not of infectious viruses. The dog died without ever having exhibited the symptoms of rabies. Rabies antigen was demonstrated in its brain by immunofluorescent microscopy, but no infectious virus was isolated (Veeraraghavan et al., 1970). There are also, from time to time, anecdotal reports of dogs without signs of disease being infectious for rabies. On balance, it is not improbable that such cases occur more frequently than adequately documented reports suggest. If infection with rabies virus were invariably fatal the disease would be in a clinical category virtually of its own. Even pneumonic plague in man, which is probably the most lethal infectious disease known to medicine and may in small populations achieve a case fatality rate of 100%, does not regularly kill all those infected in an epidemic outbreak.

There is a reasonable amount of evidence, both clinical and experimental, that animals may, after infection, develop symptoms of rabies and yet recover—some, albeit, with residual neurological damage (Johnson, 1948; Bell et al., 1971). Hattwick et al. (1972) have recorded what must be accepted as an authentic recovery from paralytic rabies in a child. Infectious diseases may become chronic, when symptoms and excretion of the agent occur for long periods, or they may become latent, when signs of both clinical disease and agent are absent, but both may become apparent when the infection is reactivated. Herpes simplex (cold sores or fever blisters) is a typical example of this type of infection. Because of the irregular and possibly long incubation period in naturally occurring rabies and after experimental introduction of street virus and because antibody may be produced before an animal becomes infectious, it is difficult to establish firmly that rabies in an animal was the result of reactivation of a latent infection. But because the nervous system is intimately involved in some of the commoner latent infections, the possibility of this type of infection occurring with rabies cannot be dismissed simply because of the difficulty of establishing it firmly.

IV. Epidemiology of Rabies

Epidemiology is the study of the distribution and determinants of disease. The epidemiology of rabies clearly depends on the spread of viruses from infected to susceptible subjects. The virus is spread predominantly by the transfer of saliva from the infected animal to the bite wound on its victim. The aerial route is important in naturally occurring infection only in circumscribed areas, such as caves heavily populated with infected bats. Infection with rabies virus does not invariably cause disease, and the appearance of clinical symptoms of rabies may, possibly, not be an invariable precursor of death. These aspects of rabies have not been quantified and, indeed, in naturally occurring rabies would be very difficult to quantify. This must, therefore, introduce a degree of uncertainty into the quantitative study of the disease, but it is considerably less than the uncertainty that exists because the information available about rabies in wildlife is incomplete.

Although all warm-blooded animals are susceptible to infection with rabies virus, some are more apt than others to spread the virus, and some species are more susceptible than others (Table I).

Those most likely to act as vectors are animals whose natural offensive or defensive activity is biting. In general, rabid herbivores, although infectious

TABLE I

Susceptibility of Animals to Infection with Rabies Virus Based on LD_{50} by the Intramuscular Route[a]

Very high[b]	High[b]	Moderate[b]	Low
Foxes	Hamsters	Dogs	Opossums
Coyotes	Skunks	Nonhuman primates	
Kangaroo Rats	Raccoons		
Cotton Rats	Domestic cats		
Field Voles	Bats		
	Bobcats		
	Guinea pigs		
	Rabbits		
	Cattle		

[a] Derived from information in the Sixth Report of the WHO Expert Committee on Rabies (1973).

[b] Epidemiological evidence suggests that jackals and wolves are very highly, mongooses and other viverridae highly, and sheep, goats and horses moderately susceptible.

because of the virus in their saliva, are very seldom responsible for the spread of the disease to fresh subjects. The animals most frequently reported as sources of exposure for man are dogs and cats and for herbivores are foxes, bats and dogs, but the picture is different in different parts of the world. In different environments, although the cause of rabies (the virus) remains the same, both distribution and other determinants may vary widely. Probably no other disease that has been extensively studied shows such differences as does rabies. These differences exist because of the large number of species able to spread the infection and the diverse ways they interact with their environments. In short, the epidemiology of rabies depends heavily on the ecology of the species involved in its propagation.

A. IMPORTANCE OF DOGS

Under some circumstances, dogs may be the most important animals in the rabies cycle. Rabies was present in Britain for centuries before it was eradicated in 1903. It seems to have been largely a disease of dogs and, less frequently, cats. In the nineteenth century, there was a high incidence of rabies in British dogs with a consequent relatively large annual number of human deaths from the disease. Dog rabies was not confined to the towns. Country dogs were also involved, but there is no good evidence that carniverous wildlife was affected, although cases in cattle, sheep and deer were not infrequently reported. If an occasional fox, for example, was infected, it never acted as a focus of infection for others. This uncomplicated epidemiology made possible the eradication of the disease by simple but rigorously enforced dog control measures.

B. SYLVATIC RABIES

On the European mainland, the history of rabies has been very different. There are early reports of rabies in foxes and wolves as well as in dogs. In the early years of the nineteenth century, rabies was enzootic in foxes, and at certain times and places, the incidence of the disease attained epizootic proportions. From about 1805, the number of rabid foxes in the Jura region of France and contiguous parts of Switzerland and Germany increased considerably, and the animals presented a distinct hazard, not only to other foxes, dogs and farm animals, but to the human population as well. This rather prolonged epizooty, which may have been promoted by the Revolutionary and Napoleonic wars, subsided by about 1830. During the 1880s, when Pasteur was engaged in his study of rabies and the development of an anti-rabic vaccine, the most important vector in France and much of Europe was the dog. Indeed, with the clear understanding of the role and importance of dogs in the natural history of rabies and a general acceptance of the so-called 'germ theory' of infectious disease, control of dogs led to a general reduction (but not abolition) of rabies in western Europe, which lasted until after the Second World War.

C. RABIES IN EUROPE

The post-war epizooty of rabies in Europe is thought to have begun in 1939, just before or at the outset of the Second World War, in the Soviet Union–Polish border areas. The animals most heavily implicated were Red Foxes (*Vulpes vulpes*), and after the war, it was noted that fox rabies was widespread in Poland. By 1947, the disease was present in East German foxes and soon thereafter was found in West Germany. It spread rapidly to, and in, central European countries during the 1950s. The westward spread of the infection was not halted. By 1963, it invaded Denmark, in 1966 was reported from Belgium, and in 1968 entered northern France from where it has been spreading southwards and westwards (see Fig. 2).

In Denmark and also the southern Länder of West Germany efforts, often considerable, have been made to control the incidence and spread of the disease by reducing the number of susceptible animals. In practice, this meant slaughtering large numbers of foxes. In some instances, the reduction in population density of foxes wrought by rabies may have been as effective in reducing the local incidence of the disease as the controlled slaughtering by health authorities. In Denmark, a rigorous policy of killing foxes eradicated the disease from south Jutland and the maintenance of a fox-free zone immediately north of the border with West Germany prevented re-entry of the disease for several years. Badgers and martens are occasionally found rabid, the former possibly infected by foxes, which sometimes use badger sets as dens, but the Red Fox is at present over-whelmingly the most important species in the European epizooty of rabies.

In any given geographical area, it is very unusual for more than one species to be important as a vector of rabies—a fact which has been remarked repeatedly but which may not be universally correct. In eastern Europe and parts of Scandinavia, the Raccoon Dog (*Nyctereutes procyanoides*) is increasingly important as a vector of rabies and seems able to co-exist in the same habitats as Red Foxes, which show no decrease in the incidence of rabies. The animal was introduced at the turn of the century from Korea into the far eastern Soviet Union as a potential fur bearer. It has since spread steadily westward and is now present in Finland, Sweden, and as far as East and West Germany. It will no doubt continue increasing its range in Europe and adding further complexity to the epidemiology of rabies in its new habitats.

The epizooty of rabies in western Europe does not advance uniformly (Toma and Andral, 1977). In some years, the average distance covered by the epizootic front may be 60–80 km, but at various points on the front the advance may be

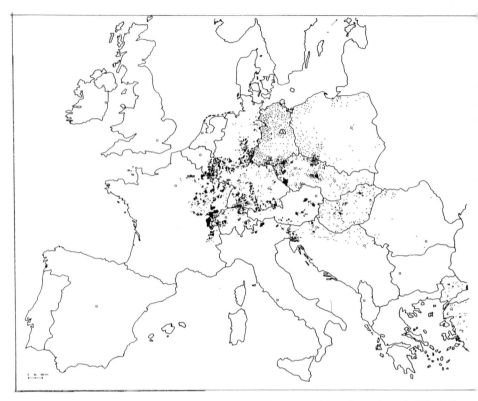

Fig. 2. Verified cases of rabies in Europe for the third quarter (July to September) of 1982; 4838 cases were reported. (Reproduced by kind permission of WHO Collaborating Centre for Rabies Research, Tübingen.)

considerably more or almost nil. The reasons for these differences must be sought not only in the behaviour of foxes but in the detailed topography of particular areas. The period of greatest advance of rabies is that of the dispersal of young foxes from the parental den. This occurs in late winter or early spring. Some young animals, preponderantly males, may move many kilometres in search of territories. Should such an animal be infected at the outset of or during its travels, it may cover much ground before developing symptoms and excreting virus. The incubation period of rabies in the Red Fox is variable and, in experimental infections with salivary gland (i.e. street) virus, the incubation period varied from 12 to 100 days (Sikes, 1962). The incubation period was inversely related to the amount of the infecting dose of virus and also apparently to less readily quantified factors, such as the strain of virus, the site of inoculation and the physical condition of the animal. Observation of foxes naturally (Sykes-Andral, 1981) and experimentally infected (Sikes, 1962) suggests that the duration of symptomatic disease is generally short, usually less than 4 days. Bearing this information in mind, the importance for the spread of rabies not only of the population density but also the behaviour of both healthy and diseased foxes is clear.

It is generally agreed by field workers that the establishment of rabies in a fox population depends largely on the density of the population (Steck and Wandeler, 1980), but other factors must also be involved. Rabies has invaded Italy from the north three times in recent years. On the first occasion the disease—presumably fox-borne—entered the south Tyrol by crossing the Krimmler Pass (2600 m), but by 1979, it had died out. The crossing of the pass was itself exceptional; mountains higher than 2000 m are generally thought to be a barrier against the movement of foxes. A second invasion was made over passes less than 2000 m high, but this invasion also, seemed not to establish itself, although the density of the fox population was probably adequate for the purpose. The third entry was from Switzerland—via the Schliring Pass (2298 m) in October 1980—and moved rapidly southwards. In the following spring, rabid foxes were found 60 km from the entry point. By the third quarter of 1982, the disease was present in four alpine regions—Lombardy, Alto Adige, Veneto and Friuli. Of the wild carnivores diagnosed as rabid, 83% were foxes and 10% badgers. Rabies was also reported in three cats and two dogs.

There is no entirely satisfactory method for determining precisely the population density of foxes. A method widely used in Europe is the hunting index of fox population density (HIPD), which is derived from the game-bag returns of hunters. The figure so derived lacks precision but is used *faut de mieux*. The second invasion into south Tyrol spread into areas with hunting indices greater than 0.2 foxes shot/km^2/year but not into areas with indices less than 0.2. Nevertheless, the disease did not thrive even in the areas with the higher indices. In the region invaded in 1980 with subsequent rapid movement, the index was 0.26.

In Germany, Switzerland, France and other countries with epizootic fox rabies, when the disease front has passed through a particular area, rabies is absent or scarce for periods of up to 5 years. This scarcity or absence is related to the low population density of surviving foxes. The populations increase over the years, and scattered foci of rabies appear from which the disease spreads in all directions, no longer only towards areas with no previous experience of the disease. At this stage, the disease has become enzootic in the fox population; a sudden increase in population density may permit it once more to become epizootic, but only in a more or less circumscribed area defined by the distribution of the susceptible population.

In Europe, the Field Vole (*Microtus arvalis*) is among the most susceptible animals to experimental infection with rabies virus. Other field rodents, e.g. the Woodmouse (*Apodemus sylvestris*) and the Bank Vole (*Clethrionomys glareolus*), are also susceptible but less so than the Field Vole. Sodja *et al.*

(1971) reported the isolation of rabies-like viruses from wild field rodents in central Europe. Schneider and Schoop (1972) confirmed the report of Sodja *et al.* (1971); about 2% of Schneider's samples yielded virus.

Sodja *et al.* (1971) found signs of infection, i.e. neutralizing antibody to rabies virus, in 22.5% of rodents from areas with enzootic rabies and in almost 13% from areas free of rabies. This finding suggests that rabies or rabies-like virus in field rodents (if it indeed exists) plays no part in the maintenance of the enzootic state. Neither Sodja *et al.* nor Schneider isolated virus directly from field material, but only after several blind passages by intracerebral inoculation of mice. Any virus present in the field material must thus have been in very low concentration, or the field rodents were latently infected. In either case, it is difficult to see how these animals can have any role in the initiation of epizooties of rabies.

Rabies is present not only in eastern European counries—Czechoslovakia, Poland, Hungary, the Soviet Union, but also in the Balkans. Much of it is wildlife rabies—mainly in foxes—but dogs and farm animals are also involved.

Rabies, which was eradicated from Britain in 1903, was re-introduced in a smuggled dog in 1919 and was not re-eradicated until 1922. The outbreak was confined to dogs; there was no evidence of foxes or other wildlife being involved. In a study of naturally occurring virus infections in British field rodents, Kaplan *et al.* (1980) did not isolate rabies virus from the brains of 269 rodents; nor were neutralizing antibodies to rabies virus present in any serum taken from a rodent. The work was done with strict precautions against inadvertent contamination of samples with rabies virus being used at the time in the laboratory. This may, perhaps, be regarded as further evidence for the absence of sylvatic rabies in Britain in the period before the eradication of the disease. Britain is still free of rabies, but there are now large urban and suburban populations of foxes in all parts of the country. (Urban foxes are a phenomenon apparently less recognised on the European mainland than in Britain.) An appreciable proportion of these foxes appear to interact amicably with dogs. The dog population of Britain has increased considerably in the past 30 years, and many of the animals appear to lead an autonomous or semi-autonomous existence. Should rabies be re-introduced now, there is no certainty that it would be confined to dogs, and there is a strong likelihood that it would enter the fox population in which it would probably become enzootic. As in the countries of mainland Europe with enzootic fox rabies, badgers would probably be involved in the epidemic process. Harris has reported that urban badgers readily fight with foxes, dogs and cats.

D. RABIES IN NORTH AMERICA

1. Terrestrial Carnivores

The North American continent provides several examples of the predominance of a particular species as a vector of rabies in a given geographical region. In the arctic and immediately sub-artic parts of Canada and Alaska, rabies is enzootic in the Arctic Fox (*Alopex lagopus*). This animal occurs within the arctic circle in Russia and Greenland as well as North America. It may at times be very numerous, when rabies appears in epizootic forms. Rabies in Arctic Foxes is closely related to outbreaks of rabies in sledge dogs. Arctic Fox territory is north of the treeline. Within the treeline, the Red Fox (*Vulpes vulpes*) finds a suitable habitat and becomes the most important vector of rabies; the disease is also enzootic in wolves.

   Although the Red Fox is found widely in North America, and as far south as the northernmost parts of South America, it is important as a vector of rabies only in the eastern part of the continent, but it may be that this importance is waning. Twenty to 30 years ago rabies in the states of New York and Tennessee was found almost entirely in foxes, but rabies is now found with increasing frequency in skunks. However, as recently as 1972, the Grey Fox (*Urocyon cinereoargenteus*) was the major host species of wild carnivore rabies in Virginia (Carey and McLean, 1978). Skunks are clearly the most important vectors in the middle western United States with an extension northwards into Manitoba and Sasketchawan, Canada, and southwards into Mexico, adjacent to Texas. Rabies in skunks occurs sparsely in the Rocky Mountain region, but significant numbers of cases occur in California. Both the Striped Skunk (*Mephitis mephitis*) and the Spotted Skunk (*Spilogale putorius*) are subject to rabies. The Striped Skunk is numerically the more important. Other terrestrial mammals are important in certain localities. The Raccoon (*Procyon lotor*) is widely distributed from southern Canada to the Isthmus of Panama. Rabies occurs only as scattered cases in most habitats of this animal. During the 1950s, however, the disease became established in Raccoons in Florida, spreading steadily throughout the state and extending northwards into Georgia (McLean, 1975). McLean and his colleagues have collected evidence that indicates that Raccoons in Florida and Georgia may provide a reservoir of rabies virus through the reactivation of latent infection in response to the appropriate environmental and physiological stimuli. The mechanism is unclear, but is thought to be related to physiological states, e.g. in the breeding season. In this connection, it is interesting to recall that Kaplan *et al.* (1980) induced the reactivation of pulmonary virus infection in 52% of captive wild rodents by dosing them regularly with the adrenocorticotrophic hormone of the pituitary gland. Among other things, this hormone causes enlargement of the adrenal cortex. It is interesting that Field Voles (*Microtus agrestis*) subjected to stress showed a marked increase in the weight of the adrenal glands and spleen and in the involution of the thymus (Clarke, 1953). Those animals treated by Kaplan *et al.* that developed pneumonia also had enlarged adrenal glands.

2. Bats

Numerically, bats are probably the largest group of American animals in which rabies is endemic. Hurst and Pawan (1931, 1932) described paralytic rabies in human beings caused by the bites of infected vampire bats on the island of Trinidad. Subsequently, Pawan (1936a,b) described rabies in both frugivorous and insectivorous bats as well as in vampires. He showed that experimentally infected fruit-eating bats could transmit the virus in their saliva by biting and that bats occasionally recovered from the acute form of the disease but continued to excrete virus in their saliva for months. The relevance of these findings to North America only became apparent in the 1950s when Venters *et al.* (1954) diagnosed rabies in an insectivorous bat in Florida that had attacked and bitten a child. Thereafter, many reports followed of rabies in insectivorous and fruit-eating bats from many of the continental United States and from Canada. Baer (1975), who has made an extensive study of bat rabies, suggested that the steady increase in the number of reports of rabid bats in North America reflects increasing scientific interest rather than indicating a widening involvement of bats and a true increase in incidence. The Mexican Freetail Bat (*Tadarida brasiliensis mexicana*)—a migrant and colonial species—is found roosting in enormous numbers in caves in Texas and New Mexico. Although rabies occurs in only about 1% of the bat population, this amounts to a large number of rabid bats since Davis (quoted by Baer, 1975) estimated that there were more than 60 million Mexican Freetail Bats in Texas alone each summer.

The concentration of rabies virus in caves inhabited by these colonial bats is great enough to make aerial infection by the virus a serious risk to terrestrial mammals, including man. At least two men are known to have contracted rabies while exploring the Frio Cave in Texas, and all of the 12 foxes and coyotes kept in Frio Cave for up to 30 days died of rabies. The animals were caged under conditions that precluded any other route of infection than the aerial. Winkler (1975), who has published experimental and observational studies on the relationship of bat rabies to enzootic and epizootic rabies in terrestrial mammals, suggested that the evidence indicates that the mechanism exists for bats to initiate outbreaks of rabies in terrestrial carnivores but that definitive proof that particular outbreaks have been caused thus is lacking.

Despite the great preponderance of colonial over solitary bats and, presumably, the greater number of colonial bats with rabies, the majority of human cases of rabies undoubtedly caused by bat bites have followed the bites of non-colonial species. This imbalance in numbers is probably caused by the different behavior of the two types when they are infected, colonial bats seldom seem to become violent, whereas solitary bats frequently appear to attack when rabid.

E. RABIES IN SOUTH AMERICA

Rabies is endemic throughout the South American continent. Most human cases are caused by the bites of rabid dogs. For example, Bolivia and Colombia each reported more than 1000 rabid dogs in 1979, whereas Brazil reported 4500.

Rabies in man resulting from bites by rabid vampire bats is also reported from time to time. However, the most important problem is *paralytic rabies in cattle* associated with the bites of vampire bats.

Vampire Bat Rabies

About 500,000 head of cattle are reported annually to die as a result of paralytic rabies in the countries of South and Central America, including Mexico. It is thought, however, that the actual loss may be as much as four times greater because of incomplete reporting. The distribution of cattle deaths is by no means uniform, varying widely not only from country to country but also within countries. Three different vampire bats occur in Central and South America. The commonest one, *Desmodus rotundus,* is found in almost all areas where bovine paralytic rabies occurs. It appears to prefer bovine blood above that of other animals. In the Trinidad outbreak, Hurst and Pawan (1931) noted that sleeping human beings tended to be bitten by *Desmodus rotundus* when cattle had been enclosed for the night in barns to protect them against feeding vampires. Those people who were bitten were generally sleeping out of doors on verandahs because of the heat. Retrospectively, because of a history of parasthesiae (abnormal sensations) in the part in the early stages of disease, it seemed that an appreciable proportion of the victims had been bitten on the great toe, which was presumably exposed during the night. The other vampires are the Hairy-legged Vampire, *Diphylla ecandata,* which is found in cooler climates than *Desmodus* and thus often at higher altitudes. It, too, prefers bovine blood, but has an almost equal liking for horse blood. The third species, *Diaemus youngi,* is rare and thought by some to prefer avian blood.

Pawan (1936a,b) found that experimentally infected *Desmodus* were able to transmit virus by bite during the incubation period; several of his experimental animals developed signs of disease as long as 1 or 2 months after demonstrating their infectivity, and occasional bats recovered after developing furious symptoms.

An important difference between the United States and Canada on the one hand and the countries of Central and South America on the other is the resources available in the two northern countries for research in and surveillance of rabies (and other infectious diseases) compared with what the poorer southern counries are able to afford. This difference inevitably means that information about the continental epidemiology of rabies in South and Central America is, unlike the North, relatively sparse. For example, with the exception of vampire bats, the extent of wildlife involvement in rabies has not been studied on anything like the scale that it has in the United States and Canada. Developed national epidemiological services generally tend to indicate affluence and are an adjunct of well-found health services, whereas in ideal circumstances epidemiology should be the basis of a health service.

F. RABIES IN AFRICA

Rabies occurs throughout Africa. In questionnaires returned annually to the World Health Organization (WHO), some of the North African countries report rats among the animals found rabid or transmitting the disease. Dogs are almost always included by most countries. Jackals and other canids are involved too, but the degree of involvement of wildlife is generally unknown. Reports of rabies in wild animals are largely qualitative although in some countries, e.g. Zimbabwe, it is known that more rabies occurred as a result of the reduction of preventive measures, such as vaccination of dogs during the period of the civil war (Foggin and Swanepoel, 1979). But even here, numbers are notably absent. More is known about the epidemiology and ecology of rabies and its causative virus in the Republic of South Africa than probably any other country on the continent. As in Europe and North and South America, this knowledge is related to the size of the gross national product.

For many years, rabies has been endemic in the central part of the Republic of South Africa, mainly in the northern part of the Cape Province and the Orange Free State. Each year, cases occur in a few human beings—usually fewer than five—and in cattle and dogs. The animals mainly responsible are a viverrid, the Yellow Mongoose (*Cynictis penicillata*) and two species frequently associated with it—the Suricate (*Suricata suricatta*) and the Ground Squirrel (*Xerus inauris*). The Genet Cat (*Genetta genetta*), although spread widely throughout the Republic, is important as a vector of rabies only in the northern part of the Cape Province and in the western part of the Transvaal on the border with Botswana. These animals are normally very shy of human beings. A common story given by the parents of little children with rabies is that their child picked up a mongoose or some other animal to play with it and was bitten. It is certainly abnormal that any one of these animals would allow itself to be approached, let alone picked up. Cattle and dogs are commonly bitten on the nose while examining such an abnormally behaving animal. For as long as observations have been made (at least for the past 40 or 50 years), there has been no major change in the species involved in this enzootic rabies; nor has there been any significant change in the geographical distribution of the disease.

From time to time, epizootic dog rabies enters the Republic from the north. The most recent incursion occurred in 1975, when rabid dogs carried the infection into Natal over its northern border with Mozambique. There were 10 known human cases of rabies, all acquired by dog bites. Apart from these cases, the circulation of the virus seems to have been confined to dogs, although there was some apprehension that the virus might be transmitted to the Banded Mongoose (*Mungos mungos*) and become enzootic in that species.

Africa is also notable for being the home of the known rabies-related viruses (see above), two of which (Lagos Bat and Duvenhage viruses) have been transmitted by bats and may be enzootic in these animals. However, adequate epidemiological and ecological studies need to be made to determine if this is so. Duvenhage virus was originally identified as rabies virus by immunofluorescent microscopy (Meredith *et al.*, 1971). Tignor *et al.* (1977) subsequently found Duvenhage virus to be distinct from rabies virus by several biological, biochemical and immunological characteristics. The differences between Duvenhage and rabies viruses were about as great as those previously shown by Shope *et al.* (1970) between rabies and Mokola and Lagos Bat viruses.

G. RABIES IN ASIA

In Asia Minor, rabies is present not only in dogs, but also in foxes, jackals and wolves, but reliable figures are lacking for most countries in the region. The situation is much the same in the rest of Asia. Some countries, e.g. Japan and some of the smaller Emirates and Sheikdoms of the Persian Gulf, are free of rabies, but most Asian countries, while admitting the presence of rabies, return to the WHO clearly inadequate reports of the numbers of rabid dogs and other animals. For example, in 1979, India reported (from the Central Research Institute, Kasauli) 72 rabid dogs and a total of 83 rabid animals, but of 2304 persons given post-attack anti-rabic treatment, 1986 were reported to have been put at risk by dogs. The many other Indian centres, which make rabies vaccine and provide treatment, did not return information. In Viet Nam in the same year, however, the National Institute of Hygiene and Epidemiology reported 33,145 rabid dogs. Indonesia, Thailand and the Philippines—in all of which rabies in human beings and dogs is not a rare event—did not return information to the WHO. In the absence of useful statistics, it is impossible to offer any cogent comment about rabies in Asia other than to point out that there is a lot of it about and to warn prospective travellers against any sort of approaches to or by dogs. Rabies is unknown in Australia, New Zealand, Papua New Guinea, Fiji and many other islands of Oceania.

V. Summary

Rabies is a hazard to the health of man and animals (both wild and domestic) in most parts of the world. In many countries, the ecology of the agent and the epidemiology of the disease it causes are well enough understood to make the control of rabies a rational undertaking, although not always an immediately successful one. In parts of the world, however, the ecology of the virus is poorly understood, largely because it has not been investigated, and the true incidence of rabies is unknown because of inadequate surveillance of disease in human and animal populations. Disease control depends on adequate quantitative information about the disease to be controlled. It is important, therefore, to propose methods for collecting and interpreting information about rabies, which can be widely applied.

References

Andral, L., and Serié, C. (1957). Etudes expérimentales sur la rage en Ethiopie. *Ann. Inst. Pasteur, Paris* **93**, 475–88.

Baer, C. M. (1975). *In* "The Natural History of Rabies" (G. M. Baer, ed.), Vol. 2, pp. 79–97. Academic Press, London.

Baer, G. M., and Cleary, W. F. (1972). A model in mice for the pathogenesis and treatment of rabies. *J. Infect. Dis.* **125**, 520–527.

Baer, G. M., Shantha, T. R., and Bourne, G. H. (1968). The pathogenesis of street rabies virus in rats. *Bull. W. H. O.* **38**, 119–125.

Bell, J. F., Gonzalez, M. A., Diaz, A. M., and Moore, G. J. (1971). Nonfatal rabies in dogs: Experimental studies and results of a survey. *Am. J. Vet. Res.* **32**, 2049–2058.

Boulger, L. R., and Porterfield, J. S. (1958). Isolation of a virus from Nigerian fruit bats. *Trans. R. Soc. Trop. Med. Hyg.* **52**, 421–424.

Carey, A. B., and McLean, R. G. (1978). Rabies antibody prevalence and virus tissue tropism in wild carnivores in Virginia. *J. Wildl. Dis.* **14**, 487–491.

Clarke, J. R. (1953). The effect of fighting on the adrenals, thymus and spleen of the vole (*Microtus agrestis*). *J. Endocrinol.* **9**, 114–126.

Crick, J., and Brown, F. (1970). *In* "The Biology of Large RNA Viruses" (R. D. Barry and B. W. J. Mahy, eds.), pp. 130–140. Academic Press, London.

Foggin, C. M., and Swanepoel, R. (1979). Rabies in Rhodesia: The current situation. *Cent. Afr. J. Med.* **25**, 98–100.

Hamparian, V. V., Hilleman, M. R., and Ketler, A. (1963). Contribution to the characterization and classification of animal viruses. *Proc. Soc. Exp. Biol. Med.* **112**, 1040–1050.

Hattwick, M. A., West, T. T., Stechschuite, C. J., Baer, G. M., and Gregg, M. B. (1972). Recovery from rabies: A case report. *Ann. Intern. Med.* **76**, 931–942.

Hurst, E. W., and Pawan, J. L. (1931). An outbreak of rabies in Trinidad without history of bites and with the symptoms of acute ascending myelitis. *Lancet* **2**, 622–628.

Hurst, E. W., and Pawan, J. L. (1932). A further account of the Trinidad outbreak of acute rabic myelitis: Histology of the experimental disease. *J. Pathol. Bacteriol.* **35**, 301–322.

Johnson, H. N. (1948). Derriengue: vampire bat rabies in Mexico. *Am. J. Hyg.* **47**, 189–204.

Kaplan, C., Healing, T. D., Evans, N., Healing, N., and Prior, A. (1980). Evidence of infection by viruses in small British field rodents. *J. Hyg.* **84**, 285–294.

Kemp, G. E., Lee, V. H., Moore, D. L., Shope, R. E., Causey, O. R., and Murphy, F. A. (1970). Kotonkan, a new virus related to Mokola virus of the rabies serogroup. *Am. J. Epidemiol.* **98**, 43–49.

Kissling, R. E., and Reese, D. R. (1963). Anti-rabies vaccine of tissue culture origin. *J. Immunol.* **91**, 362–368.

McLean, R. G. (1972). Rabies in raccoons in the South-eastern United States. *J. Infect. Dis.* **123**, 680–681.

McLean, R. G. (1975). *In* "The Natural History of Rabies" (G. M. Baer, ed.), Vol. 2, pp. 53–77. Academic Press, London.

Meredith, C. D., Roussou, A. P., and van Praag Koch, H. (1971). An unusual case of human rabies thought to be of chiropteran origin. *S. Afr. Med. J.* **45**, 767–769.

Miyamoto, K., and Matsumoto, S. (1965). The nature of the Negri body. *J. Cell Biol.* **27**, 677–682.

Murphy, F. A., Bauer, S. P., Harrison, B. S., and Winn, W. C. (1973). Comparative pathogenesis of rabies and rabies-like viruses. *Lab. Invest.* **28**, 361–376.

Pasteur, L., Chamberland, C., Roux, E., and Thuiller, L. (1882). Nouveaux faits pour servir à la connaisance de la rage. *C. R. Hebd. Séances Acad. Sci.* **92**, 1187–1192.

Pawan, J. L. (1936a). The transmission of paralytic rabies in Trinidad by vampire bat (*Desmodus rotundus murinus* Wagner, 1840). *Ann. Trop. Med. Parasitol.* **30**, 101–130.

Pawan, J. L. (1936b). Rabies in the vampire bat of Trinidad with special reference to the clinical course and the latency of infection. *Ann. Trop. Med. Parasitol.* **30**, 401–422.

Porterfield, J. S., Hill, D. H., and Morris, A. D. (1958). Isolation of a virus from the brain of a horse with 'staggers' in Nigeria. *Br. Vet. J.* **114**, 25–33.

Remlinger, P. (1933). Sur la comportement du virus rabique en A.O.F. et en A.E.F. *Bull. Soc. Pathol. Exot.* **26**, 941–946.

Schmidt, J. R., Williams, M. C., Lule, M., Mivule, A., and Mujomba, E. (1965). Viruses isolated from mosquitoes collected in the Southern Sudan and Ethiopia. *East Afr. Virus Res. Inst. Rep.* **15**, 24–26.

Schneider, L. G., and Schoop, U. (1972). Pathogenesis of rabies and rabies-like viruses. *Ann. Inst. Pasteur, Paris* **123**, 469–476.

Shope, R. E., Murphy, F. A., Harrison, A. K., Causey, D. R., Kemp, G. E., Simpson, D. I. H., and Moore, D. L. (1970). Two viruses serologically and morphologically related to rabies virus. *J. Virol.* **6**, 690–692.

Sikes, R. K. (1962). Pathogenesis of rabies in wildlife. I. Comparative effect of varying doses of rabies inoculated into foxes and skunks. *Am. J. Vet. Res.* **23**, 1042–1047.

Smith, W. B., Blenden, D. C., Fuh, T.-H., and Hiler, L. (1972). Diagnosis of rabies by immunofluorescent staining of frozen sections of skin. *J. Am. Vet. Med. Assoc.* **161**, 1495–1497.

Sodja, I., Lim, D., and Matouch, O. (1971). Isolation of rabieslike virus from small wild rodents. *J. Hyg. Epidemiol., Microbiol., Immunol.* **14**, 271–277.

Sokol, F., Kuwert, E., Wiktor, T. J., Hummeler, K., and Koprowski, H. (1968). Purification of rabies virus grown in tissue culture. *J. Virol.* **2**, 836–849.

Steck, F., and Wandeler, A. (1980). The epidemiology of fox rabies in Europe. *Epidemiol. Rev.* **2**, 71 96.

Sykes-Andral, M. (1981). Le comportement des animaux sauvages enragés. Paper delivered at Joint CNER-WHO Scientific Meeting on Animal Rabies on the occasion of the tenth anniversary of the Centre National d'Etudes sur la Rage.

Tierkel, E. S. (1959). Rabies. *Adv. Vet. Sci.* **5**, 183–226.

Tierkel, E. S. (1975). *In* "The Natural History of Rabies" (G. M. Baer, ed.), Vol. 2, pp. 123–136. Academic Press, London.

Tignor, G. H., Murphy, F. A., Clarke, H. F., Shope, R. E., Madore, P., Bauer, S. P., Buckley, S. M., and Meredith, C. D. (1977). Duvenhage virus: Morphological, biochemical, histopathological and antigenic relationships to the rabies group. *J. Gen. Virol.* **37**, 596–611.

Toma, B., and Andral, A. (1977). Epidemiology of fox rabies. *Adv. Virus Res.* **21**, 1–36.

Veeraraghavan, N. Gajanawa, H., Rangasam, R., Osnnunni, P. T., Saraswatti, C., Devarraj, R., and Hallan, K. M. (1970). "Studies on the Salivary Excretion of Rabies Virus by the Dog from Surundai," Sci. Rep., 1969. Pasteur Institute of South India, Coonoor.

Venters, H. D., Heffert, D. R., Scatterday, J. E., and Hardy, A. V. (1954). Rabies in bats in Florida. *Am. J. Public Health* **44**, 182–185.

Winkler, W. G. (1975). *In* "The Natural History of Rabies" (G. M. Baer, ed.), Vol. 2, pp. 115–120. Academic Press, London.

World Health Organization Expert Committee on Rabies (1973). *WHO Tech. Rep. Ser.* **153**, 12.

Multispecies Rabies in the Eastern United States

2

Andrew B. Carey

Forest Service,
United States Department of Agriculture,
Olympia, Washington

I. Rabies Surveillance in the United States

A. REPORTING OF LABORATORY-CONFIRMED CASES OF RABIES IN SUSPECT ANIMALS

Rabies was first recognized in the United States in Virginia in 1753. However, surveillance programs were not initiated by individual states until 1925–1950, and a national program of compiling rabies incidence data was not begun until 1938. The current assignment of the surveillance program to the Centers for Disease Control began in 1960 (McLean, 1970, 1975). The national program consists of compiling state reports; state reports consist of summaries of suspect animals submitted by citizens, physicians, veterinarians, and public health workers to state laboratories for diagnosis of rabies. Long-term systematic field surveillance (objective collecting of animals for examination) has not been attempted.

Policies for submitting and reporting suspect animals are highly variable among states and even vary among health department jurisdictions within states. A common policy is to test principally only those suspect animals that have potentially exposed humans to rabies. Unfortunately, reports of laboratory-confirmed rabid animals usually fail to identify the animal's species precisely. For example, two species of foxes are common in the eastern United States—the Red Fox (*Vulpes vulpes*) and the Gray Fox (*Urocyon cinereoargenteus*). Even though the two species differ in their ecologies and in their involvement with rabies in particular geographic areas (Carey, 1982), they were still lumped into the category "foxes" in the most recent (1978) annual rabies summary for the United States (Centers for Disease Control, 1981a). Likewise, there is the category "skunks" that includes the Striped Skunk (*Mephitis mephitis*), the Hooded Skunk (*Mephitis macroura*), the Spotted Skunk (*Spilogale putoris*), and the Hognosed Skunk (*Conepatus leuconotus*). Thirty of the 39 species of bats in the United States have been found to be infected with rabies, and all are assigned to the category "bats." Such loose categorizations are sometimes followed in research reports, e.g., Sikes (1962) used rabies virus isolated from a "fox" salivary gland to inoculate both Red Foxes and Gray Foxes, which were indiscriminately mixed in treatment groups, to determine "fox" susceptibility to rabies.

B. SPECIES OF ANIMALS PROMINENT IN SURVEILLANCE REPORTS

Since the beginning of the surveillance program in 1938, the total number of reported cases of rabies has declined by more than 50%; most of this decline occurred in the 1950s with the reduction, through vaccination, of dog rabies (McLean, 1970; see Table I). With the decline of rabies in dogs, attention became focused on rabies in wild animals. Rabid foxes predominated in the reported cases of rabies in wild animals until 1957, when skunks predominated. Reports of rabid foxes gradually declined (but with a sharp increase in 1964–1965), but reports of skunks increased to 1909 in 1964 and have remained at high levels with peaks in 1971–1972 (>2000 cases) and 1980 (4040 cases). Rabid Raccoons (*Procyon lotor*) accounted for only an incidental portion of reported wildlife rabies until 1962 to 1964 (160–175 cases); reports of rabid Raccoons gradually increased to 393 cases in 1980. Cases of rabid bats continued to increase until they were second only to skunks in 1974 (McLean, 1970, 1975; Centers for Disease Control, 1981b; see Table I).

TABLE I

Approximate Numbers of Laboratory-confirmed Cases of Rabies in Groups of Animals Commonly Infected during 1955–1980 in the United States in 5-Year Intervals[a]

	Animal groups					
Year	Foxes	Skunks	Raccoons	Bats	Dogs	Farm animals
1955	1223	580	37	14	2657	924
1960	915	725	47	88	697	645
1965	1038	1582	99	484	412	625
1970	771	1235	254	296	185	399
1975	276	1226	190	514	129	200
1980	207	4040	393	723	247	398

[a] Principally compiled from Centers for Disease Control (1981a,b) and McLean (1975).

C. GEOGRAPHIC PATTERNS IN REPORTED CASES

1. Rabies in Foxes

Rabies epizootics were reported in the northeastern United States in 1812 (Massachusetts), 1934 (Maine), 1936 (Massachusetts), and 1943–1950 (New York). Red Foxes were more abundant than Gray Foxes in New York and were considered the principal host species for rabies, although the Gray Fox and Striped Skunk were also significantly involved (Fig. 1). Epizootics in foxes were reported in the Southeast in 1762 (North Carolina), 1890 (Alabama), 1940–1945 (Georgia and Alabama), and 1953–1958 (Florida). Gray Foxes were implicated throughout the Southeast, but Red Foxes, though much less numerous than Gray Foxes, also were implicated in Georgia and Alabama. An epizootic took place in the whole Appalachian region (southern New York to northern Georgia, including parts of Kentucky, Tennessee, Virginia, and West Virginia) in 1947. West of the Appalachian region, epizootics were reported in Wisconsin in 1938 and in Ohio in 1948. Gray Foxes appear to have been the primary species involved in the Appalachian and Ohio epizootics. Rabies has persisted as an enzootic disease only in the Appalachian region (the Valley and Ridge Province and Appalachian Plateau in Fig. 1) (Carey, 1982). Temporary extensions of enzootic fox rabies have occurred in Texas and Missouri (Ozark Plateau) (McLean, 1970).

2. Rabies in Skunks

Rabid skunks have been reported in 33 states. In the eastern United States, rabies is commonly reported in skunks in Ohio, Kentucky, Tennessee, and westward through the Central Lowland (Fig. 1) and south through Missouri, Oklahoma, and Texas. The eastern range of skunk rabies overlaps the western range of fox rabies, particularly in Tennessee and Kentucky; epizootics in skunks

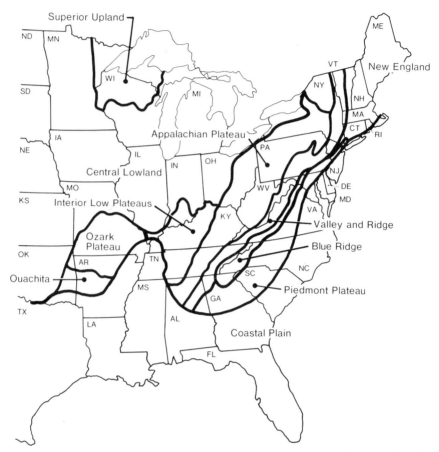

Fig. 1. Physiographic provinces in the eastern United States of America. State name abbreviations for states mentioned in text. AL, Alabama; GA, Georgia; FL, Florida; KY, Kentucky; ME, Maine; MA, Massachusetts; MO, Missouri; NY, New York; NC North Carolina; OH, Ohio; OK, Oklahoma; TN, Tennessee; TX, Texas; VA, Virginia; WV, West Virginia; WI, Wisconsin.

also were noted in New York. The Striped Skunk is the species of skunk most often found infected with rabies (Parker, 1975; Winkler, 1975).

3. Rabies in Raccoons

Raccoons have been found infected with rabies in most eastern states. The Raccoon, however, has been prominent in case reports only in the Southeast, especially in Florida where Raccoons were found infected with rabies in 1947 and where cases have been reported continuously since 1953. The number of rabid Raccoons reported from Florida increased during 1954–1962, with an accompanying northward spread into Georgia. Rabies in Raccoons has been reported from Florida and Georgia since 1962. By 1971, Raccoon rabies had spread to South Carolina (McLean, 1975). Cases were subsequently reported in Alabama, and in 1981, an epizootic occurred in northwestern Virginia and adjacent West Virginia (Centers for Disease Control, 1981c). New York reported an epizootic of Racoon rabies during 1946–1952 that was concurrent with an epizootic in foxes, but it appears that that outbreak was a temporary phenomenon. Texas has reported low levels of Raccoon rabies since 1956; the cases in Texas may be spillover infections from rabies infections among Brazilian Free-tailed Bats (*Tadarida brasiliensis*) (McLean, 1975).

4. Rabies in Bats

Rabies was first reported in bats in the United States in 1953 in *Lasiurus intermedius* and *L. seminolus* (Baer, 1975b). Since 1953 rabies has been found in all the common, indigenous bats (Constantine, 1979). In general, in the United States, bats have been found to be infected with rabies wherever anyone has looked for rabies in bats. Rabid bats were reported from 46 of the 48 contiguous states in 1980 (Centers for Disease Control, 1981b).

D. CHANGES IN INCIDENCE PATTERNS

Initial surveillance data suggested that rabies was prevalent in two major groups of terrestrial mammals, i.e., foxes and skunks. Rabies was commoner in skunks to the west of the Appalachians, whereas rabies was commoner in foxes in the Appalachians and eastward (Parker, 1975; Tierkel, 1959; Sikes and Tierkel, 1960). Subsequently, exceptions to the geographic zonation became apparent in Florida, Tennessee, and New York.

1. Florida

The significance of rabies in wild animals in Florida was not recognized until 1948 when rabies epizootics were eliminated in dogs. During 1948–1958, one-third of all reported cases of rabies were linked to a rabies epizootic in Gray Foxes (Jennings *et al.,* 1960). Rabies had been enzootic in Gray Foxes for at least 20 years and epizootics in foxes had been reported in 1949 and 1953–1958. These epizootics were concentrated in northwest Florida, but some cases were also reported from central Florida. Of the confirmed cases of rabid wild animals reported during 1951–1958, 53% were Gray Foxes; 29% Raccoons, 14% bats, and 3% skunks. The cases in Raccoons were sporadic and were confined to peninsular Florida (Scatterday *et al.,* 1960). Wood and Davis (1959) failed to find rabies in 299 Raccoons captured in northern Florida and Georgia, but 3% of 1026 Red Foxes and Gray Foxes were infected with rabies. By 1959, Raccoons had become the most commonly reported rabid wild animal in Florida, and rabies in Gray Foxes had declined (McLean, 1975). The number of rabid Raccoons continued to rise. In 1961 rabid Raccoons were reported in northern Florida, in 1965–1966 an epizootic in Raccoons was reported in central Florida, and in 1966–1971 epizootics were occurring throughout Florida and southern Georgia. Raccoon rabies continues to spread while reports of rabies in Gray Foxes remain low (Centers for Disease Control, 1981c).

Rabies was first diagnosed in bats in Florida in 1953; at least six species of bats have been found rabid in Florida since then (Baer, 1975b). Rabid bats are now second only to rabid Raccoons in the frequency of their case reports (Centers for Disease Control, 1981a). Scatterday *et al.* (1960) examined case histories of rabid animals (dogs, cats, foxes, Raccoons, bats, and skunks) in Florida, but found no general explanation for isolated cases. Epizootics of rabies in foxes and endemic rabies in Raccoons could explain most cases, but some cases in pets were most logically explained by their unnoticed exposure to infected bats. In a study of Raccoon rabies, McLean (1975) discounted the idea of bats as a reservoir species of rabies and concluded that rabies in Raccoons was endemic and would persist independently of other species.

2. Tennessee

Hall (1978) compiled case data for northeastern Tennessee and adjacent Virginia and North Carolina for 1946–1976. Dogs accounted for 1227 (86%) of the reported cases during 1946–1955; rabies was probably enzootic in foxes (presumably Gray Foxes); 97 (6% of total cases) rabid foxes were reported. In 1955, 16 rabid foxes made up 29% of reported cases and the incidence of rabid foxes began to rise. Epizootics of rabies in foxes occurred, and in 1964–1965, 501 rabid foxes accounted for 78% of reported cases. Thereafter, the incidence of fox rabies declined; during 1971–1976 only 12 rabid foxes (8% of total cases) were reported. Reports of rabid skunks (presumably Striped Skunks) were sporadic during 1946–1968 (15 cases; 0.5% of total cases). During 1969–1976, epizootics were reported in skunks; 37% of 350 reported cases were skunks. Skunks have dominated the case reports since 1971. Hall (1978) felt that dogs were the initial source for fox rabies in Tennessee and that persistent (1952–1956) fox rabies in southwestern Virginia provided the opportunity for skunks to be exposed to rabies at rates that were sufficient to eventually establish a strain of the virus in the skunk population. Subsequent to the establishment of enzootic rabies in skunks, epizootics of rabies occurred with a resulting geographic expansion. The change in the geographic pattern of case reports was accompanied by changes in the temporal (seasonal) pattern of reported cases. Hall (1978) felt that the changes in patterns of reported cases during 1946–1976 reflected major shifts in the principal host species and were not merely a change in species suffering epizootics after exposure to inapparent reservoirs such as mustelids (other than Striped Skunks) and bats. Hall (1978) found a high prevalence of antibody in Virginia Opossums (*Didelphis virginiana*) (17% of 608 cases during 1973–

1976), a species relatively resistant to rabies (Sikes and Tierkel, 1960). Hall argued against the antibody being a result of skunk bite exposure to rabies and suggested exposure through ingestion of infected skunk carcasses. The salivary glands of 10 Virginia Opossums were tested for rabies virus; one opossum was infected with rabies (it also had antibody). On this evidence, Hall suggested the possibility of another major host shift, to Virginia Opossums by rabies virus. However, Hall did not feel that Virginia Opossums would become the predominant species in reported cases. Rather, he suggested an inapparent role.

Rabid bats were first reported in Tennessee in 1961 and small numbers have been reported regularly since; at least four species of bats have been found to be infected with rabies (Fredrickson and Thomas, 1965). These authors postulated that the geographic localization of fox rabies in middle and eastern Tennessee was a result of rabies being transmitted from bats to foxes in caves used as bat roosts, as caves were more abundant in the fox–rabies area than elsewhere in western Tennessee. Fischman (1976) reported a similar geographic correspondence between the distribution of caves and the occurrence of fox rabies in the United States. Mahan (1973) captured bats and terrestrial carnivores around a number of caves, examined these animals for rabies, and compared the distribution of caves to the pattern of reported cases of fox rabies in Tennessee and concluded that there was no relationship between fox rabies and the bat rabies. Carey (1982) presented a counter argument to Fischman's (1976) thesis that was based on the inappropriateness of rabies incidence data for the statistical methods used by Fischman.

3. New York State

Friend (1968) compiled the history of rabies in New York. Human rabies cases have been reported since 1851, but rabid animals were not systematically recorded until 1899. Thereafter, dogs dominated case reports until 1945; since then, cases of rabies in dogs decreased due to vaccination programs. The first rabid fox was reported in 1941; this report was followed by another in 1943, and 15 in 1944. An epizootic in foxes in southwestern New York occurred in 1944 and was followed by one in south central New York in 1945. The incidence of rabid foxes climbed from 50 in 1945 to 309 in 1946 and then remained at a high level through 1950 (497 cases). During 1951–1965, the incidence of fox rabies fluctuated from 25 to 186 cases/year, with peaks at 5-year intervals. Rabies persisted in southern New York until 1961 and then declined until 1966. An epizootic occurred in northern New York in 1961 and continued through 1969 (McLean, 1970). Both Red Foxes and Gray Foxes are found in New York and both species were presumably involved in the epizootics. Single isolated cases of rabid skunks were reported in 1929, 1934, 1937, and 1942. Rabies in Striped Skunks began a slow increase in 1948 and rapidly increased during 1960–1965. The initial rapid increase in rabid Striped Skunks coincided with an epizootic in foxes in southwestern New York. Since then rabies in Striped Skunks has been widely reported from much of New York State. Fox rabies and skunk rabies epizootics exhibited no evidence of association and seemed largely independent of one another. An epizootic of rabies in Raccoons also followed the fox rabies epizootics in southern New York in 1944–1945. After 1952, only sporadic, widely distributed cases of Raccoon rabies were reported; Friend (1968) concluded that the incidence of rabid Raccoons reflected rabies in other terrestrial carnivores.

The first rabid bat in New York was reported in 1956. Since then, all 10 species of indigenous bats have been found to be infected with rabies. Although the total number of rabid animals has declined since 1972, cases of rabid bats have remained relatively high (Trimarchi and Debbie, 1977; Centers for Disease Control, 1981a,b). Friend (1968) concluded that rabies in bats was independent of rabies in other wild animals.

II. Patterns of Disease in Principal Hosts

A. FACTORS INFLUENCING THE COURSE OF INFECTION

The outcome of an exposure to rabies virus is highly variable and depends not only on the strain of the virus but also on the dose, route of exposure (intramuscular injection, ingestion of infected material, inhalation of aerosolized virus), site of exposure (neck, hind leg, oral mucosa, nasal mucosa), inter- and intra-specific genetic differences among the animals inoculated, and the age, sex, and physiological status of the individual inoculated (Nathanson and Cole, 1971; Winkler *et al.,* 1972; Murphy and Bauer, 1974; Baer 1975a; Bell, 1975; Ramsden and Johnston, 1975; Charlton and Casey, 1979a,b).

B. COMPARATIVE PATHOGENESIS

Laboratory studies generally have indicated that foxes are more susceptible to rabies virus than skunks, Raccoons are less susceptible than both, and Virginia Opossums are the least susceptible (Table II). Sikes and Tierkel (1960) listed the relative susceptibilities as <5, 500, 1000, and $>80,000$ (number of mouse LD_{50} required to kill 50% of the animals inoculated intramuscularly). Caution must be exercised in extrapolating an animal's susceptibility to experimental inoculations to its susceptibility under natural conditions. The amount of virus found in salivary glands and its concentration in saliva varies among species; for example, the amount of virus in the saliva of infected Striped Skunks greatly exceeds that found in foxes. For example, Sikes (1962) found that 67% of the Striped Skunks

TABLE II

The Susceptibilities of Terrestrial Species Commonly Found Naturally Infected with Rabies to Experimental Infections with Rabies Virus from Salivary Glands

Species inoculated	Site of inoculation[a]	Source of inoculum	Dose of inoculum[b]	N dying (N inoculated)	Median lethal dose (MLD$_{50}$)	References
Red and Gray Foxes	Neck	Fox	1.1–4.1	24 (28)	<1.1	Sikes (1962)
Red and Gray Foxes	Neck	Fox	2.2–2.6	9 (10)	<2.2	Schmidt and Sikes (1968)
Red Fox	Hind leg	Fox	1.2–4.7	32 (34)	<1.2	Black and Lawson (1970)
Red Fox	Hind leg	Fox	2.4	1 (5)	>2.4	Winkler et al. (1975)
Red Fox	Neck	Skunk	0.9–5.0	23 (23)	<0.9	Parker and Wilsnack (1966)
Gray Fox	Neck	Bat[c]	2.9–3.6	2 (2)	<2.9	Constantine (1966a)
Gray Fox	Neck	Bat[d]	2.9–4.2	2 (2)	<2.9	Constantine et al. (1968)
Striped Skunk	Neck	Fox	2.1–5.1	18 (31)	2.1–3.1	Sikes (1962)
Striped Skunk	Neck	Skunk	0.9–5.0	25 (29)	0.9	Parker and Wilsnack (1966)
Striped Skunk	Neck	Bat[c]	2.9–3.6	1 (2)	>2.9	Constantine (1966a)
Raccoon	Neck	Fox	0.2–9.7	11 (24)	2.2	Sikes and Tierkel (1962)
Raccoon	—	Raccoon	3.5–4.0	8 (15)	3.9	Sanderson, in McLean (1975)
Virginia Opossum	Neck	Fox	4.2–4.9	0 (13)	>4.9	Sikes and Tierkel (1960)

[a] Winkler (1975) reported that R. L. Parker (unpublished data) found that a rabies vaccine strain killed 80% of foxes inoculated in the neck but only 20% of the foxes inoculated in the hind leg.

[b] A consensus finding is that the latent period and the presence of virus in saliva is inversely proportional to the dose of inoculum in foxes. Dosages are log$_{10}$ of the dose required to kill 50% of mice inoculated intracerebrally (MICLD$_{50}$).

[c] Tadarida brasiliensis mexicana.

[d] Macrotus waterhousii; virus from three other species of bat failed to kill animals with doses of five MICLD$_{50}$.

he infected excreted more than 100 LD_{50} (up to 10,000 LD_{50}) of virus in their saliva, whereas 92% of the foxes he infected excreted less than 100 LD_{50}. Concentrations of virus in inoculum as low as 14 LD_{50} were sufficient to infect all the foxes in a treatment group, whereas 1400 to 14,000 LD_{50} was required to infect all the Striped Skunks in a treatment group. How well intramuscular injection in the neck or hind leg mimics natural bite exposure is not known. One would presume, however, that under natural conditions there would be selection for dosages and virulence, which would facilitate intraspecific spread of the virus. High dosages of virulent virus in saliva could easily preclude bite transmission among animals by killing infected animals before they become infective.

Both the length of the latent period and the presence of virus in the saliva are inversely proportional to the dose of inoculum; it appears that the other factors affecting susceptibility also affect the length of the latent period. Of particular interest in Table III are the latent periods observed in naturally infected animals; these tend to be longer than the latent periods in experimentally infected animals.

Clinical signs of rabies are quite variable and may be absent until shortly before death; virus may appear in the saliva 1–8 days before the onset of signs in foxes, skunks, and Raccoons (McLean, 1975; Parker, 1975; Winkler, 1975). Foxes may exhibit aggressive signs, paralysis, or both. Rabid foxes in captivity rarely exhibit the extreme aggression that characterizes more than 50% of the cases of human exposure from foxes under natural conditions. Foxes exhibiting furious behavior are those most likely to attack people or to draw people's attention; thus, reports on the behavior of rabid foxes ''under natural conditions'' are presumably biased towards foxes exhibiting extreme behavior. Normally, clinical onset begins with restlessness, abnormal pacing around the cage, and loss of appetite, and these symptoms are followed by a characteristic deep-toned bark and paralysis (Winkler, 1975). Signs in both naturally infected and experimentally infected skunks range from extreme aggressiveness (47% of cases) to no signs prior to death (Parker, 1975); 33–47% of naturally infected Raccoons exhibit aggressive behavior, and 7–38% are uncoordinated or appear ill (McLean, 1975). Most colonial bats do not exhibit furious rabies; many solitary bats do (Baer, 1975b). Once signs are apparent, it usually is not long before the animal dies (Table III). Commonly, illness lasts 1–3 days in foxes, 4–9 days in Striped Skunks, and 3–8 days in Raccoons.

C. SURVIVAL AFTER EXPOSURE

Not all animals naturally exposed to rabies die of the disease, just as not all experimentally exposed die (Table II). Virus prevalence in foxes trapped in the southeastern United States ranged from none in 13 areas to 3–11% in six areas; overall prevalence in 1026 foxes was 3% (Wood and Davis, 1959). In the southeast, Sikes (1962) found antibody in 3–4% of 174 foxes in areas reporting

TABLE III

Latency, Morbidity and Presence of Virus in Saliva in Terrestrial Animals Commonly Found Naturally Infected with Rabies

Species	Time from exposure to illness or death		Morbidity (days)	Virus in saliva (N)	References
	(N)	Days			
Red and Gray Foxes	24[a]	12–109	1–3	10	Sikes (1962)
Red and Gray Foxes	10	19–48	—	—	Schmidt and Sikes (1968)
Red Fox	1	105	—	—	Winkler et al. (1975)
Red Fox	58	15–153	—	—	Black and Lawson (1970)
Red Fox	23	21–68	2–17	9	Parker and Wilsack (1966)
Fox[b]	3	>275–450	—	—	Schmidt and Sikes (1968)
Gray Fox	2	9–11	<1	2	Constantine (1966a)
Gray Fox	2	22–29	6–11	1	Constantine (1966a)
Gray Fox[c]	2	14–15	<1	0	Constantine (1966b)
Striped Skunk	18	14–88	1–3	15	Sikes (1962)
Striped Skunk	25	14–172	1–18	15	Parker and Wilsnack (1966)
Striped Skunk[b]	11	19–49+	1–16	—	Gough and Niemeyer (1975)
Raccoon	11	10–42	<1–13	7	Sikes and Tierkel (1960)
Raccoon	8	10–66	—	1	Sanderson, in McLean (1975)
Raccoon[b]	2	>39–79	3–8	2	McLean (1975)
Virginia Opossum[d]	1	30	1	0	Sikes and Tierkel (1960)

[a] Additional foxes survived inoculation and developed antibody; results not reported by species.

[b] Naturally infected; foxes' taxa not reported; 1 skunk developed rabies 7 weeks after capture and 1 initiated an epizootic in a laboratory colony, which killed 10 Striped Skunks.

[c] Infected by bite of experimentally infected Brazilian Free-tailed Bat.

[d] Eighteen additional Virginia Opossums survived; none died from intramuscular inoculations; one of three died from intracranial inoculation.

rabies. In epizootic areas in Virginia, Carey and McLean (1978) found that 5% of 40 Gray Foxes were infected and that 8% of 94 had antibody; none of 25 Red Foxes were infected, but 2% of 47 had antibody. Virus prevalence was 8% of 268 Striped Skunks and 4% of 52 Spotted Skunks in Iowa (Hendricks and Seaton, 1969); a later study found that 68% of 82 Striped Skunks and 26% of 19 Spotted Skunks had antibody (Gough and Dierks, 1971). Virus prevalences in Raccoons in epizootic areas in Florida were 3–36%, whereas antibody prevalences were 17–22% (McLean, 1975). In enzootic areas, virus prevalences were often less than 1%, but antibody prevalences averaged 7.2%. McLean (1975), after holding Raccoons captured during an epizootic for 2 years, concluded that 8 of 10 Raccoons survived after receiving natural exposures sufficient to induce antibody. In New York, 3% of 278 Big Brown Bats (*Eptesicus fuscus*) were infected, and 10% of 187 had antibody; less than 1% of 333 Little Brown Bats (*Myotis lucifugus*) were infected, but 2% had antibody (Trimarchi and Debbie, 1977).

III. Rabies Ecology

A. MULTISPECIES INVOLVEMENT

1. Surveillance Reports

Surveillance reports generally have been interpreted as implicating one principal terrestrial carnivore species as the source of most concurrent cases in other species. Rabies in bats has been interpreted as a separate phenomenon. Because of the general policy for examining suspect animals only if humans have been exposed to them, surveillance programs are probably good indicators of the existence of epizootics. But it would be unwise to try to draw many inferences about the incidence of enzootic rabies from these reports. During epizootics, individuals of many species are reported to be infected with rabies. During fox rabies epizootics in New York, more than 20 species were found to be infected with rabies (Friend, 1968). Cases in domestic animals paralleled the rise and fall of fox rabies; cases in cattle were approximately the same magnitude as the reported cases in foxes. Cases in Raccoons also were correlated with cases in foxes. Cases in bats and in Striped Skunks, however, did not reflect the cases in foxes. A similar pattern occurred in Tennessee, but with far less involvement of cattle. More than 20 species have been found infected with rabies in Virginia, but case reports during 1963–1969 were dominated by 360 Gray Foxes (92% of the rabid foxes) and 132 cattle, with a smaller number (31) of Red Foxes found rabid (Prior, 1969).

2. Field Investigations

Several field investigations have been conducted to determine, with less bias than pertains to rabies surveillance programs, the species of wild animals that were involved with rabies. While surveillance programs have the peculiar bias of having greater proabilities of detecting rabid animals exhibiting the most extreme signs (e.g., aggressive behavior of "sick" animals), programs of capturing wild animals would be biased toward animals that are behaviorally normal (i.e., respond to olfactory or food stimuli).

a. **Fox–Rabies Areas.**   Wood and Davis (1959) examined 2148 wild animals in the southeastern United States. There was no statistically significant difference between the prevalence of rabies virus in Gray Foxes and Red Foxes (see Table IV). No infected Raccoons, Virginia Opossums, or Eastern Cottontails were found. A few Bobcats (*Felis rufus*), Striped Skunks, and bats were infected. Serological surveys found that many (4.6–18.5%) of the terrestrial carnivores in areas of recent rabies outbreaks in foxes had antibody to rabies (see Table IV), but none of 300 animals from areas that had not reported rabies had antibody (Tierkel, 1959). Prior (1969) reported that none of 25 Gray Foxes, 15

TABLE IV

Prevalence of Rabies Virus Infections and Rabies-neutralizing Antibody in Wild Mammals Trapped in Areas of Rabies Outbreaks in the Southeastern United States[a]

Species	Rabies infections		Rabies antibody[b]	
	Number tested	Number infected (%)	Number tested	Number with antibodies (%)
Gray Fox	909	2.8	262[c]	4.6
Red Fox	117	1.7	—	—
Bobcat[d]	89	1.1	27	18.5
Striped Skunk	144	0.7	48	14.5
Raccoon	299	0.0	196	5.6
Virginia Opossum	215	0.0	185	1.8
Eastern Cottontail[e]	123	0.0	0	—
Bats[f]	252	0.8	0	—

[a] Adapted from Wood and Davis (1959).

[b] None of 300 animals from areas that had not reported rabies had antibody.

[c] Includes both Gray Foxes and Red Foxes.

[d] *Felis rufus.*

[e] *Sylvilagus* spp.

[f] One of one *Lasiurus seminolus* and one of 71 *Myotis austroriparius* were infected.

Red Foxes, 56 Striped Skunks, 75 assorted rodents, 11 insectivores, and 47 bats captured in a fox–rabies enzootic area in Virginia were infected with rabies. More than 1000 rodents were examined in New York and Georgia but none were found to be infected (Tierkel, 1959).

b. Skunk–Rabies Areas. Hendricks and Seaton (1969) examined 1634 animals in Iowa; Striped Skunks and Spotted Skunks were infected with rabies, but none of six other carnivore species were infected (see Table IV). In Iowa, Niemeyer (1973) found high prevalences of antibody in Striped Skunks and Spotted Skunks and moderate prevalences in Raccoons and Virginia Opossums (see Table V), but he cautioned that nonspecific reaction may have inflated the results. Gough and Jorgenson (1976) found antibody in the sera of 23% of predatory birds ($N = 65$) and 2.9% of nonpredatory birds ($N = 278$) in Iowa. It is unlikely that birds are reservoirs of rabies. Antibody to rabies was induced in a Great Horned Owl (*Bubo virginianus*) by feeding it an infected Spotted Skunk carcass (Jorgenson *et al.,* 1976). In Illinois, 8.6% of Striped Skunks ($N = 362$) were infected with rabies, but none of 26 Red Foxes or 48 Gray Foxes were infected (Verts and Storm, 1966). Hall (1978) found that 17% of Virginia

TABLE V

Prevalence of Rabies Virus Infections and Rabies Antibody in Areas of Rabies Outbreaks in Skunks in Iowa

Species	Rabies infections[a]		Rabies antibody[b]	
	Number tested	Number infected (%)	Number tested	Number with antibodies (%)
Striped Skunk	268	7.8	82	68.3
Spotted Skunk	52	3.8	19	26.3
Mink[c]	377	0.0	—	—
Fox	365	0.0	—	—
Raccoon	219	0.0	301	7.6
Virginia Opossum	208	0.0	84	1.2
Coyote[d]	65	0.0	—	—
Badger[e]	7	0.0	—	—
Weasel[f]	1	0.0	—	—

[a] From Hendricks and Seaton (1969).
[b] From Niemeyer (1973), who cautioned that non-specific reactions may have inflated prevalences.
[c] *Mustela vison.*
[d] *Canis latrans.*
[e] *Taxidea taxus.*
[f] *Mustela* spp.

Opossums ($N = 608$) had antibody to rabies in areas of skunk–rabies epizootics in Tennessee.

3. Theoretical Explanations

Three manifestations of multispecies rabies are common throughout the eastern United States. First, rabies virus seems to be maintained concurrently, but independently, in bats and in one common terrestrial carnivore (e.g., Striped Skunk, Gray Fox, Red Fox, or Raccoon). Second, during epizootics in terrestrial carnivores, up to 20 species may be infected. Cases in these additional species are "spillovers" from the major species. But the degree of involvement of these other species has been particularly high in Virginia Opossums, Bobcats, and Spotted Skunks. Third, changes in the major terrestrial carnivore species suffering epizootics may occur over time.

A major deficiency in studies of rabies in wildlife has been the failure to investigate enzootic rabies. It is difficult to muster the resources necessary to adequately sample carnivore populations with rabies prevalence of less than 1% (epizootic prevalences are commonly 1–5%). Several hundred animals would have to be trapped to obtain reliable estimates of the prevalence in any particular population. In my experience, adequate sample sizes could be obtained with six professional trappers, supported by three technicians (to do necropsies and laboratory tests). It is beyond the ability of most health agencies to devote such an effort solely to the study of rabies in wild carnivores in a relatively restricted geographic area. Theoretical explanations, then, must be largely speculative. For example, it is not possible to confidently postulate that rabies has been maintained in a balanced host–parasite relationship with any of the terrestrial carnivores associated with rabies. An equally likely explanation is that rabies virus is an adaptable parasite. Once introduced into a species population, rabies virus may persist at low (enzootic) incidence, undergo cycles of epizootic abundance (e.g., with an amplitude of 3–5 years) and persist indefinitely, or the virus may cause drastic declines in host populations that disrupt the continuity of transmission. Sometime in the course of the association, the virus may become established in another species population. Hall (1978) termed such parasites "dynamic disease entities." An elaboration on this pattern entails changes in the virus virulence that, while disrupting the extant host–parasite association, facilitates transfer to a new host species. The first case, the balanced association, implies coadaption, whereas the second only implies genetic variability in the virus. These hypotheses, however, are not mutually exclusive. It is not possible to say whether the major decline in reported cases of fox rabies in the past decade was due to an achievement of enzootic balance or to a disappearance of rabies virus from the fox populations. Likewise, the idea that an inapparent reservoir (e.g., in mustelids, bats, or felids) provides virus for epizootics in other species cannot be discarded without intensive studies of rabies during enzootic periods.

B. ZOOGEOGRAPHIC AND LANDSCAPE EFFECTS

There seems to be little relationship between the distribution of the major hosts (bats, Red Fox, Gray Fox, Striped Skunk, and Raccoon) and the primary host in a particular area. All are widely distributed across the eastern United States. Within a geographic area, persistent rabies may be confined to particular landscapes. Carey et al. (1978) discussed the relationship between rabies in Gray Foxes and the landscape in Virginia; Carey (1982) discussed the fox–rabies patterns in the eastern United States. Fox rabies persisted in areas of rugged topography with a mixture of farms and forests, despite equally high fox populations in the Piedmont and Coastal Plain areas. Discontinuity of environments preferred by foxes and patchiness in fox population density were postulated as a mechanism that forestalls depletion of susceptible foxes by rapid epizootic spread. The host shifts from fox to skunk, in New York and Tennessee, were first noted in such areas of persistent fox rabies, but rabies in skunks did not thereafter remain confined to those regions.

C. VIRUS VIRULENCE AND HOST RESISTANCE

Differences in susceptibility and amount of virus secreted in saliva were postulated as mechanisms whereby rabies was maintained in a primary host species (Sikes and Tierkel, 1960). The argument was as follows: foxes excrete too little virus to infect Striped Skunks; Striped Skunks excrete a quantity of virus that kills foxes before they become infective (i.e., secrete virus in their saliva); Raccoons are more resistant to rabies than skunks or foxes (Raccoons were not major hosts of rabies before 1960). Differences in virus strains (street strains adapted to a particular species) were also suggested to play a role. Sanderson et al. (1967) felt that ecological and behavioral barriers among species further contributed to limiting rabies to one primary species. It is likely that changes in virus virulence do occur in natural populations. Epizootics may, in part, reflect a change towards increased virulence and thus facilitate transfer from foxes to skunks or Raccoons. Likewise, enzootic maintenance in Striped Skunks could produce a lower virulence virus that could serve to precipitate an epizootic in foxes. Pantropism (Carey and McLean, 1978; Debbie and Trimarchi, 1970; Howard, 1981), or the presence of virus throughout the organs of the body, could play a role in infecting (or immunizing) animals that consume infected tissues, as Hall (1978) suggested had occurred in Virginia Opossums. But these are speculations; the actual importances of these mechanisms are not known.

The presence of virus-neutralizing substances (often interpreted as antibody and implying immunity) in the blood of hosts of rabies suggests that a balance between susceptible and immune animals may interact with environmental quality (and the resultant species population density) to contribute to enzootic maintenance of the virus (Carey, 1982), but it would not seem to be an important influence on multispecies complexes. The implication of immunity seems justified because such virus-neutralizing substances have been induced experimentally and have conferred resistance to further, massive inoculations of rabies virus. Sanderson *et al.* (1967) and McLean (1970) felt that virus could be maintained in latent form in major host species until stress (due to population density or physiological status such as pregnancy or lactation) served to suppress the immune system and cause a recrudescence of the latent infection. Here again, antibody-related mechanisms are speculations.

D. CONCLUSIONS

Multispecies rabies in the United States is manifested in three ways: (1) independent cycles in bats and terrestrial carnivores, (2) spillover infections from epizootics in a primary species, and (3) apparent shifts of major host species with time. But field data are lacking and elucidation of the ecology of rabies virus must await further research.

References

Baer, G. M. (1975a). Pathogenesis to the central nervous system. *In* "The Natural History of Rabies" (G. M. Baer, ed.), Vol. 1, pp. 181–198. Academic Press, New York.

Baer, G. M. (1975b). Rabies in nonhematophagous bats. *In* "The Natural History of Rabies" (G. M. Baer, ed.), Vol. 2, pp. 79–97. Academic Press, New York.

Bell, J. F. (1975). Latency and abortive rabies. *In* "The Natural History of Rabies" (G. M. Baer, ed.) Vol. 1, pp. 331–354. Academic Press, New York.

Black, J. G., and Lawson, K. F. (1970). Sylvatic rabies studies in the silver fox (*Vulpes vulpes*). Susceptibility and immune response. *Can. J. Comp. Med.* **34,** 309–311.

Carey, A. B. (1982). The ecology of red foxes, gray foxes, and rabies in the eastern United States. *Wildl. Soc. Bull.* **10,** 18–26.

Carey, A. B., and McLean, R. G. (1978). Rabies antibody prevalence and virus tissue tropism in wild carnivores in Virginia. *J. Wildl. Dis.* **14,** 487–491.

Carey, A. B., Giles, R. H., and McLean, R. G. (1978). The landscape epidemiology of rabies in Virginia. *Am. J. Trop. Med. Hyg.* **27,** 573–580.

Centers for Disease Control (1981a). "Rabies Surveillance Annual Summary 1978." U.S. Dept. of Health and Human Services, Atlanta, Georgia.

Centers for Disease Control (1981b). Rabies—United States, 1980. *Morbid Mortal. Wkly. Rep.* **30,** 147.

Centers for Disease Control (1981c). Rabies in raccoons—Virginia. *Morbid Mortal. Wkly. Rep.* **30,** 353–355.

Charlton, K. M., and Casey, G. A. (1979a). Experimental oral and nasal transmission of rabies virus in mice. *Can. J. Comp. Med.* **43,** 10–15.

Charlton, K. M., and Casey, G. A. (1979b). Experimental rabies in skunks: Oral, nasal, tracheal and intestinal exposure. *Can. J. Comp. Med.* **43,** 168–172.

Constantine, D. G. (1966a). Transmission experiments with bat rabies isolates. Reaction of certain carnivora, opossum, and bats to intramuscular inoculations of rabies virus isolated from free-tailed bats. *Am. J. Vet. Res.* **27,** 16–19.

Constantine, D. G. (1966b). Transmission experiments with bat rabies isolates: Bite transmission of rabies to foxes and coyote by free-tailed bats. *Am. J. Vet. Res.* **27,** 20–23.

Constantine, D. G. (1979). An updated list of rabies-infected bats in North America. *J. Wildl. Dis.* **15,** 347–349.

Constantine, D. G., Solomon, G. C., and Woodall, D. F. (1968). Transmission experiments with bat rabies isolates: Response of certain carnivores and rodents to rabies virus from four species of bats. *Am. J. Vet. Res.* **29,** 181–190.

Debbie, J. G., and Trimarchi, C. V. (1970). Pantropism of rabies virus in free-ranging rabid red fox, *Vulpes fulva. J. Wildl. Dis.* **6,** 500–505.

Fischman, H. R. (1976). Consideration of an association between geographic distribution of caves and occurrence of rabies in foxes. *J. Am. Vet. Med. Assoc.* **169,** 1207–1213.

Fredrickson, L. E., and Thomas, L. (1965). Relationship of fox rabies to caves. *Public Health Rep.* **80,** 495–500.

Friend, M. (1968). History and epidemiology of rabies in wildlife in New York. *N.Y. Fish Game J.* **15,** 71–97.

Gough, P. M., and Dierks, R. E. (1971). Passive haemagglutination test for antibodies against rabies virus. *Bull. W.H.O.* **45,** 741–745.

Gough, P. M. and Jorgenson, R. D. (1976). Rabies antibody in sera of wild birds. *J. Wildl. Dis.* **12,** 392–395.

Gough, P. M., and Niemeyer, C. (1975). A rabies epidemic in recently captured skunks. *J. Wildl. Dis.* **11,** 170–176.

Hall, H. F. (1978). The ecology of rabies in northeastern Tennessee. Ph.D. Dissertation, University of Tennessee, Knoxville.

Hendricks, S. L., and Seaton, V. A. (1969). Rabies in wild animals trapped for pelts. *Bull. Wildl. Dis. Assoc.* **5,** 231–234.

Howard, D. R. (1981). Transplacental transmission of rabies virus from a naturally infected skunk. *Am. J. Vet. Res.* **42,** 691–692.

Jennings, W. L., Schneider, N. J., Lewis, A. L., and Scatterday, J. E. (1960). Fox rabies in Florida. *J. Wildl. Manage.* **24,** 171–179.

Jorgenson, R. D., Gough, P. M. and Graham, D. L. (1976). Experimental rabies in a great horned owl. *J. Wildl. Dis.* **12,** 444–447.

McLean, R. G. (1970). Wildlife rabies in the United States: Recent History and current concepts. *J. Wildl. Dis.* **6,** 229–233.

McLean, R. G. (1975). Raccoon rabies. *In* "The Natural History of Rabies" (G. M. Baer, ed.), Vol. 2, pp. 53–77. Academic Press, New York.

Mahan, W. E. (1973). An evaluation of the relationship between cave-dwelling bats and fox rabies in Appalachia. M.S. Thesis, University of Georgia, Athens.

Murphy, F. A., and Bauer, S. P. (1974). Early street rabies virus infection in striated muscle and later progression to the central nervous system. *Intervirology* **3,** 256–268.

Nathanson, N., and Cole, G. A. (1971). Immunosuppression: A means to asses the role of the immune response in acute virus infections. *Fed. Proc., Fed. Am. Soc. Exp. Biol.* **30,** 1822–1830.

Niemeyer, C. C. (1973). An ecological and serological survey of rabies in some central Iowa mammals. M.S. Thesis, Iowa State University, Ames.

Parker, R. L. (1975). Rabies in skunks. *In* "The Natural History of Rabies" (G. M. Baer, ed.), Vol. 2, pp. 41–51. Academic Press, New York.

Parker, R. L., and Wilsnack, R. E. (1966). Pathogenesis of skunk rabies virus: Quantitation in skunks and foxes. *Am. J. Vet. Res.* **27,** 33–38.

Prior, E. T. (1969). A study of rabies incidence in western Virginia. M.S. Thesis, Virginia Polytechnic Institute, Blacksburg.

Ramsden, R. O., and Johnston, D. H. (1975). Studies on the oral infectivity of rabies virus in Carnivora. *J. Wildl. Dis.* **11**, 318–324.

Sanderson, G. C., Verts, B. J., and Storm, G. L. (1967). Recent studies of wildlife rabies in Illinois. *Bull Wildl. Dis. Assoc.* **3**, 92.

Scatterday, J. E., Schneider, N. J., Jennings, W. L., and Lewis, A. L. (1960). Sporadic animal rabies in Florida. *Public Health Rep.* **75**, 945–953.

Schmidt, R. C., and Sikes, R. K. (1968). Immunization of foxes with inactivated-virus rabies vaccine. *Am. J. Vet. Res.* **29**, 1843–1847.

Sikes, R. K. (1962). Pathogenesis of rabies in wildlife. I. Comparative effect of varying doses of rabies virus inoculated into foxes and skunks. *Am. J. Vet. Res.* **23**, 1041–1047.

Sikes, R. K., and Tierkel, E. S. (1960). Wildlife rabies in the southeast. *In* "Proceedings of the 64th Annual Meeting of the U.S. Livestock Sanitary Association," pp. 268–272. MacCrellish & Quigley Co., Trenton, New Jersey.

Tierkel, E. S. (1959). Rabies. *Adv. Vet. Sci.* **5**, 183–226.

Trimarchi, C. V., and Debbie, J. G. (1977). Naturally occurring rabies virus and neutralizing antibody in two species of insectivorous bats of New York States. *J. Wildl. Dis.* **13**, 366–369.

Verts, B. J., and Storm, G. L. (1966). A local study of prevalence of rabies among foxes and striped skunks. *J. Wildl. Manage.* **30**, 419–421.

Winkler, W. G. (1975). Fox rabies. *In* "The Natural History of Rabies" (G. M. Baer, ed.), Vol. 2, pp. 3–22. Academic Press, New York.

Winkler, W. G., Schneider, N. J. and Jennings, W. L. (1972). Experimental rabies infection in wild rodents. *J. Wildl. Dis.* **8**, 99–103.

Winkler, W. G., McLean, R. G., and Cowart, J. C. (1975). Vaccination of foxes against rabies using ingested baits. *J. Wildl. Dis.* **11**, 383–388.

Wood, J. E., and Davis, E. E. (1959). The prevalence of rabies in populations of foxes in the southern states. *J. Am. Vet. Med. Assoc.* **135**, 121–124.

Mongoose Rabies in Grenada

3

C. O. R. Everard
J. D. Everard
Leptospira Laboratory,
Medical Research Council,
Collymore Rock,
St. Michael, Barbados

I. Introduction

Mongooses are indigenous to Africa and most of the Middle and Far East, where they are important reservoirs of rabies. The small Indian mongoose (*Herpestes auropunctatus*) was introduced into many of the Caribbean islands in the 1870s and 1880s to combat rats in the sugar cane fields. Within 10–15 years, the mongoose had itself become an agricultural pest and the object of numerous unsuccessful attempts at eradication, but it now commands little attention in most of the islands to which it was introduced. The exceptions are those islands where it is a known reservoir and vector of rabies (Grenada, Puerto Rico, Cuba and the Dominican Republic). On Grenada, *Herpestes* is known to be the direct or indirect source of the majority of rabies cases recorded on that island, and where the source is not known, *Herpestes* is the probable cause.

POPULATION DYNAMICS OF RABIES IN WILDLIFE

The Caribbean mongoose was first positively incriminated as a rabies vector in 1950 in Puerto Rico (Tierkel *et al.,* 1952), and subsequently in Grenada, Cuba and the Dominican Republic. Rabies was present in dogs in Puerto Rico at least in 1841 (that is, before the mongoose was introduced) (Colon, 1930), but when it first appeared in Grenada, and whether it came in with the mongoose on one of several importations or was introduced by dogs, bats or some other source, is not known. However, records from 1902 indicate the suspect behaviour of mongooses and domestic animals, and there are reports of rabies cases in the 1940s, but the disease was not laboratory confirmed until 1952, when a cow died of it (Murray, 1968). In 1953 another cow died of rabies, but this one was known to have been bitten by a mongoose. It is not possible now to say what course the epizootic took, when it reached its peak, or how many cyclic fluctuations of rabies there have been since its first appearance, which may have been in the last century. In the 1960s, the situation on Grenada was particularly disturbing and led to the setting up, in 1968, of a full-time research and surveillance programme. The problem was also costly, and Everard (1975) calculated that in 1973 rabies cost the Grenada Government 0.4% of its entire revenue for that year, and this sum did not include expenditure by foreign agencies.

Between 1952 and 1967, cases of rabies in Grenada were reported sporadically. They comprised 3 humans, 1 bat, 88 dogs, 3 cats, 100 livestock animals, 142 mongooses and 21 unknowns (total 358). Between 1968, when the full-time surveillance and research programme was initiated, and 1977, there were 699 cases of rabies comprising 1 human, 2 bats, 541 mongooses, 1 opossum, 29 dogs, 12 cats and 113 livestock animals. The cumulative record shows that at least 1057 rabies cases were recorded on the 120-square mile island in the 26 years between 1952 and 1977 (Everard *et al.,* 1979a). The surveillance data are summarized below according to the different categories of victim.

II. Surveillance

A. HUMANS

Three young people died of rabies in 1962–1963, two of whom had been bitten by dogs and one by a cat. A 7-year-old boy died of rabies in 1970, but neither he nor his parents could explain how the exposure to rabies virus had occurred. Although this was the only known fatality in the 10 years of the surveillance programme, the number of people needing treatment for bites or contact with rabid animals was relatively high. In all, 208 individuals were treated, over one-half of them (57%) for mongoose bites (Table I). Treatment prompted by dog and cat bites constituted the next largest categories (22 and 7%, respectively). Most of the people treated for livestock contact had handled the animals and had not been bitten.

TABLE I

Post-exposure Antirabies Treatment of Humans on Grenada

Year	Human contact											
	Mongoose	Dog	Cat	Bovine	Human	Donkey	Goat	Rat	Bat	Total	Unknown	Total
1968[a]	12	3	—	2	—	—	—	1	—	18	11	29
1969	11	8	3	—	—	—	—	—	—	22	—	22
1970	22	15	4	2	2	—	—	—	—	45	—	45
1971	18	6	1	—	—	—	—	—	—	25	—	25
1972	15	1	1	—	—	—	1	—	—	18	—	18
1973	7	4	4	6	—	1	—	—	—	22	—	22
1974	12	—	1	—	1	1	—	—	1	16	—	16
1975	5	—	—	—	—	—	—	—	—	5	—	5
1976	8	4	—	1	—	—	—	—	—	13	—	13
1977	9	4	—	—	—	—	—	—	—	13	—	13
Total	119	45	14	11	3	2	1	1	1	197	11	208
Percentage of all contacts	57	22	7	5	1	1	0.5	0.5	0.5	95	5	100

[a] There are no detailed records of human antirabies treatment before 1968.

B. DOGS AND CATS

The 132 cases of dog and cat rabies recorded between 1952 and 1977 are shown by year in Table II. Table III shows the numbers of dogs immunized in major vaccination campaigns, in recent years using ERA vaccine (which has a known 4-year period of conferred immunity in dogs) or suckling mouse brain vaccine. In addition, 339 cats were immunized in 1976. The decline in dog rabies seen in 1972–1975 was probably a consequence of the many dogs vaccinated in 1971 and the follow-up immunization of 7350 dogs in 1973. There was a corresponding reduction in human treatments for dog bite in the same period. However, the five cases in 1976 and two in 1977, and the numbers of human treatments for dog contact in those years, showed that too few dogs were being immunized. The overall effectiveness of the dog vaccination campaigns was shown by comparing the numbers of dog rabies cases in the 13-year period of 1965–1977 (39 or an average of 3/year) with those in the earlier 10-year period of 1955–1964 (78 or 8/year). The existence of a large stray dog population and the freedom allowed to domesticated dogs and cats afford ample opportunity for contact with mongooses. Most of the potential cases of dog rabies arose from dogs attacking disorientated rabid mongooses, rather than from intraspecific contact between dogs, as is the case in most of Central and South America. For example, in 1973, 21 of 39 laboratory-confirmed rabid mongooses were killed while fighting with dogs. Every unvaccinated dog is a potential threat because of

TABLE II

Cases of Rabies in Dogs, Cats and Livestock on Grenada[a]

Year	Dog	Cat	Bovine	Goat	Sheep	Pig	Equine	Total	Unknown	Total
1952	—	—	1	—	—	—	—	1	—	1
1953	—	—	4	—	—	—	—	4	—	4
1954	—	—	—	—	—	—	—	0	—	0
1955	4	—	6	1	—	—	—	11	—	11
1956	1	—	1	1	2	—	4	9	—	9
1957	19	—	—	—	—	1	3	23	—	23
1958	4	—	4	—	—	—	—	8	—	8
1959	9	—	8	—	—	—	—	17	—	17
1960	4	—	4	—	—	—	1	9	—	9
1961	3	—	3	1	—	—	—	7	8	15
1962	5	—	4	—	—	—	—	9	9	18
1963	18	3	14	2	—	2	—	39	—	39
1964	11	—	8	—	—	—	—	19	3	22
1965	6	—	5	1	4	—	—	16	—	16
1966	3	—	3	—	2	—	—	8	1	9
1967	1	—	5	1	1	1	2	11	—	11
1968	7	—	9	2	—	1	—	19	—	19
1969	2	3	2	2	—	3	—	12	1	13
1970	5	4	6	—	—	—	1	16	—	16
1971	4	1	7	2	4	2	—	20	—	20
1972	1	1	4	2	3	—	—	11	—	11
1973	2	2	13	8	4	—	5	34	—	34
1974	—	1	3	1	1	—	1	7	—	7
1975	1	—	8	—	—	1	1	11	—	11
1976	5	—	5	1	2	3	—	16	—	16
1977	2	—	3	1	—	1	—	7	—	7
Total	117	15	130	26	23	15	18	344	22	366
Percentage of 366	32	4	36	7	6	4	5	—	6	—
Total 1968–1977	29	12	60	19	14	11	8	153	1	154
Percentage of 154	19	8	39	12	9	7	5	—	1	—

[a] The figures include some cases not laboratory-confirmed but with a high index of suspicion.

its close association with man and its innate tendency to attack and bite, especially domestic animals. Also, considering the numbers of cases of cat rabies and the human death caused by a cat bite, cat vaccination should be standard policy on Grenada. There is probably more cat–mongoose contact on the island than generally supposed.

TABLE III

Antirabies Immunization of Dogs on Grenada

Year	No. of dogs immunized
1956	5,290
1965	8,963
1967	1,371
1968	8,087
1969	3,598
1971	11,384[a]
1972	531
1973	7,350[b]
1975	1,001
1976	3,240

[a] These include 200 immunized privately.
[b] The dog population in 1973 was estimated at 35,000.

C. LIVESTOCK

Because people value their domestic animals, it would be reasonable to suppose that all cases of rabies in this category are discovered and that the numbers of reported cases approach a true value. However, a poor farmer in a remote area whose cow has died may not be able to report the death, since communication in Grenada is often difficult and tedious. He may also fear that the authorities will require him to slaughter his other animals or pay for vaccinations. For much of the time in the earlier years of the epizootic, there were few veterinarians (sometimes none at all) to give advice or to diagnose rabies, and there was many a farmer who, having seen his cow bitten by a mongoose, slaughtered it and sold the carcass for human consumption. Indeed, this became such a problem that advice on immediate slaughter and the excision of wounds prior to sale had to be given officially. Almost certainly, therefore, the recorded numbers of cases of livestock rabies are too low.

Of the 234 livestock rabies cases recorded (Table II), 130 (56%) occurred in bovine animals, 26 (11%) in goats and 23 (10%) in sheep. Mongooses were directly responsible for the great majority of cases where the source was known. There were four substantiated reports of livestock being bitten by mongooses on a known day and subsequently dying of rabies. The number of days between the biting incident and death ranged from 20 to 40. Where no firm dates were available, casual reports indicated that the biting incident usually took place 3–4 weeks before the death of the animal. Clinical signs of the disease in livestock were usually observed at least 5 days before death. There was one recorded failure of pre-vaccination. There were three instances where unvaccinated live-stock animals were followed up after they had been bitten by mongooses, and their owners refused to slaughter them. The rabies serum neutralizing (SN) antibody titres of blood samples collected from these animals 1 month or more after the biting incident ranged from 1 : 5 to 1 : 32. (Titration endpoints are expressed as the highest dilution inhibiting the reaction. A titre of 1 : 5 or higher is considered to be positive.)

The small size of Grenada, its rural nature and the ubiquity of the mongoose have provided an environment in which there is ready contact between man and domestic animals on the one hand and mongooses on the other. The com-paratively high cattle losses recorded can probably be attributed to the almost invariable practice of tethering cows in pastures or scrub woodland, where they are easily bitten and unable to avoid persistently attacking rabid mongooses. Sheep and goats are more usually tethered by roadsides or in back gardens and are not attacked so often. The high number of cases in 1973 may be attributed in part to better reporting and surveillance following the appointment of a veteri-nary advisor. During 1973, approximately 1500 cattle, equines and other farm animals were vaccinated against rabies, and an even better response was achieved in 1976 when vaccination was not charged to the farmer. In this year, the livestock vaccination programme, which ran concurrently with the dog and cat campaign, was especially well publicised, and 2311 animals comprising 575 bovines, 828 goats, 721 sheep, 182 donkeys, 3 horses and 2 mules were immu-nized.

D. WILDLIFE

Besides bats, the terrestrial fauna of Grenada includes five species of amphibi-an, 8 lizard species, 6 snake species, and 12 mammalian species of which 7 are rodents (Groome, 1970). The other five are *Marmosa mitis* (opossum), *Didelphis marsupialis* (opossum), *Dasypus novemcinctus* (armadillo), *Cercopithecus mona* (monkey) and *Herpestes auropunctatus* (mongoose). Among these, other than *Herpestes*, there is one recorded (unconfirmed) case of rabies in a *Didelphis* opossum. This record is probably spurious, taking into account the circumstances surrounding the report, the species' high resistance to rabies infection (Beamer *et al.*, 1960), and the fact that *Didelphis* is highly aggressive when cornered, spitting and hissing in a manner which might indicate rabies to the inexperienced observer.

1. Bats

There are 13 bats species on Grenada, all of which are fruit or insect eating. One *Molossus sp.* was found rabid in 1961 by fluorescent antibody (FA) micros-copy (though mouse inoculation tests were inconclusive) (Murray, 1968). Two cases of rabies in *Artibeus jamaicensis* were reported in 1974, but only one was laboratory confirmed. Price and Everard (1977) collected 411 Grenadian bats belonging to six species. These were *Anoura geoffroyi, Artibeus cinereus, A. jamaicensis, Glossophaga longirostris, Molossus molossus* and *Sturnira lilium.* Tests for rabies virus were negative, but SN antibodies were found in 27 of 353 (7.6%) examined. Positives occurred in each of the six species sampled. Seventeen of 42 *A. jamaicensis* examined (40%) were positive for SN antibodies, 14 of 25 of them coming from a single cave. According to Jones and Phillips (1970), *A. jamaicensis* is widely distributed on every major island in the Caribbean. It is a fruit-eating bat of medium size, frequents gardens with fruit trees at night, and often roosts during the day under the eaves of houses, so that the potential exists for exposure of humans, pets and livestock. The rabies cycles in Grenadian bats and mongooses are almost certainly independent of one another, and rabies can exist in bats for long periods, as in Trinidad, without transmission to available carnivore hosts. However, the presence of a rabies reservoir in bats from which mongooses could be reinfected (either by being bitten or, more likely, through eating moribund or disorientated rabid bats) should not be overlooked. Indeed, it is possible, though unprovable, that the present mongoose rabies enzootic originated in this way.

2. Mongooses

Where possible, brain material from mongooses that attacked humans, domestic pets or livestock without provocation was examined for rabies by FA microscopy according to the method of Dean (1966). Attacking mongooses could not always be retrieved, but since a close correlation was shown between unprovoked attack and laboratory confirmation (Jonkers *et al.,* 1969), rabies could be presumed with a very high degree of certainty. Because mongooses are normally quick-moving, furtive and well able to avoid vehicles, brain material from those found run over on the roads was also examined. The numbers of rabid mongooses in all three categories (laboratory confirmed, suspect and run-over) are shown in Table IV. There was a large number of attacking mongooses reported in 1973, paralleling the large number of domestic animal cases. There are no reports of mongooses attacking other mongooses. It is reasonable to assume that relatively few rabid mongooses are seen by people, and that even fewer come to the attention of individuals who are able to report them, so that the numbers of reported cases are only a small proportion of the actual cases. Because the figures in all the categories in Table IV are dependent on the presence of a human and/or domestic animal population, they cannot be used in calculating the prevalence of the disease in mongooses.

The prevalence of mongoose rabies was monitored by maintaining a trapping programme and examining the brains of trapped animals by FA microscopy. Between 1968 and 1977 trapping usually took place 5 days a week at least 45 weeks a year, but its organization did not come within the jurisdiction of the research programme. For logistic reasons it was not possible to expend the same

TABLE IV

Cases of Rabies or Presumed Rabies in Attacking Mongooses and Those Run Over on the Road

Year	Attacking mongooses with confirmed rabies		Attacking mongooses presumed rabid	Rabid mongooses run over	Total
	Categories combined				
1952	0				
1953	3				
1954	0				
1955	7				
1956	9				
1957	4				
1958	15				
1959	8				
1960	5				
1961	4				
1962	5				
1963	20				
1964	9				
1965[a]	4		16		20
1966[a]	4		0		4
1967[a]	7		0		7
1968	22[b]		12	1	35
1969	18		11	0	29
1970	14		17	2	33
1971	30		15	1	46
1972	18		11	1	30
1973	39		24	0	63
1974	26		13	0	39
1975	20		25	0	45
1976	16		13	0	29
1977	17		19	0	36
Total	235	89	176	5	

[a] Taken from Jonkers *et al.* (1969).
[b] Includes one rabid mongoose of two specimens examined by Jonkers *et al.* (1969).

trapping effort throughout the island and in every month of the year; more trapping took place on the western side of the island than on the eastern side. Among the factors that influence the catch in this type of investigation are weather (since mongooses prefer not to forage in the wet), skill of the trapper, the trapping history of the area, the length of time spent in an area, trap spacing, vegetation and terrain. However, because of the long duration of the study and the large numbers of animals involved, the overall effects of these factors can be discounted. Table V shows the numbers of mongooses trapped annually between

TABLE V

Wild-caught Mongooses on Grenada with Rabies or Rabies Serum Neutralizing Antibody

Year	No. of mongooses examined for rabies	No. positive for rabies (%)		No. examined for SN antibody	No. positive for SN antibody (%)
1965[a]	75	2	(2.7)		
1966[a]	191	8	(4.2)		
1967[a]	262	12	(4.6)		
1968[b]	705	26	(3.7)		
1969	1,019	11	(1.1)		
1970	1,727	9	(0.5)		
1971	1,742	61	(3.5)	149	31 (20.8)
1972	1,404	28	(2.0)	818	197 (24.1)
1973	780[c]	6	(0.8)	546	200 (36.6)
1974	828[d]	5	(0.6)	162	70 (43.2)
1975	1,140	6	(0.5)		
1976	1,108	2	(0.2)		
1977	1,464	2	(0.1)		
1978[e]	1,000 approx.	2	(0.2)		
1979[e]	292	2	(0.7)		
1980[e]	1,343	18	(1.3)		

[a] Taken from Jonkers et al. (1969).

[b] These include seven rabid mongooses of 72 (9.7%) examined by Jonkers et al. (1969).

[c] These numbers are low because a poisoning campaign necessitated a reduction in trapping effort.

[d] These numbers are low because political difficulties caused the trapping effort to be reduced.

[e] Personal communication from Andrew C. James, Public Health Department, Grenada.

1965 and 1980 and the numbers and percentages found positive for rabies virus. Few of the positive animals showed behavioural signs of disease.

Of 11,917 mongooses caught between 1968 and 1977, 156 or 1.3% were rabid (range, 0.1–3.7%). There was a marked trend towards a reduction in the numbers of trapped rabid mongooses during the second half of the period. Following the fluctuation in 1968–1972 (during which years the annual proportions of trapped mongooses found rabid averaged 2.0% and ranged from 0.5–3.7%), there was a steady decline in rabies among trapped mongooses from the second half of 1972. Between January and mid-June of 1972, 24 of 651 (3.7%) trapped mongooses were positive, a slight increase over 1971, but by mid-August only 28 of 924 (3.0%) mongooses examined were positive. No trapped animals were found positive for rabies in September to December, and the final figure for the year was 28 of 1404 (2.0%). The drop continued during 1973 to 0.8% by the end of the year. Between 1973 and 1977 the percentages of trapped mongooses found rabid averaged only 0.4% (range, 0.14–0.8%). There is no totally satisfactory explanation for the apparent discrepancy between the reduced proportion of trapped mongooses found rabid and the increased number of reported rabies cases in 1973, though improved reporting is probably responsible for the most part of it.

Of the 34 cases of rabies in domestic animals and 69 in mongooses (all categories) for 1973, 22 and 56, respectively, were from the three western parishes, as were 17 of 22 humans given antirabies treatment in that year. In February 1973 a mongoose poisoning campaign was undertaken in the west, so that fewer resources were available for trapping and the catch was consequently much reduced. Trapping in that year was mainly confined to the north coast and to those western areas where poison was not laid, for example, near human habitations or livestock grazing grounds. In a few cases, trapping followed poisoning to "mop up" mongooses that the poison had missed. Political problems in 1974 also resulted in a smaller trapping effort and a consequently reduced catch.

Mongoose control campaigns (by poisoning–trapping) were undertaken in 1955–1956, 1959, 1965, 1968–1969 and 1973, but all were terminated prematurely (Malaga-Alba, 1955; Cocozza, 1956; Murray, 1968; Presnall, 1965, 1966, 1968, 1969; Sikes et al., 1968; Winkler, 1971; Everard et al., 1972; Everard, 1975). At best, they produced marked reductions in mongoose population density in some areas of the island and a concommitant reduction in mongoose-transmitted rabies, but these gains were temporary, and further control programmes were needed. The poisoning campaign of 1973 was the most thorough and probably destroyed one-third to two-thirds of the mongoose population in the western areas during that year. There appeared to be a marked reduction in the prevalence of rabies in the western side of the island immediately after poisoning, but at the same time the decline in the proportion of trapped rabid mongooses, which started in 1972, could not have been wholly the result of the campaign. The fall in numbers of rabies cases could not be attributed simply to the smaller numbers of contacts in a reduced population because trapping was undertaken mainly in areas where poison had not been laid. Further, it was evident from the proportions of mongooses with rabies SN antibody in 1973–1974 (see next section) that the contact rate had been high. The mongoose population was thought to have recovered within 6–9 months in most areas, so that those populations that had been poisoned at the start of the campaign could have returned to their original density, or even exceeded it, by the beginning of 1974.

Although there is no evidence that rabies is consistently more prevalent in any one area of the island than another, it appears that there is considerable local variation. Thus, there were no cases of mongoose rabies from the southwest dry zone during 1970 (though there may well have been rabies activity in the area;

see Section III,A). In 1971 9 of 107 cases (8.4%) were from this area or close to it, as were 5 of 58 (8.6%) in 1972. In 1973, 26 of 69 reported and trapped rabid mongooses (37.7%) were taken from this zone, and five of the six rabid mongooses trapped in that year came from here before poison was laid in the area. Trapping was relatively intensive in this zone, and the area's large human population made reporting more likely, but the increase in mongoose rabies in the area (from 0 to 38% of recorded cases) is valid despite the overall decline in rabies prevalence. Figure 1 shows the southwest dry zone of Grenada and the distribution of mongoose rabies cases for 1971–1973.

In most years of the study, the numbers of trapped rabid mongooses were too small to allow inferences to be drawn about any possible seasonal variation, and data from 1968, 1971 and 1972 alone are insufficient for the purpose. Further, the uneven trapping effort and local variation would introduce error. Casual observation did not suggest that mongoose rabies was more prevalent at any particular time of year, and it would be difficult to show that it is so. Several factors could theoretically influence the seasonal rate of rabies transmission. These include the following: (1) the possibility that males travel larger distances during the main breeding months and that contact rates are increased during that time, (2) increases in population size following births, (3) the reluctance of mongooses to forage during wet weather, and (4) a possible shortage of food during the dry season leading to foraging at greater distances. The geographic

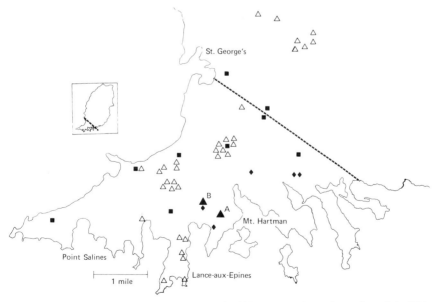

Fig. 1. The distribution of reported and trapped rabid mongooses in southwest Grenada in 1971 (■), 1972 (♦) and 1973 (△). Closed triangles (▲) represent grids A and B.

effects of the seasons are not uniform throughout the island, and it is possible that if there is seasonal variation in rabies transmission rates it would be more marked in the southwest dry zone than elsewhere. However, because vegetation is sparser during the dry season and mongooses are therefore more noticeable, a higher reporting rate could be expected at this time, particularly in the southwest dry zone.

Table V shows that the proportions of rabid mongooses on Grenada ranged between 0.1% and less than 5%, while Steck and Wandeler (1980) report that 30 to 60% of fox populations in Europe may be rabid at any one time (year interval). For this reason and because in Europe the numbers of rabid foxes are considerably larger than numbers in other wildlife species, rabies is often considered to be more ''serious'' in foxes than in mongooses. However, if an acre of land supports between 1 and 2.5 mongooses (see Section IV), 0.14–3.70% of which are rabid, the numbers of rabid mongooses per square-kilometre range between 0.34–0.86 and 9.1–22.9. Steck and Wandeler (1980) found the highest incidence of fox rabies in Europe to be in the frontwave of the epizootic, amounting to 0.7–1.8 rabid foxes per km^2 per year. Thus, considering numbers of rabid animals alone, Grenadians and their domestic animals are at far greater risk from rabid mongooses than Europeans are from rabid foxes.

III. Immune Response in Mongooses

A. PROPORTIONS OF MONGOOSES WITH RABIES OR SN ANTIBODY

Table V shows that of the 4754 mongooses examined during the 4-year period 1971–1974, 100 (2.1%, range 0.6–3.5%) were rabid. 1675 of these 4754 were tested for rabies SN antibody, and 498 (29.7%) were found to be positive (Everard et al., 1981). The data for 1971–1974 are presented in Figs 2a and 2b as percentages and transformed arcsine scales to show the relationship between the proportions of trapped rabid mongooses and those with SN antibody during a declining rabies cycle. The correlation between the proportions of those with SN antibody and those with rabies virus during the 4-year period is 0.96, which is significant at the 0.05 level. On the arcsine scale, the transformed quadratic regression equation is $Y = 61.9 - 2.87X + 0.035X^2$, where Y is the percentage of rabid mongooses and X is the percentage with SN antibody. However, the linear transformed regression line ($Y = 21.6 - 0.43X$) is a significantly better fit: here, with extrapolation, for a value of $X = 59.2\%$ with rabies SN antibody (arcsin 50.3), $Y = 0\%$ rabid in the population. Conversely, when $X = 0\%$ with SN antibody, $Y = 13.5\%$ (arcsin 21.6) of the population rabid. This suggests that almost 60% of mongooses would have rabies SN antibodies at the end of a cycle

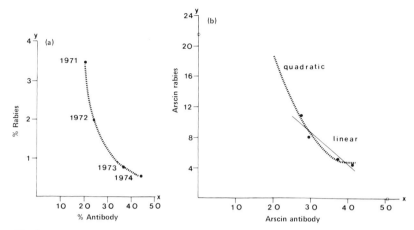

Fig. 2.   The relationship over a 4-year period between rabies-positive and SN antibody-positive mongooses on (a) a percentage scale and (b) an arcsine scale.

before transmission ceased and no rabies was present in the population. Conversely, as much as 13.5% of the mongoose population could become rabid if no antibodies were being developed during an epizootic peak on Grenada. Obviously, extrapolating beyond the range $X = 26$ to $X = 42$ is unwise since only four points are available; nevertheless, after 1974, the proportion of rabid mongooses in the population continued to fall (Table V). Theoretically, when 0.16% of the population is rabid, exactly 50% of mongooses will have rabies SN antibody.

High proportions of mongooses with rabies SN antibody were found in localized areas. Figure 3 shows the 19 areas in which 993 mongooses were captured from late 1972 to 1974. The percentages of mongooses with rabies SN antibody in the different areas ranged from 9% (3 of 33) to 55% (30 of 55) but were usually between 22 and 52%. In four localities, the numbers of animals were too small to give a meaningful percentage.

McLean (1975) showed that even for routine surveillance, SN antibody determination can be a more sensitive test than virus isolation for rabies activity in Raccoons. On Grenada, one study found five of 88 mongooses at Mt. Rodney (Fig. 3) were positive for rabies SN antibody, but none were positive for rabies virus by FA microscopy examination. Tests for virus alone would have been misleading in showing no rabies activity in the area. The data for 1971–1974 (Table V) show that considerably fewer animals need to be examined for rabies SN antibody than for rabies virus to show rabies activity. The fact that the animals do not need to be killed is a further advantage of the use of SN antibody determination as a screening technique.

Little laboratory work has been done so far on the level of immunity conferred

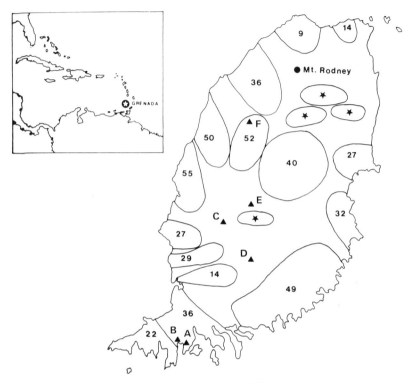

Fig. 3. Map of Grenada showing areas of capture of 993 mongooses, and the percentages with rabies SN antibody. Inset: location of Grenada in the Caribbean. Triangles represent grids; stars indicate that numbers are too small to give a meaningful percentage.

on mongooses by naturally-acquired rabies SN antibody, but, judging by studies on other animals, the assumption that mongooses with SN antibody are immune is reasonable. The data suggest that high rabies SN antibody prevalence rates can be obtained as a result of natural exposure; but as the number of rabid mongooses decreases, the chances of contact between rabid and susceptible animals lessen so that figures of 60% and over of mongooses with antibody (for nil transmission) may never be achieved naturally, except in localized areas. The rabies cycle in many species of wildlife probably follows the sequence of high antibody/low rabies prevalence–low antibody/high rabies prevalence, because after the dispersal or death of the immune individuals in the population, more susceptibles are available to promote a resurgence of the disease. As an immune population builds up, the cycle is repeated. The fluctuation in wildlife rabies inherent in the natural cycle of virus transmission, antibody development, build-up of an immune population, population turnover and recruitment of young susceptibles suggests an eventual resurgence of rabies activity. Since 1979, the rabies surveillance programme on Grenada has been much reduced, but mongoose trapping has continued. Tentative figures for 1978–1980 shown in Table V (A. James, personal communication) suggest that the resurgence of rabies has started.

The fox is highly susceptible to rabies virus, and probably not more than 8% of a population becomes immune (Steck and Wandeler, 1980). These authors believe that the rabies cycle in European foxes is caused by the death (through rabies) of a large proportion of the population and hence to fewer opportunities for transmission. This causes a drop in rabies prevalence, but as the population builds up and contacts increase, there is a resurgence of rabies. Rabies activity in European foxes has been shown to peak about every 3 years. Rabies has not been consistently monitored in Grenada long enough to allow positive conclusions to be reached, but it appears that the phase of low rabies prevalence may be considerably longer than 3 years. The fox and the mongoose have certain characteristics in common: both are carnivores tending to the omnivorous, capable of building large populations, and highly adaptable, even to the point of becoming semi-urbanized scavengers. Their life-spans in the wild are probably comparable; so are the numbers of young produced by a female in a year, so that it seems reasonable to suspect that the extended cycle in the mongoose (if indeed it is such) may be the result of the immunity factor and that the high proportions of immune animals attainable account for the long recovery period. Fluctuations in population density and rabies prevalence will therefore be less marked in mongooses than in foxes. Mortality in foxes through rabies may be as high as 50% (Steck and Wandeler, 1980), but the presence of large proportions of antibody-protected mongooses leads to the conclusion that considerably smaller proportions of mongoose populations are reduced by the disease.

Steck and Wandeler (1980) state that in view of the small population of immune foxes and the simultaneous high population turnover, it is very unlikely that naturally acquired immunity is of epidemiological importance and that the lack of immunity and rapid recovery of a reduced population even appear to be essential factors in maintaining the endemicity of rabies. Although immunity may not be of epidemiological importance in foxes, this is not true for mongooses, and data from Grenada indicate that it cannot be true that lack of immunity is essential in maintaining endemicity. However, it may well be that rabies can disappear spontaneously from populations with high proportions of immune individuals, and the possibility that there have been unrecorded rabies infections, which have died out in mongoose populations, cannot be discounted. A possible case in point is Barbados: rabies was present there in at least 1866 (Times Newspaper of Barbados, 1866a,b), though the island is at present rabies free. Not long after the introduction of the mongoose Feilden (1890) wrote that the coloured people of Barbados dreaded its bite, many fearing that it could bring on rabies in individuals. Feilden had no proof of the matter, but it is at least possible that mongoose rabies was known in the island at that time.

Implications for Rabies Control

The object of mongoose poisoning campaigns is to reduce the transmission rate of the disease, but a high transmission rate is necessary to produce high proportions of antibody-protected animals. Further, poisoning removes immune mongooses as well as susceptibles, and since high proportions of mongooses can circulate rabies SN antibody, control campaigns may defeat their own purpose, especially as overtly rabid animals would be unlikely to enter traps for food or take baits. It is a matter for speculation whether the campaign of 1973 was largely responsible for the subsequent 4-year drop in rabies prevalence or whether, had it not been carried out, even larger proportions of mongooses would have developed rabies SN antibody, leading in any case to a drop in rabies prevalence. A thorough mongoose poisoning campaign would take a minimum of 2–3 years on Grenada, but given the island's limited financial and material resources it would not be feasible at present to implement and sustain a campaign on the necessary scale. Taking into account public antagonism towards poisoning campaigns, the relatively huge resources required to conduct large-scale poisoning might be better utilized otherwise since the long-term effectiveness of mongoose reduction in rabies control is questionable. Alternative methods of rabies control in mongooses are needed, and the animal's ready immune response, both to naturally-acquired rabies virus and to ERA vaccine (Everard *et al.*, 1981) suggests that it is an ideal candidate for immunization in the field. This should be carried out soon after an epizootic peak has occurred, when the proportion of mongooses with rabies SN antibody is highest and the theoretical figure of 60% SN antibody for nil rabies would be most easily attainable.

B. DURATION OF RABIES SN ANTIBODY IN MONGOOSES

The levels of rabies SN antibody of 20 wild-caught mongooses were monitored for varying periods up to 35 months by withdrawing blood directly from the heart while the animal was anaesthetised and examining it by the rapid fluorescent focus inhibition test (RFFIT) of Smith *et al.* (1973). This work is described by Everard *et al.* (1981). The titres and numbers of days after capture on which the blood was taken are shown in Table VI. Four mongooses (Nos 5, 7, 14, 20) were monitored for less than 1 year, seven (Nos 2, 3, 4, 9, 10, 11, 19) for between 12 and 18 months, two (Nos 6, 8) for between 18 months and 2 years, two (Nos 1, 13) for between 2 and $2\frac{1}{2}$ years, and five (Nos 12, 15, 16, 17, 18) for over $2\frac{1}{2}$ years. In all but two mongooses, antibody was still circulating when

TABLE VI

Change in Rabies SN Antibody Titres of Captive Wild-caught Mongooses in Grenada[a]

Mongoose no.,[b] sex and date captured	SN antibody titres and number of days after capture (in parentheses)									
	Bleeding									
	1st	2nd	3rd	4th	5th	6th	7th	8th	9th	10th
1 ♀ (C1)	56	45	54							
16.4.73	(3)	(647)	(840)							
2 ♀ (C2)	11	11	11							
6.6.74	(1)	(231)	(425)							
3 ♂ (C3)	50	50	13							
6.6.74	(1)	(232)	(425)							
4 ♂ (C4)	250	440	230							
21.6.74	(3)	(216)	(409)							
5 ♂ (C5)	14	21	45							
21.8.74	(2)	(155)	(348)							
6 ♂ (A1)	>25	25	25	11	died					
4.9.74	(2)	(141)	(427)	(671)						
7 ♀ (C6)	1400	1400	625							
25.9.74	(1)	(119)	(313)							
8 ♀ (A2)	625	>280	250	280	died					
25.9.74	(1)	(311)	(407)	(559)						
9 ♀ (A3)	25	11	11	8						
18.3.75	(2)	(137)	(233)	(477)						
10 ♂ (A4)	56	56	56	45						
21.3.75	(3)	(134)	(230)	(474)						
11 ♂ (A5)	280	280	250	280						
21.3.75	(3)	(134)	(230)	(474)						
12 ♀ (A6)	>60	56	50	56	25	11	11	8	8	8
4.4.75	(3)	(121)	(217)	(369)	(461)	(560)	(756)	(867)	(1008)	(1072)
13 ♂ (A7)	250	250	200	200	200	56	56	19	died	
4.4.75	(3)	(121)	(217)	(369)	(461)	(560)	(756)	(867)		
14 ♀ (C7)	625	125								
15.4.75	(2)	(109)								
15 ♂ (A8)	8	6	6	6	<5	<5	<5	<5	<5	<5
6.6.75	(3)	(57)	(152)	(304)	(396)	(495)	(691)	(802)	(943)	(1007)
16 ♂ (A9)	11	6	11	11	11	<5	<5	<5	<5	<5
10.6.75	(1)	(53)	(149)	(301)	(393)	(492)	(715)	(826)	(967)	(1031)
17 ♂ (A10)	280	250	250	250	250	60	56	42	56	40
19.6.75	(1)	(44)	(139)	(291)	(383)	(482)	(678)	(789)	(930)	(994)
18 ♂ (A11)	280	>250	200	200	56	56	11	33	40	died
19.6.75	(1)	(44)	(139)	(291)	(383)	(482)	(678)	(789)	(930)	
19 ♂ (A12)	9	9	9	9						
20.6.75	(3)	(43)	(139)	(383)						
20 ♀ (A13)	56	56	56							
16.10.75	(3)	(20)	(264)							

[a] Adapted from Everard *et al.* (1981).

[b] Original numbers in parentheses.

monitoring ceased. These two animals (Nos 15 and 16) had very low titres on capture (1 : 8 and 1 : 11, respectively), but even these titres were maintained for over 300 days. The highest titre recorded on capture was 1 : 1400 (No 7), but an earlier study recorded a mongoose with a naturally-acquired titre of 1 : 5900 (Everard *et al.*, 1974), and a titre of 1 : 34800 has been induced by vaccination (Everard *et al.*, 1981).

Figure 4 shows the fall in antibody titres in mongooses plotted against time $[\log_{10}T_1$ (original titre) $- \log_{10}T_2$ (final titre) $= Y$ (abscissa); time in months $= X$ (ordinate)]. There is a significant correlation at the 0.001 level ($r = 0.774$). Mongooses 4 and 5 were omitted because they showed rising titres (which suggest very recent exposure to virus, with the continuing formation of antibody), and mongoose No 14 because it was monitored for only 109 days, but the line includes four mongooses (Nos 2, 11, 19,20) which showed no loss in titre. For comparison, Fig. 5 shows values for $\log_{10}T_1$ (original titre) plotted against $\log_{10}T_0$, where T_0 is the titre after approximately 1 year. Titres of 1 : 5 (log

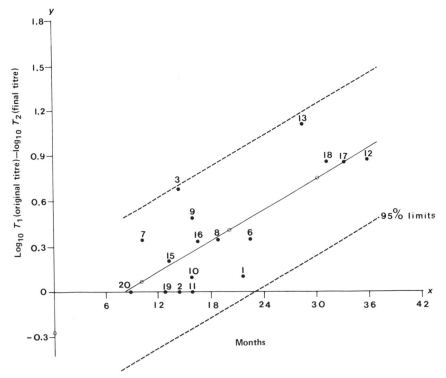

Fig. 4.   Changes in rabies SN antibody titre in mongooses with time ($y = 0.0343 \times -0.27$).

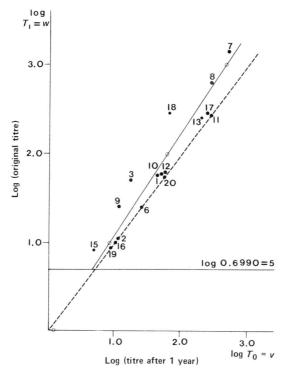

Fig. 5. Calculated loss of naturally-acquired rabies SN antibody in mongooses after 1 year (the broken line indicates no loss of antibody).

0.6990) or less should be considered as negative on the regression line $V(T_0) = 0.0870 + 0.8664W(T_1)$.

The loss in titre for a given period can be estimated (see Fig. 4). At 20 months, $\log (T_1/T_2) = (0.0343 \times 20) - 0.2702 = 0.4158 = $ (antilog) 2.605. So $T_1/T_2 = 2.605$, or $T_1/2.605 = T_2$; using the reciprocal, $0.38T_1 = T_2$. Thus, after 20 months, the final titre would be 38% of the original, and after 12 months, it would be 72% of the original. The regression line of Fig. 4, which cuts the X axis at 7.87, confirms that some mongooses would not lose titre for 7 or 8 months.

The data have an exponential distribution in that higher titres are reduced at a greater rate than lower ones. Figure 5 shows that a mongoose with an initial titre of 1 : 1000 ($\log_{10} = 3$) would lose titre by just over 51% in 1 year. For an initial titre of 1 : 100, the reduction would be 34% and for 1 : 10 about 10%. High titres from mongooses in any given area would therefore suggest recent rabies activity, but low titres can be maintained for some time in these animals. In 18 of 20 mongooses, antibody was still circulating when monitoring ceased, so that, presumably, antibody can be maintained beyond the recorded times. Further, how long before capture exposure to rabies virus actually occurred is not known, so antibody may well have been circulating, especially in mongooses with low titres, for some time before monitoring started.

Probably only 10–15% of wild mongooses survive into their third year on St. Croix, where rabies is not a mortality factor (Nellis and Everard, 1983). Data on tooth wear given by Pearson and Baldwin (1953) for *Herpestes auropunctatus* on Hawaii indicate that most mongooses probably do not survive beyond 4 years in the wild. Since rabies antibody can be detected in mongooses for at least 35 months and probably longer, most, if not all, of those found in the wild without antibody were probably never exposed to rabies virus and therefore never lost titre to the point where it could not be measured. Further, if the life-span in the wild is not much more than 3 years, immunity to rabies is probably maintained for life.

IV. Ecology of the Mongoose

There are no major ecological studies of *Herpestes auropunctatus* in its native habitat (Iraq, through Iran, Pakistan and India, to the Malay Peninsula and South China—Hinton and Dunn, 1967), though the animal has been studied in Hawaii, Fiji, St. Croix, Puerto Rico, Trinidad and Grenada, all islands to which it was introduced and on which it has had considerable impact (Tomich, 1969; Tomich and Devick, 1970; Pimentel, 1955a,b; Pearson and Baldwin, 1953; Baldwin *et al.,* 1952; Gorman, 1976; Nellis and Everard, 1983).

Grenada, at 12°N, 61°41′W, is the most southerly of the Windward Islands. It comprises about 31,079 ha (120 square miles) with a length and breadth nearing 26×16 km exclusive of contours. There is a central mountain mass rising to 838 m. Much of the land has been cleared for cultivation, and the human population numbers just over 100,000. Mongooses are found throughout the island, from the remotest central hilly areas of thick rain forest where the annual rainfall may be over 4064 mm (160 in.) to the dry scrub of the southwest peninsulas where rainfall may be less than 1016 mm (40 in.). The dry zones are the mongoose's preferred habitat, but these comprise less than one-tenth of the island. Rainfall is seasonal; the early months of the year are dry and maximum rainfall is in November in most of the island, July in the southwest dry zone.

Herpestes auropunctatus is diurnal and terrestrial, though it may scramble after lizards along low tree branches or tangles of vines and it can jump to a height of about 1.5 m. It lives, probably singly, among rocks, in simple burrows, or in cavities among tree roots etc. Although a carnivore, it tends to the omnivorous and can adapt to a wide variety of food. The bulk of its diet normally consists of insects and spiders, any other small animals which it can overpower (such as rats, birds, lizards, snakes, frogs and toads), and some plant matter.

Crabs and fish are commonly taken in littoral zones, but contrary to popular belief snakes are an unimportant part of its diet. The animal is small, the mean weight of non-pregnant adult females in Grenada being 434 g, and of adult males 662 g. The average head and body length of Grenada specimens studied was 303 mm for females and 340 mm for males. *Herpestes auropunctatus* may show boldness and curiosity, making it an easy animal to trap. At the same time, it is quick and furtive, shy when approached, aggressive when cornered, and difficult to domesticate. Specimens which approach humans, do not run away, and attack unprovoked are almost certainly rabid, and activity at night can also indicate rabies.

Mongoose movement on Grenada was studied by mark-and-release on grid B (Fig. 1) (Nellis and Everard, 1983). The mean distances travelled between successive recaptures by 45 marked mongooses were 220 m for males and 241 m for females, but the difference between the sexes was not statistically significant. The mean distance travelled between successive recaptures by both sexes combined was 229 m, with a maximum of 579 m. The mean distance travelled by a male mongoose which was captured 13 times in 12 weeks was 166 m, while the area it utilized was between 5.7 ha and 8.5 ha calculated by the exclusive and inclusive boundary strip methods, respectively, of Stickel (1954). All these figures are almost certainly minimum values because even grid B, with an area of 30.1 ha and a diagonal of 777 m, was probably too small. Resources were not available to service a larger grid or to use radio-tracking. Two marked mongooses were caught accidentally in the routine trapping programme; the shortest distance they could have travelled was between 1524 m and 1737 m. One animal was caught twice on grid A (Fig. 1), three times on grid B, and killed by a dog at Lance-aux-Epines 26 months after first capture and 2103 m from grid A by the shortest route. However, it proved to be rabid so that its movements may have been abnormal. Studies in Trinidad gave greater values for movement and home range than on Grenada (Nellis and Everard, 1983), and Tomich (1969) on Hawaii thought that a daily range might be 0.25 mile (402 m) for males and 0.10 mile (161 m) for females, with a maximum of about four times the daily figures. However, distances moved may be smaller in denser populations. Had a larger grid been used in Grenada, differences between the sexes in distances travelled might have been observed.

Male *H. auropunctatus* reach sexual maturity at about four months and females by about nine months of age (Pearson and Baldwin, 1953). Pregnant females were found in Grenada during all months of 1970, 1971 and 1972, though mainly between January and October (Nellis and Everard, 1983). The November period of heaviest rainfall in the greater part of the island coincides with the time of minimum breeding. Comparable data were obtained in Hawaii and Puerto Rico (Baldwin *et al.*, 1952; Pearson and Baldwin, 1953; Pimentel, 1955a), but considering information from Fiji (in the southern hemisphere) it would appear that the season of breeding is dependent on day length (Gorman, 1976). The data from Grenada suggest that there must be at least two litters a year, and maybe even three in some cases, depending on age, month of birth, and onset of first breeding season. On Grenada the mean number of embryos carried by pregnant females was 2.17 and the range was from 1 to 5, but 5 was recorded only once among 255 pregnant females examined, and 63% had two embryos developing at the same time. The gestation period is approximately 7 weeks. Sexing embryos was not attempted on Grenada, but the sex ratio at birth of the few litters examined was approximately 1 : 1. Trapping results indicated a ratio of 1 : 2.6 (female to male) on Grenada and 1 : 1.2 on Trinidad, and ratios as high as 1 : 7 have been observed on Grenada. Female mongooses have never been observed greatly to outnumber males in any area; there is a consistent difference in sex ratio with males predominating, sometimes substantially so. There is insufficient evidence in the literature or from Grenada to determine whether this reflects an inherent sex ratio in favour of males or is the result of female trap-shyness or females being eliminated more frequently by natural events at some time after their birth.

Other pathogens, namely leptospires and salmonellae, have been found in high proportions of Grenadian mongooses (Everard, 1975; Everard et al., 1976, 1979b, 1980, 1983). So far, there is no proof that either organism is seriously pathogenic for mongooses, though leptospires probably are. Two of 12 Trinidadian mongooses were found to have *Toxoplasma* agglutinins, but none of 287 from Grenada was positive (Nellis and Everard, 1983). A search for pulmonary viruses was negative, and searches for external parasites showed Grenadian mongooses to be remarkably clean (Nellis and Everard, 1983). Among fleas, only the cat flea (*Ctenocephalides felis felis*) was found, and among mites only free-living and plant-parasitic forms which had adhered accidentally to the fur. Among ticks, larvae and nymphs of only *Amblyomma* and *Ornithodorus* were recorded, while Trinidadian specimens carried larvae and nymphs of *Amblyomma sp.* and *Rhipicephalus sanguineus*. This is interesting in view of the possibility that ticks can transmit rabies virus. No blood parasites were found in 2300 mongooses examined, and among macro-endoparasites there were only three genera of small intestinal nematodes (though there may well be protozoa) (Nellis and Everard, 1983). Other workers have reported relatively few parasites and pathogens from mongooses elsewhere. On the present evidence, therefore, it seems that natural fluctuations in the mongoose population, over and above those due to environmental factors such as weather and food shortage, are more likely to be due to rabies than to other diseases.

Grenadian mongooses have no natural enemies other than domestic dogs, possibly cats, and man. Since the mongoose pelt is of no commercial value, the flesh is not eaten, and the animal is rarely hunted for sport, man's predations are limited to occasional control campaigns. The few other small mammals, including *Didelphis* opossums, cannot be considered serious competitors for the food available. Mongooses have adapted to the semi-urbanization of their habitat, and they forage near human habitations, even scavenging near dustbins and on rubbish heaps in urban areas. Their great adaptability, few parasites and pathogens, and their near omnivorous habit mean that mongooses can build up very dense populations and individuals can be long-lived. Mongoose density on Grenada was studied between 1970 and 1973 (Everard, 1975) by mark-and-release on grids according to the methods of Schnabel(Krumholz) and Schumacher-Eschmeyer (Davis, 1963). Six grids (A–F in Fig. 3) were laid out in different representative habitats, and they varied in size from 12.4 acres (5 ha) to nearly 75 acres (30.4 ha). Population estimates for the areas sampled gave a calculated range of not less than 1.0 mongoose per acre to 5.1 (2.5–12.6 per ha), with an overall mean of 2.5 per acre (6.2 per ha). This is thought to be near the carrying capacity of the land, and densities of over 3 per acre are probably peak populations of short duration.

In Trinidad, rabies is present in bats but absent in the mongoose population. A much lower density of mongooses was recorded on that island than on Grenada (0.3–2.2 per acre, mean 0.8), with populations confined to the savannahs and flat agricultural areas (Everard, 1975). Just over one-fifth of all marked mongooses were recaptured on Trinidad, while one-half were recaptured on Grenada, suggesting that overpopulation and limitations of space on the latter island caused the animals to return more frequently to the traps for food. Further, the time interval within which recaptures were made on Grenada was considerably shorter than on Trinidad. It appears from past literature (reviewed by Everard, 1975) that mongooses were formerly a serious pest in Trinidad, but there is no certain explanation for the decline in numbers which appears to have occurred. If there was an epizootic of rabies or any other disease in mongooses, it passed unrecorded. However, the heavy and prolonged floods, which occur in some years in the central plain of Trinidad, could account for sudden drops in the mongoose population; with the bush fires which are a common feature of the dry season in that island, they create a more precarious habitat for the mongoose than is found in Grenada. The absence of mongooses from the forests of Trinidad, where an abundant food supply would have been available, implies that the low density of the mongoose population in the savannahs has not given rise to those overpopulation pressures, which, in Grenada, initiated dispersal to the less characteristic environment of forest. It is possible that the lower population density of mongooses in Trinidad has kept them free from rabies.

The relationship between mongoose population dynamics and cyclic fluctuations of rabies is still largely a matter for conjecture. This is partly because it is not possible to accurately census wild animal populations, so that density figures are always, at best, a good guess; partly because knowledge of the population structure of mongooses is still incomplete and partly because detailed information needs to be collected over many decades. Also, population densities may fluctuate greatly even in the absence of epizootics. One of the frustrations of the Grenada study was that in 10 years not one dead mongoose was found by the trappers except for the few run over on the roads, so that an important source of information was lost. No doubt the rapid decay of corpses in the tropics, destruction by ants, the small size of the animal and the rugged, overgrown nature of the terrain were responsible. Some of the ecological data most relevant to the study of rabies in wildlife are the most difficult to collect, and age-grading and the estimation of life-spans of small mammals in the wild are some of the numerous problems that face biologists. One of the objectives of the study on Grenada was the estimation of the minimum mongoose population density required to maintain rabies (the threshold level). This objective was not realized because, with the limited resources available, mongoose density could not be maintained low enough, for long enough, to give this information.

There is little doubt that rabies is a density-dependent disease, though it is not clear whether a high density simply provides more opportunities for transmission of the virus or whether, as argued by several authors including Johnson (1965) and McLean (1975), stress resulting from overcrowding brings out a latent rabies infection. Whichever the case, lower population densities appear to mitigate the mongoose's importance as a rabies vector elsewhere. The reporting of rabies data from many territories is often sporadic and incomplete, but it is interesting that in southern India only 27 of 485,608 people given antirabies treatment between 1908 and 1971 were bitten by mongooses (N. Veeraraghavan, personal communication), whereas on Grenada, with its small size and population, 119 of 208 people (57%) received antirabies treatment following mongoose bites in the decade 1968–1977 alone, and mongooses accounted for over 77% of the rabies cases on the island. The relationship between rabies and rabies SN antibody in Grenada mongooses was determined for a population of 1.0–2.5 per acre under small island conditions. Under mainland and large island conditions, where mongoose populations of considerably less than 1.0 per acre can be expected, antibody and rabies prevalence figures are likely to be lower.

H. N. Johnson (personal communication) believes that mustelids (martens, stoats, weasels, skunks) and viverrids (mongooses, civets, genets) are the true natural reservoirs of rabies, while canines (wolves, dogs, foxes, jackals) are aberrant hosts. He believes that many mustelids and viverrids can maintain rabies virus without the occurrence of epizootics and that the study of sporadic cases provides the key to the location of the reservoir host system (Johnson, 1966). The findings on rabies SN antibody in mongooses lend weight to this view, because it seems reasonable that a true natural reservoir of the virus would have a ready defence against it. However, whether (as Johnson believes) mongooses can maintain symptomless infections while shedding virus in their saliva remains to be shown, and although in India cases of mongoose rabies appear to be sporadic, there is no doubt that mongoose rabies has reached epizootic proportions in Grenada. Since Johnson himself (1966) says that on the basis of our knowledge of the epidemiology of parasitic diseases of wildlife we would not expect to observe epidemics of rabies in the long-term natural wildlife host of rabies virus, it is evident that further study of the problem is needed.

Acknowledgements

The contents of this chapter include data and illustrations already published (but now updated and modified) in 1981 in *Transactions of the Royal Society of Tropical Medicine and Hygiene,* **75,** 654–666.

The data on dog, cat and livestock rabies and immunization in Section II,B were provided by the Government of Grenada and veterinarians D. W. Dreesen and S. N. Watson of the Pan American Health Organization. Dr. Watson also provided data on the poisoning campaign of 1973 cited in Section II,D,2.

References

Baldwin, P. H., Schwartz, C. W., and Schwartz, E. R. (1952). Life history and economic status of the mongoose in Hawaii. *J. Mammal.* **33,** 335–356.
Beamer, P. D., Mohr, C. O., and Barr, T. R. B. (1960). Resistance of the opossum to rabies virus. *Am. J. Vet. Res.* **82,** 507–510.
Cocozza, J. (1956). "Report on the Rabies Problem" (unpublished document). Ministry of Health, Grenada.
Colon, E. D. (1930). "Datos sobre la historia de la Agricultura de Puerto Rico antes 1898." Privately Printed, San Juan, Puerto Rico.
Davis, D. E. (1963). Estimating the numbers of game populations. *In* "Wildlife Investigational Techniques" (H. S. Mosby, ed.), pp. 89–118. Wildlife Society, Washington, D.C.
Dean, D. J. (1966). The fluorescent antibody test. *W.H.O. Monogr. Ser.* **23,** 59–68.
Everard, C. O. R. (1975). The ecology of the mongoose, *Herpestes auropunctatus,* in Grenada and Trinidad, with special reference to its importance as a vector of disease. Ph.D. Thesis, University of London.
Everard, C. O. R., Murray, D., and Gilbert, P. K. (1972). Rabies in Grenada. *Trans. R. Soc. Trop. Med. Hyg.* **66,** 878–888.
Everard, C. O. R., Baer, G. M., and James, A. (1974). Epidemiology of mongoose rabies in Grenada. *J. Wildl. Dis.* **10,** 190–196.
Everard, C. O. R., Green, A. E., and Glosser, J. W. (1976). Leptospirosis in Trinidad and Grenada, with special reference to the mongoose. *Trans. R. Soc. Trop. Med. Hyg.* **70,** 57–61.
Everard, C. O. R., James, A. C., and DaBreo, S. (1979a). Ten years of rabies surveillance in Grenada, 1968–1977. *Bull. Pan. Am. Health Organ.* **13,** 342–353.
Everard, C. O. R., Tota, B., Bassett, D., and Ali, C. (1979b). *Salmonella* in wildlife from Trinidad and Grenada, W.I. *J. Wildl. Dis.* **15,** 213–219.
Everard, C. O. R., Sulzer, C. R., Bhagwandin, L. J., Fraser-Chanpong, G. M., and James, A. C. (1980). Pathogenic *Leptospira* isolates from the Caribbean islands of Trinidad, Grenada and St. Vincent. *Int. J. Zoonoses* **7,** 90–100.

Everard, C. O. R., Baer, G. M., Alls, M. E., and Moore, S. A. (1981). Rabies serum neutralizing antibody in mongooses from Grenada. *Trans. R. Soc. Trop. Med. Hyg.* **75,** 654–666.

Everard, C. O. R., Fraser-Chanpong, G. M., Bhagwandin, L. J., Race, M. W., and James, A. C. (1983). Leptospires in wildlife from Trinidad and Grenada. *J. Wildl. Dis.* **19,** 192–199.

Feilden, H. W. (1890). Notes on the terrestrial mammals of Barbados. *Zoologist* **14,** 52–55.

Gorman, M. L. (1976). Seasonal changes in the reproductive pattern of feral *Herpestes auropunctatus* (Carnivora: Viverridae), in the Fijian Islands. *J. Zool.* **178,** 237–246.

Groome, J. R. (1970). "A Natural History of the Island of Grenada, W.I." Caribbean Printers, Trinidad.

Hinton, H. E., and Dunn, A. M. S. (1967). "Mongooses, their Natural History and Behaviour." Oliver & Boyd, Edinburgh and London.

Johnson, H. N. (1966). Sporadic cases of rabies in wildlife: Relation to rabies in domestic animals and character of virus. *In* "Proceedings of the National Rabies Symposium," pp. 25–30. National Communicable Disease Center, Atlanta, Georgia.

Johnson, H. N. (1965). Rabies Virus. *In* "Viral and Rickettsial Infections of Man" (F. L. Horsfall, Jr. and I. Tamm, eds.), 4th ed., pp. 814–840. Lippincott, Philadelphia, Pennsylvania.

Jones, J. K., and Phillips, C. J. (1970). Comments on systematics and zoogeography of bats in the lesser Antilles. *Stud. Fauna Curacao Other Caribbean Islands* **32,** 131–145.

Jonkers, A. H., Alexis, F., and Loregnard, R. (1969). Mongoose rabies in Grenada. *West Indian Med. J.* **18,** 167–170.

McLean, R. G. (1975). Raccoon rabies. *In* "The Natural History of Rabies" (G. M. Baer, ed.), Vol. 2, pp. 53–57. Academic Press, New York.

Malaga-Alba, A. (1955). "Report and Recommendations for Control of Rabies in Grenada" (unpublished document). Ministry of Health, Grenada.

Murray, D. (1968). Rabies in Grenada; its epidemiology and control; and a discussion on some more recent advances in forms of treatment. Thesis for Diploma in Tropical Public Health, University of London.

Nellis, D. W., and Everard, C. O. R. (1983). The biology of the mongoose in the Caribbean. *Stud. Fauna Curacao Other Caribbean Islands* LXIV **195,** 1–162.

Pearson, O. P., and Baldwin, P. H. (1953). Reproduction and age structure of a mongoose population in Hawaii. *J. Mammal.* **34,** 436–447.

Pimentel, D. (1955a). Biology of the Indian mongoose in Puerto Rico. *J. Mammal.* **36,** 62–68.

Pimentel, D. (1955b). The control of the mongoose in Puerto Rico. *Am. J. Trop. Med. Hyg.* **4,** 147–151.

Presnall, C. C. (1965). "Control of Rabies Among Mongooses in Grenada, W. I." (unpublished document). PAHO, AMRO-0701, Washington, D.C.

Presnall, C. C. (1966). "First Year Progress Report, Grenada Rabies Control Program" (Unpublished document). PAHO, Washington, D.C.

Presnall, C. C. (1968). "Summary and Partial Analysis of Mongoose Data, Grenada, W.I. 1968" (unpublished document). Ministry of Health, Grenada.

Presnall, C. C. (1969). "Rabid Mongoose Control, Grenada, W.I. January 6th to April 6th, 1969" (unpublished document). PAHO, Washington, D.C.

Price, J. L., and Everard, C. O. R. (1977). Rabies virus and antibody in bats in Grenada and Trinidad. *J. Wildl. Dis.* **13,** 131–134.

Sikes, R. K., Malaga-Alba, A., and Presnall, C. C. (1968). "Grenada Rabies Control Program" (unpublished document). PAHO, Washington, D.C.

Smith, J. S., Yager, P. A., and Baer, G. M. (1973). A rapid reproducible test for determining rabies neutralizing antibody. *Bull. W.H.O.* **48,** 535–541.

Steck, F., and Wandeler, A. (1980). The epidemiology of fox rabies in Europe. *Epidemiol. Rev.* **2,** 71–96.

Stickel, L. F. (1954). A comparison of certain methods of measuring ranges of small mammals. *J. Mammal.* **35,** 1–15.

Tierkel, E. S., Arbona, G., Rivera, A., and de Juan, A. (1952). Mongoose rabies in Puerto Rico. *Public Health Rep.* **67,** 274–278.

Times Newspaper of Barbados (1866a). Report on Hydrophobia, August 8th.

Times Newspaper of Barbados (1866b). Letter to the Editor on Hydrophobia, August 11th.

Tomich, P. Q. (1969). Movement patterns of the mongoose in Hawaii. *J. Wildl. Manage.* **33,** 576–584.

Tomich, P. Q., and Devick, W. S. (1970). Age criteria for the prenatal and immature mongoose in Hawaii. *Anat. Rec.* **167,** 107–114.

Winkler, W. G. (1971). "Evaluation of Rabies Control Program in Grenada (3–18 February, 1971)" (unpublished document). PAHO, Washington, D.C.

The Biological Basis of Rabies Models

4

David W. Macdonald
Department of Zoology,
University of Oxford,
Oxford, England

Dennis R. Voigt
Wildlife Branch,
Ontario Ministry of Natural Resources,
Maple, Ontario, Canada

I. Introduction

The most common mode of transmission of the rabies virus is by injection of infected saliva via a bite wound. Members of the Order Carnivora have dentition and behavior that adapt them to predation, and the same traits facilitate intra-specific transmission of rabies via bite wounds. In comparison to other mammals, many species of carnivores are both susceptible to rabies and wide-ranging, and so they tend to predominate among lists of wild species diagnosed as rabid. These qualities are shared by several species of predatory bats (Order Chiroptera), which are heavily involved in sylvatic rabies in some regions. The overall result is that in some ecological communities there are several important wild vectors of rabies, whereas in other communities there is a single principal vector.

One ecological distinction is between communities of different vectors, and another is between different populations of the same vector. We will illustrate the first by a comparison of the multivector community of eastern Canada with the single-vector community of central Europe. We will illustrate the second by a

71

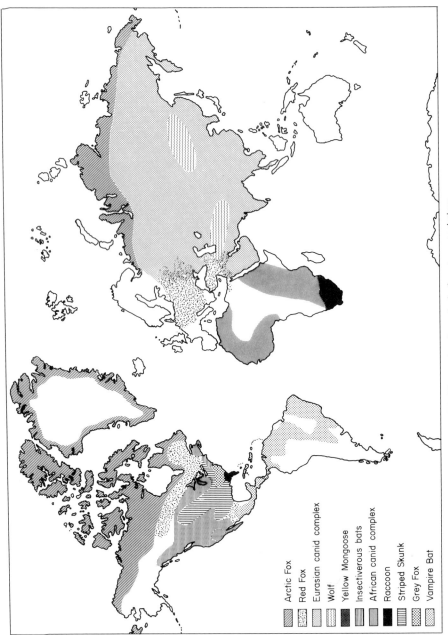

Arctic Fox

Red Fox

Eurasian canid complex

Wolf

Yellow Mongoose

Insectiverous bats

African canid complex

Raccoon

Striped Skunk

Grey Fox

Vampire Bat

Fig. 1. World map showing principal vector associations.

comparison of different populations of Red Foxes (*Vulpes vulpes*), an important vector of rabies throughout much of the northern temperate zone. The purpose of these comparisons and of this chapter is to provide those interested in mathematical aspects of the epizootiology of rabies with a biological basis for their models. We will emphasise that the epizootiology of rabies reflects the vectors' behaviour and that behaviour patterns vary, both between and within species. Such variation is important to models of rabies spread and to the control of the disease. We will argue that variations in rabies epizootiology reflect the different ecological circumstances, and thus the behaviour, of populations of vectors. Those differences affect the most fundamental biological ingredient of a rabies model—the contact rate. The *contact rate* for a population is the average number of susceptible individuals infected by each diseased animal (See Bailey, 1975). Contact rate is not a constant, but a complex function of the social organisation and density of the vectors, and thus of the frequency of meetings amongst them. It is easy to demonstrate deterministically that contact rate must be 1.0 or greater in order for rabies to remain enzootic (May, 1983). However, in the stochastic world of complex animal populations, measurement of contact rate is notoriously difficult; the frequency of meeting between individuals, and hence the potential contact rate of the disease, is a reflection of their population density, social organisation and their ecology. But we do know that the spatial organisation of vectors influences the local rate of contact, the reintroduction and the long-range dispersal of vectors and, thus, rabies. Hence, to the biologist, the studies of rabies transmission and its control are closely linked to the study of the social behaviour of its vectors (e.g. Wandeler, 1980a; Macdonald and Bacon, 1982).

II. Sylvatic Rabies Worldwide

More than a millennium has passed since Acteon the hunter chanced to encounter the goddess Diana and her nymphs while they bathed. The chroniclers of ancient Greece recorded that the divine punishment for his voyeurism was to be savaged by his own hounds, magically made rabid at Diana's command. Fear of rabies, or hydrophobia, and knowledge of the danger of dog bites have been recorded for more than 2000 years (Steel, 1975). Today, although it is absent from many islands, rabies (together with similar members of the rhabdovirus group, such as Mokola, Duvenhage and Lagos bat virus) is virtually pandemic, being absent only from Australia and the Antarctic.

The principal assembleges of wild vectors vary worldwide (Fig. 1 and Table I) as do the relative roles of wild and domestic species, although everywhere domestic dogs and cats remain a major link to man. In each community, species may differ in their susceptibility and/or exposure to the disease (Sikes, 1962; Parker and Wilsnack, 1966). In the Arctic, where Eskimos have been familiar for

TABLE I

Wild Species Diagnosed as Rabid in Each of Four Major Epizootiological Zones

North America	Europe
Carnivora	Carnivora
Red Fox, *Vulpes vulpes*	Red Fox, *Vulpes vulpes*
Arctic Fox, *Alopex lagopus*	Arctic Fox, *Alopex lagopus*
Grey Fox, *Urocyon cinereoargenteus*	Wolf, *Canis lupus*
Wolf, *Canis lupus*	Jackal, *Canis aureus*
Coyote, *Canis latrans*	Raccoon Dog, *Nyctereutus pro-*
Striped Skunk, *Mephitis mephitis*	*cyonoides*
Spotted Skunk, *Spilogale* spp.	Wildcat, *Felis sylvestris*
American Badger, *Taxidea taxus*	Badger, *Meles meles*
Fisher, *Martes pennanti*	Weasels, *Mustela* spp.
Weasels, *Mustela* spp.	Ardiodactyla
Raccoon, *Procyon lotor*	Red Deer, *Cervus elephas*
Black Bear, *Ursus americanus*	Roe Deer, *Capreolus capreola*
Polar Bear, *Ursus maritimus*	Chamois, *Rupicapra rupicapra*
Cougar, *Felis concolor*	Mouflon, *Ovis musimon*
Artiodactyla	Ibex, *Capra ibex*
White-tailed Deer, *Odocoileus virgi-*	Perissodactyla
nianus	Wild Boar, *Sus scrofa*
Bison, *Bison bison*	Rodentia
Elk, *Cervus elaphus*	Field Vole, *Microtus agrestis*
Moose, *Alces alces*	House Mouse, *Mus musculus*
Caribou, *Rangifer tarandus*	Red Squirrel, *Sciurus vulgaris*
Rodentia	Muskrat, *Ondatra zibethicus*
Woodchuck, *Marmota monax*	Lagomorpha
Black Squirrel, *Sciurus carolinensis*	Hare, *Lepus europaeus*
Muskrat, *Ondatra zibethicus*	Insectivora
Meadow Vole, *Microtus pensylvanicus*	Shrew, *Sorex* spp.
Porcupine, *Erethizon dorsatum*	Hedgehog, *Erinaceus europaeus*
Beaver, *Castor canadensis*	
Chiroptera	Southern Africa
Mexican Free-tailed Bat, *Tadarida*	
brasiliensis	Carnivora
Vampire Bat, *Desmodus rotundus*	Silver-backed Jackel, *Canis meso-*
Big Brown Bat, *Eptesicus fuscus*	*melas*
Little Brown Bat, *Myotis lucifugus*	Golden Jackal, *Canis aureus*
Hoary Bat, *Lasiurus cinereus*	Side-striped Jackal, *Canis adustus*
Silver-haired Bat, *Lasionycteris noc-*	Cape Fox, *Vulpes chama*
tivagens	Bat-eared Fox, *Otocyon megalotis*
Eastern Pipestrelle Bat, *Pipistrellus*	Yellow Mongoose, *Cynictis pe-*
subflavus	*niscillata*
Red Bat, *Lasiurus borealis*	Grey Meerkat, *Suricata suricatta*
Eastern Long-eared Bat, *Myotis keenii*	Slender Mongoose, *Herpestes san-*
	guineus
	Water Mongoose, *Atilax paludinosus*

TABLE I *(Continued)*

	Latin America
Banded Mongoose, *Mungos mungo*	
African Civet, *Viverra civetta*	Carnivora
Genets, *Genetta* spp.	Colpeo Fox, *Dusicyon culpaeus*
Honey Badger, *Mellivora capensis*	Crabeating Fox, *Cerdocyon thous*
Cape Polecat, *Ictonyx striatus*	Small-eared Dog, *Atelocynus microtis*
Wildcat, *Felis libyca*	Bush Dog, *Speothos venaticus*
Black-footed Cat, *Felis nigripes*	Small Indian Mongoose, *Herpestes*
Serval, *Felis serval*	*auropunctatus*
Caracal, *Felis caracal*	Coati, *Nasua nasua*
Leopard, *Panthera pardus*	Chiroptera
Cheetah, *Aonyx jubatus*	Vampire Bat, *Desmodus robundus*
Spotted Hyaena, *Crocuta crocuta*	*Diphylla ecaudata*
Aardwolf, *Proteles cristatus*	*Diaemus youngi*
Artiodactyla	Free-tailed Bat, *Molossus major*
Kudu, *Tragelephus strepsiceros*	Fruit Bat, *Artibus jaamaicensis*
Eland, *Taurotraqus oryx*	Rodentia
Rodentia	Rats, *Rattus* spp.
Ground Squirrel, *Xerus inauris*	Paca, *Cuniculus paca*

centuries with a form of rabies called Arctic dog disease, or Polar madness, Arctic Foxes (*Alopex lagopus*) are an important wild vector, as are wolves (*Canis lupus*). Further south, the Red Fox is heavily implicated; in much of Europe, the Red Fox is the significant wild vector, although further to the east the Raccoon Dog (*Nyctereutus procyonoides*) complicates the epizootiological picture. In contrast, enzootics in several parts of North America are typified by complex guilds of vectors. In most of eastern Canada, the Red Fox and Striped Skunk (*Mephitis mephitis*) are involved but with local variation in the species which plays the principal role. In the southern United States, the Spotted Skunk (*Spilogale putorius*) is implicated, and in the eastern states the Grey Fox (*Urocyon cinereoargenteus*) mingles with the Red Fox. In the southeastern United States and recently the New England states, Raccoons (*Procyon lotor*) are increasingly important. The rapid spread of Raccoon rabies through Virginia, Maryland, Pennsylvania and Washington, D.C., poses new problems because the species is numerous in many urban areas. In the southern states, the Mexican Free-tailed Bat (*Tadarida brasiliensis*) is involved (Constantine, 1971). In South America, Vampire Bats (*Desmodus rotundus*) are important vectors, and amongst the carnivores the various little known species of *Dusicyon* and *Cerdocyon* foxes are involved (Gomez Orosco, 1981; Acha, 1982). At least, one species of Viverrid, the Small Indian Mongoose (*Herpestes auropunctatus*) is known to develop antibodies to rabies after exposure. This species lives feral on the Caribbean island of Grenada, where about one-half of the mongooses are immune to rabies (Everard *et al.*, 1979, Chapter 3, this volume). On Grenada, rabies also occurs in a frugivorous bat (*Artebeus jamaiciensis*) as well as in an insectivorous one (*Molossus major*) (Everard *et al.*, 1974). In Europe, the rarity of reported cases of rabies in bats is conspicuous; there have been eight positive diagnoses since 1954, the most recent in Germany in 1982, following a 12-year hiatus. Monoclonal antibody tests hint that these bats carried a strain of virus that may have hailed from Africa; the strain is different to that infecting European Red Foxes. Throughout Africa, jackals (*Canis* spp.) and foxes (*Vulpes* spp.) are important rabies vectors; in southern Africa, for instance, the Silver-backed Jackal (*C. mesomelas*) and the Cape Fox (*V. chama*) together with the Yellow Mongoose (*Cynictis penicillata*) and the Suricate Meerkat (*Suricata suricatta*), and at least a dozen other small carnivores form a complex and little-understood guild of vectors (Meredith, 1982; Barnard, 1979; Zumpt, 1976). It is noteworthy that rabies amongst a similar community of carnivores in Zimbabwe appears to be maintained not by wildlife but by feral dogs (Cumming, 1982).

Worldwide, the one mammalian family most commonly implicated in sylvatic rabies is the Canidae. Even where data are scarce, Canids are reputedly important vectors, e.g. in the eastern part of the Euro-Asian land mass, where wolves and jackals are often implicated. In 1982, 9 wolves out of 32 reported cases in wild species were diagnosed rabid in Turkey (1982 WHO Bulletin); the wild species included 1 fox and, intriguingly, 22 house mice!

Just as domestic stock are susceptible to rabies, so can wild artiodactyls contract the disease. An outbreak of rabies among semi-tame Red Deer (*Cervus elaphus*) in Richmond Park was a notorious case in England. On continental Europe, Roe Deer (*Capreolus capreolus*) regularly appear, in low numbers, amongst cases diagnosed in wild species (2.7% of 14,759 wild animal cases in Europe in 1981; 3.9% of 16,231 cases in 1982). Locally, deer may be more important: 287 out of 3934 (7.3%) cases of wildlife rabies in the first 10 months of 1982 in West Germany. The most striking outbreak among wild ungulates was that in south West Africa/Namibia among Kudu (*Tragelephus strepsiceros*), where 15,000 to 20,000 Kudus are estimated to have died since the outbreak began in 1977 (Hassel, 1982). They are thought to pass on the disease by transmucosal infection during mutual grooming. The Kudu populations expanded prior to that outbreak, due to changing farm practice and destruction of their predators. In North America, rabies in wild artiodactyls is extremely rare. However, several cases among White-tailed Deer (*Odocioleus virginianus*) in Ontario have resulted in human exposure to rabies. Cattle are the most common domestic livestock infected by wild vectors. In general, artiodactyles are regarded as 'dead end' hosts, in the sense of their being unlikely to pass the disease to other species. In areas of fox rabies, such as Ontario, cattle account for over 20% of diagnosed cases. In Europe, cattle made up 8.6% of 21,488 cases in

1982. Those records of bovine rabies provide some rudimentary data for epizootiological analysis because incidence patterns of rabies in cattle seem to mirror temporal and spatial patterns in fox rabies in Ontario, although transmission within herds of cattle, sheep and horses is known. In South America, the cattle–vampire bat rabies association has been much publicized but that epizootiology will not be addressed here.

The nature and magnitude of the menace posed by rabies differs regionally. Historically, rabies has killed humans throughout its range, but today in developed countries it poses more of a threat to peace of mind than to human life. Nevertheless, some authorities believe that 15,000 people may die annually from rabies, of which up to three-quarters of this number are from India. Acha (1966) recorded 2350 human deaths between 1954–1965 in South America. In the 11 years 1970–1980, some 2755 people died of rabies in Latin America, and annually some 300,000 people are given postexposure treatment (as are 18,000 dogs) (Acha, 1982). In human deaths per million inhabitants, this means rates of 2.5 in Ecuador, 2.4 in El Salvador, 1.3 in Honduras and 1.0 in Mexico. The Philippines has amongst the highest recorded rates of fatalities with seven human deaths per million (Beran *et al.*, 1972).

In contrast, there were only 17 human deaths from rabies contracted in 11 countries of western and central Europe from 1970 through 1979, and during the same period, there were 22 deaths in the United States and only one in Canada. The most recent case directly attributable to wildlife in Europe was a German who died after being bitten by a rabid vixen in June, 1974. In Michigan (United States), a girl died of rabies in 1983 (the first case in that state since 1948), probably following a bite from a bat. The last known human death from rabies in Canada was reported in 1971 in Nova Scotia after exposure to a bat. A total of 21 persons are known to have died from rabies in Canada since 1925. The last death in Ontario was in 1967 when a young girl died after exposure to a stray rabid cat. Since then, 1500–2200 people have been treated annually after exposure to rabid animals, without a fatality. According to a report by the Pan American Zoonoses Centre, in the period 1970–1979, there were 2796 human deaths from rabies in 23 countries in North and South America. Brazil alone recorded 1140. In 95% of the cases, an animal bite was the source of infection. That the threat to people in affluent regions is minimal is almost entirely due to expensive medical prophylactic schemes, vaccination of dogs and cats, public education, and adequate provision for post exposure treatment.

Rabies can be an important economic problem, not only because of the cost of prophylaxis, but also due to agricultural losses. In South America, losses of cattle, due to confirmed and suspected vampire bat rabies are a significant burden on agriculture, and rabies accounts for from 3 to 60% of annual losses of cattle (Baer, 1975). Even in France, the vaccination of cattle has a measurable cost to farmers (to the extent that it is often cheaper to insure a herd rather than to vaccinate it, an anomaly which militates against the success of vaccination schemes). In Ontario alone, the loss from the fur harvest due to rabies of Red Foxes (based on highest harvests before rabies and on current pelt prices) is estimated at over US $1.2 million annually. Additionally, rabies is estimated to cost Ontario US $20 million annually, including the yearly treatment of up to 2200 people, pet vaccination and diagnoses (Tinline *et al.*, 1982). Cattle are seldom vaccinated there, but it is estimated that to achieve herd immunity would cost US $14 million annually.

In the next section, we will briefly outline the rabies situation in Europe and in North America in order to put in context our more detailed descriptions of, first, temperate central and western Europe, and second, eastern Canada. Those two regions merit comparison because of similarities in incidence of rabies and fox involvement, but differences in detail of epizootiology and fox ecology.

III. Epizootiology

A. EUROPE

Rabies has swept through Europe periodically throughout recorded history, and the twentieth century has witnessed one such wave. Since its original diagnosis in Poland in 1939, the present epizootic has spread westward across over 1400 km of Europe at a rather constant pace of 20–60 km per year (Toma and Andral, 1977), and, with wide variation, at an average of 4.8 km per month (Bogel *et al.*, 1976). Intriguingly, there were several local epizootics of fox rabies in the late eighteenth and early nineteenth centuries, but for some reason those episodes died out (Artois, 1976). In the present epizootic, rabies reached West Germany in 1950, France in 1968 and Italy in 1977 (Fig. 2). The route has been influenced by major topographical features, for instance the epizootic front faltered at, but eventually crossed, the Elbe, the Rhine and the Alps. The species that were reported to be rabid varied between countries and with the time that had elapsed since the epizootic arrival. In 1977, Wachendorfer recognised three groups of countries on the basis of the species reported as dying of rabies between 1972–1976: (A) sylvatic rabies in 11 countries of central Europe, where 82% of cases were in wildlife (B) domestic dog rabies, principally around the Mediterranean, but also in Greenland, where only 0.3% of recorded cases were in wildlife and (C) a rather indistinct category including East Germany, Rumania, Yugoslavia and Russia, where dog rabies predominated but was interspersed with foci of sylvatic rabies and where 9% of cases were in wildlife. Between 1972–1976, there were over 63,000 cases in the sylvatic zone and nine locally contracted human cases. In contrast, in the dog rabies zone, there were 13,477 cases in animals and 284 human deaths. For the most part, that pattern has

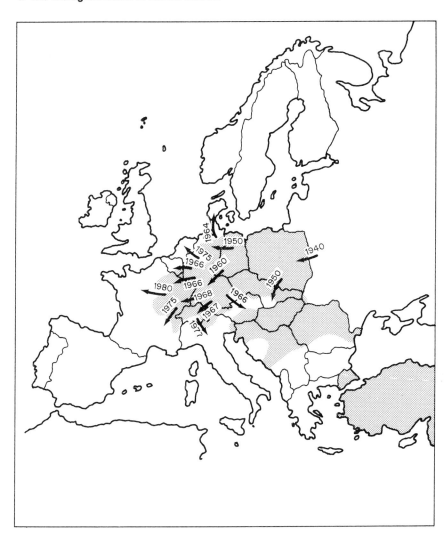

Fig. 2. History of the present European rabies epizootic. Stippled region indicates western frontiers of European rabies in 1983, and dates with arrows are the dates the epizootic crossed national borders.

persisted. Figure 3 shows the 11 countries that Wachendorfer originally grouped in the sylvatic zone. We have updated his analysis: the annual total of reported cases has stabilized with a total of 72,140 non-human cases reported in the 5 years of 1977–1981 (Fig. 3). Of those, 87% were in wildlife, and most of those were in Red Foxes. In Hungary, 99% of reported wildlife cases were among Red Foxes. In the decade 1972 through 1981, Red Foxes comprised 75% of all

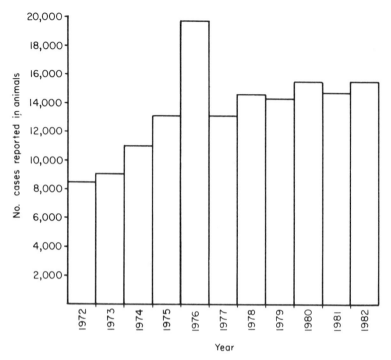

Fig. 3. The annual incidence of non-human rabies in 11 European countries typified by sylvatic (Red Fox) rabies. The countries are Austria, Belgium, Switzerland, Czechoslovakia, West Germany, East Germany, France, Hungary, Luxembourg, Poland and the Netherlands (the Netherlands had been free of rabies since 1977 until 1983 when one fox was registered near Groningen). (Data from WHO Collaborating Centre for Rabies Surveillance and Research, Tübingen, 1973–1983).

reported cases in the sylvatic zone. In 1982, 13,971 foxes were reported rabid in that zone.

Within the zone of sylvatic rabies, the composition of species that were diagnosed rabid shows a characteristic change with time after the arrival of the disease front. During the early years domestic cases predominate, but as prophylaxis and public awareness increase, the relative importance of wildlife escalates. For example, in Poland, 29% of the early cases were in wild animals, whereas by the 1970s, this figure approached 70%, and for 1977–1981, an average of 81% of all reported cases in Poland were in wild species, with the majority in Red Foxes. Turkey typifies an area where dog rabies predominate. From 1977 to 1981, the number of recorded cases in Turkey increased steadily from 1482 to 2260, but each year the number of wild animals that were diagnosed rabid remained constant and never exceeded 25 cases (wildlife averaged 1.3% of reported cases). Wachendorfer's third category (dog rabies with wildlife foci) seems less robust today and may represent an historial stage in dog control and case monitoring. Yugoslavia and Italy were previously classed as a dog

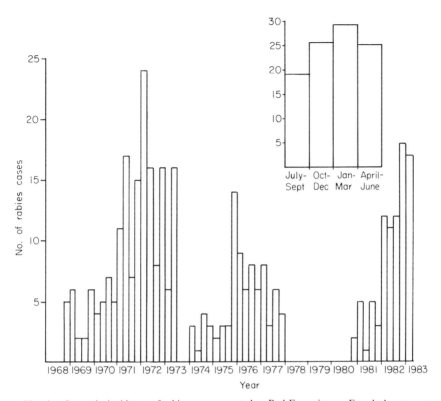

Fig. 4. Quarterly incidence of rabies cases reported in Red Foxes in one French department, Ardennes, which was amongst the first to be invaded by the original epizootic in 1968. The inset shows the percentage of all cases that were reported during each quarter of the year. (Data from WHO Collaborating Centre for Rabies Surveillance and Research, Tübingen).

rabies zone. In the past 5 years, over 95% of reported cases in Yugoslavia and over 99% of those in Italy have been from wildlife. These countries now seem typical of the sylvatic zone where Red Foxes are important. It is difficult to know to what extent this shift mirrors (1) the efficiency of preventative measures with regard to domestic animals, (2) the effectiveness of monitoring cases of rabies in wildlife or (3) a genuine epizootiological phenomenon. It is also notable that national figures may obscure regional differences, e.g. in Yugoslavia sylvatic rabies is confined to the north, and it represents the southern limit of European fox rabies; central and southern Yugoslavia are infected by urban dog rabies.

In each region, the pattern of rabies in foxes approximates a similar course; as the rabies front arrives, there is an epizootic peak in reported cases. That is followed by a silent phase of 2–3 years before another small peak in incidence occurs, and thereafter secondary peaks recur at 4- to 5-year intervals. That pattern is illustrated in Fig. 4 for one department, Ardennes, in France. Data on rabies are often collated at a national level, and thus the fox populations statistics from

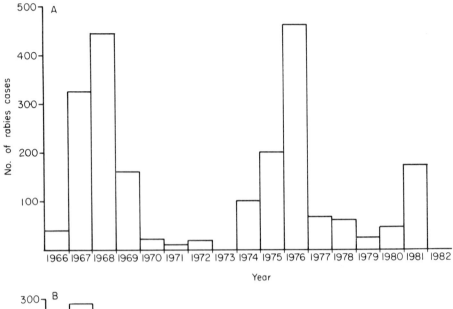

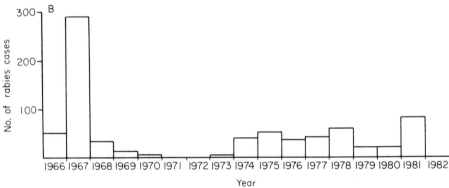

Fig. 5. The annual incidence of rabies (mostly in Red Foxes) in (A) Belgium and (B) Luxembourg.

various habitats and at different phases of the epi- and/or enzootic cycles. Hence, the periodicity of case occurrence is often obscured. However, the data for smaller countries, such as Belgium and Luxembourg, often show the pattern of epizootic wave to cycles (Fig. 5).

Locally, the incidence of rabies varies with time. Bogel *et al.* (1976) showed that among three regions in West Germany the change in the mean annual number of reported rabid foxes per km^2 (0.044–0.065) varied in the same direction as the change in mean number of foxes shot annually per km^2 (0.7–1.5). However, there was no relationship between either of those two variables

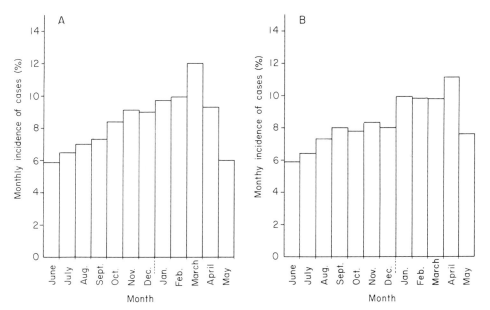

Fig. 6. Seasonal variation in the monthly percentage of recorded cases of rabies in foxes in (A) West Germany and (B) southern Ontario. The graph for West Germany was calculated for data from 3,059 cases in 12 months of 1968–69 as presented in Toma and Andral (1977), whereas that for southern Ontario is based on 12,402 cases recorded between 1958–80.

and the mean distance of new cases ahead of the previous month's front line (4.70–4.98 km). The authors concluded that hunting tallies mirrored fox population densities, which in turn affected rabies incidence but not front-line velocity (but see Ball, Chapter 11, this volume).

Finally, there tends to be a seasonal peak in the cases of fox rabies in the late winter and a trough in mid-summer. That tendency is weakly evident in the quarterly data for the Ardennes (see inset Fig. 4) but is more convincing on Fig. 6. Across Europe, this seasonal peak is emphasised by comparison between quarterly Red Fox case incidence for October–December versus January–March, e.g. 3908 versus 4993, an increase of 27% during the winter 1982–83. There is a similar peak in the mean monthly velocity of the front line (Bogel and Moegle, 1980).

B. NORTH AMERICA

The history and current distribution of rabies in North America shows a complex epizootiology. The role of species affected by rabies varies greatly from area to area as does the incidence of the disease. Rabies occurs throughout the contiguous United States, and in the last decade there have been 42,376 laboratory diagnosed cases of rabies. This total includes 1,972 dogs, 1,607 cats, 3,804 domestic stock and 34,993 wild animals. During that period, the proportion of rabies cases in wildlife has increased in comparison to domestic species and wild species are considered to be the primary source of infection in most areas of the United States. The assemblage of wildlife vectors is most complex in the eastern United States, where Red Foxes, Grey Foxes, Raccoons, and Striped Skunks are the species most often diagnosed rabid. The intriguing feature there is that foxes, skunks and Raccoons are common throughout the area, but the role of each species varies greatly in different regions. (That multivector community is described by A. Carey in Chapter 2, this volume.) In the southeastern United States of Georgia, South Carolina and Florida, the Raccoon is the major vector, accounting for 77% of the cases in those states in the last 10 years. An outbreak of rabies in Raccoons has occurred in the more northern states of Virginia, Maryland and Pennsylvania. Throughout most of the central plains of the United States, the Striped Skunk is the major wildlife species diagnosed with rabies. Skunks are also important in California, but bats are at least as important there and southward towards Mexico. A large area of skunk rabies in the central states extends northward into the southern parts of Canada's prairie provinces. That extension of rabies occurred during the 1960s and is distinct from a far more dramatic spread of rabies that occurred earlier in Canada, which largely involved Red Foxes. The latter invasion in many ways parallelled the rabies invasion that swept Europe this century. The invasion of rabies from the North American arctic into southern Canada occurred, perhaps by chance, at the same time (the late 1940s) as the European fox rabies invasion. Following that, epizootic rabies has become enzootic in eastern Canada, whereas the incidence of the disease had been previously restricted, for the most part, to the domestic species. We will review that epizootic and then describe the current status of rabies in foxes, which are enzootic in Ontario, where 91% of the total rabies cases in Canada are recorded annually.

The Invasion of Rabies from the Canadian Arctic

In a review of the history and epizootiology of rabies in Canada, Tabel *et al.* (1974) demonstrated that wildlife played a minor role in the epizootics of rabies in Canada from 1900–1940. During that period, the dog was the major vector and accounted for 60–90% of the cases in various small, localized outbreaks. However, a distinct epizootic began in 1945 in the arctic regions of Canada and Alaska. Historically, it seems that rabies had been present in the Arctic for a long time. The description by a Moravian priest of an outbreak of "dog disease" in the Ungava of Quebec in 1795 was probably rabies. From 1900 throughout the 1940s, there were several instances of native people being bitten by foxes or wolves. The arctic dog disease reported in the Canadian arctic was believed to occur in sled dogs, Arctic Foxes, wolves and ermine (*Mustela* spp.), and rabies was confirmed in Alaska in foxes, dogs and wolves during the mid-1940s. The foxes involved included both Arctic Foxes and Red Foxes. In 1947, rabies was diagnosed across the Arctic from Baffin Island in the east to Alaska in the west. The disease became more prevalent and spread southward through the Northwest Territories of Canada, where reports of rabies in Red Foxes became more common. During 1951–52, rabies spread into Manitoba, Saskatchewan and Alberta. It spread from northern to southern Alberta, a distance of over 700 miles, in 8 months. During that period coyotes were diagnosed with rabies, and the possibility that coyotes were capable of more extensive movements than foxes was mooted as an explanation for that rapid spread. Concurrently, rabies was spreading in foxes through northern Manitoba on the west coast of Hudsons Bay and through Quebec on the east coast of Hudsons Bay. By 1954 rabies was diagnosed in Ontario near Moosonee at the south end of James Bay. Two years later rabies was epizootic in southern Ontario, and by 1958, 2204 cases of rabies had been diagnosed there. Subsequently, rabies spread southward into New York State in the early 1960s, and eastward to the Maritime Provinces of Canada, reaching there in the mid-1960s. In all those invasions, Red Foxes accounted for about 50% of all the laboratory diagnosed cases. In southern Ontario, 1–2 years after the initial invasion, Striped Skunks began to be diagnosed as rabid, and in some small, urban areas, they now account for more than 60% of all the cases, although provincially they average less than 25%. Since the invasion, rabies has remained enzootic in southern Ontario. The annual number of cases of rabies diagnosed has varied from 240 cases just after the first peak to over 2000 cases in some years during the 1970s and 1980s. The average number of cases per year is 1400, and wildlife comprise 60% of those cases. Cattle are the major domestic species infected by wildlife and account for over 20% of the total cases diagnosed. In total, from 1958 to 1980, there have been 17,310 cases of rabies diagnosed in wildlife (62.4%) and 10,437 cases in domestic species (37.6%) in Ontario (see Table II). The incidence of the disease, although lower than rabies incidence as reported in Europe, is nonetheless the highest density for any jurisdiction of comparable area in North America. Rabies has become relatively uncommon elsewhere in Canada with the exception of the skunk epizootics in the prairie provinces. In the last decade, there have been only a few cases diagnosed in northern Ontario and only 1300 cases in all the provinces east of Ontario. Thus, in eastern Canada, the disease is enzootic in the agricultural farmland of southern Ontario but is uncommon or absent elsewhere. In addition to the high incidence of the disease and its restriction to the southern part of the province, rabies in Ontario is also unique in North America in that Foxes and skunks are both heavily involved. In the eastern United States, where rabies in foxes is most common, the number of cases in skunks is much lower, whereas in the prairie states where skunk rabies is most common, Red Foxes are rarely diagnosed as rabid. The enzootic rabies in skunks in the prairie states and provinces of North

TABLE II

Total Rabies Cases Diagnosed in Ontario between 1958–1980

Animal	Number	Percentage
Domestics	10,437	37.6
Cow	5,796	20.8
Dog	1,715	6.1
Cat	1,388	5.0
Sheep	608	2.2
Horse	540	1.9
Pig	320	1.1
Goat	63	0.2
Rabbit	6	—
Donkey	1	—
Wildlife	17,308	62.4
Red Fox	12,402	44.7
Striped Skunk	4,361	15.7
Bat	206	0.7
Raccoon	147	0.5
Wolf and Coyote	151	0.5
Woodchuck	22	—
White-tailed Deer	5	—
Black Bear	4	—
Muskrat	4	—
Bison	2	—
Elk	1	—
Black Squirrel	1	—
Fisher	1	—
Weasel	1	—
Total	27,745	

America has a different history from that of the rabies invasion into Ontario, where the role of the Red Fox was obvious and where skunks were not reported rabid for 1–2 years after the initial invasion (see Section 4,2).

With the exception of the areas with Raccoon rabies in the eastern United States, no wild species other than foxes and skunks are commonly diagnosed rabid in eastern North America. Certainly, there is abundant contact between several of the rabies vectors. Fox, skunk, Raccoon, Porcupine (*Erethizon dorsatum*) and woodchuck (*Marmota marmota*), all use the same burrows, even during the same years (D. R. Voigt, unpublished data). Despite the fact that home ranges, activity and travel of these species overlap both temporally and spatially in many areas, involvement by each species varies regionally. Factors causing this variation are poorly understood. For example, the role of bats in the complex epizootiology of rabies in foxes remains unknown. Preliminary results from monoclonal antibody studies of rabies virus isolates suggest that there are differences between bat strains and fox strain, although the work is inconclusive. However, bats could play an uncommon but important role in rabies transmission even in temperate areas. There are records of foxes entering bat caves, and rabid bats have been found lying in grass, unable to fly but squeaking (C. D. Mac-Innes, personal communication), which could doubtless attract foxes. In Ontario, seven species of bats have been diagnosed with rabies, but only one species is commonly found rabid. The Big Brown Bat (*Eptesicus fuscus*) accounted for 95% of all bat cases. Some species of bats in Canada migrate south annually and are known to roost colonially with southern species that are more often found rabid, such as the Mexican Free-tailed Bat (Schowalter, 1980). In Canada, rabies west of the Rocky Mountains has been diagnosed in bats but not in terrestrial mammals with the exception of one cat. The cat was known to catch and 'play' with bats. Bats could also play a role in the long-range movement of virus in the reintroduction of rabies into an area and in transmission of rabies to humans. Several cases of rabies in humans in Canada occurred after exposure to bats; Big Brown Bats often roost in, or near, human habitation, and in many areas the potential for contact with humans is high.

C. A COMPARISON

The following features are shared by the wildlife epizootics of central Europe and eastern Canada:

1. The present epizootics occured after many decades during which rabies in wildlife had been absent.

2. Prophylactics have restricted the disease largely to wildlife. Although more than 30% of cases in Ontario are in domestic animals (mostly unvaccinated cattle), the persistent source of the disease is in wild animals; in Europe over 87% of diagnosed rabid animals are of wild species.

3. In spite of attempts at control in foxes and other vectors, the disease front advanced steadily from the Arctic to southern Canada, and in Europe the advance continues today, although it may just have stopped in France. Similarly, conventional control by culling wild animals has not extirpated rabies once it has become enzootic, except perhaps locally and temporarily. Worldwide, the eradication of rabies in wildlife by culling of vectors has failed (Baer, 1975; Macdonald, 1980b). The extent to which culling has contained the disease is debatable. In Europe it appears to have little affect on the speed at which the epizootic advances, but it may affect the number of foxes that contract the disease and hence threaten humans. Certainly, the fox toll during rabies control schemes has been immense and, to the extent that it has been ineffective, this is regrettable. The arguably unsuccessful 1953 campaign in Alberta is notorious: in 18 months

the approximate toll was 50,000 Red Foxes, 35,000 Coyotes, 4,200 wolves, 7,500 Lynx, 1,850 bears, 500 Striped Skunks, and 164 Cougars (Ballantyne and O'Donoghue, 1954). Rabies persists there today albeit from a different invasion. Culling has only been successful in isolated areas, such as the Danish peninsula, where the risk of reinvasion is reduced by the narrow access route (Muller, 1971). Even there, the effect was temporary. After being free of rabies since 1970, a new outbreak occurred in 1977 and was eliminated in foxes in 1981 (Westergaard, 1982). Between 1981 and 1982, the rabies front in France appeared to stop without any obvious cause; during 1982 the quarterly incidence of wild animal cases steadily and atypically fell from the first to the last quarter (from 817 to 518) but rose to 668 in early 1983, whereas the total annual loss of domestic stock was the highest (874 cases) since the epizootic began (Andral, 1982). Today, there are grounds for optimism that vulpine rabies can be controlled by oral vaccination (Steck *et al.*, 1982).

4. In Europe, rabies occasionally appears to leap ahead of the advancing wave front by distances of up to 100 km. In Alberta and Ontario, such leaps occurred during the initial invasion. Some such leaps are beyond the known limits of a single healthy fox's dispersal; for example, in 1982 in Yugoslavia, a focus of vulpine rabies broke out in Croatia, some 400 km ahead of the front wave. These leaps may represent as yet unidentified sources of rabies or an undetected series of infections by normal dispersal.

5. The overall direction of the front is influenced by major topographical barriers such as mountains, major rivers or large lakes.

6. In the wake of initial epizootics, secondary peaks in the annual incidence of rabies among foxes recur periodically at intervals of 3–5 years. In that sense, the foci of enzootic rabies move around. Since rabies areas in nearby regions are usually out-of-phase with each other, reintroduction from another region is probable.

7. Within each year, there is a seasonal peak in the late winter in the numbers of foxes diagnosed rabid and a minimum during June and July. Bogel *et al.* (1974, 1976) noted that in Germany the velocity of the front accelerates in February whereas the incidence of rabies does not start to increase until March. They concluded that it was the greater area encompassed by the accelerating front that lead to a subsequent increase in cases.

8. In May–June, sub-adult foxes comprise a smaller proportion of those reported dying from rabies than they do of those dying from other causes (although the difficulty of finding dead rabid cubs probably biases these data).

9. A greater proportion of rabid foxes is made up of juvenile males in autumn and adult females in spring.

In contrast, the two epizootics differ in the following respects:

1. In the sylvatic zone of Europe, the Red Fox makes up 87% of the reported rabid individuals among wild species; the Eurasian Badger (*Meles meles*), and

Beech Marten, (*Martes foina*) play numerically smaller roles. For example, Badgers and other mustelids comprised 7.2% of 5490 cases reported among wild animals (80.4% foxes) in 1982 in West Germany. In Ontario, 72% of the reported cases among wildlife are in Red Fox, 25% are in Striped Skunks, and many other species are involved at a low level.

2. Rabies in skunks occurs throughout the enzootic area in Ontario, varying locally from 10 to over 60% of diagnosed cases. In many urban areas, skunks are the major wildlife species reported rabid. In Europe, no carnivore, other than the Red Fox, is so involved. There, the tight knit social structure of Badgers may ensure that the disease decimates their numbers so effectively that they play a lesser role in sustaining epizootics.

3. The epizootic front travels at an average of about 40 km per year in Europe, whereas in Ontario during the initial invasion, rabies spread at rates of over 100 km per year.

4. In Europe, it is widely held that the disease can be extirpated if the number of foxes killed annually during 'routine' hunting falls below 0.3 per km² (Bogel *et al.*, 1974, 1976; Bogel and Moegle, 1980). Note that a common misrepresentation of this figure is as the density of foxes rather than the reported numbers killed (see below). In Ontario, enzootic rabies persists where indices of fox density are much lower. There, even the highest harvest areas only average about 0.3 foxes killed annually per km²; most districts have much lower harvests (0.01–0.1 fox per km² per annum), and rabies nevertheless persists. In Ontario, incidence of rabies is lower in areas of both the highest and the lowest fox pelt harvests, and it is higher where the harvests are intermediate. This finding indicates not only a complex interaction between rabies incidence and "control" (i.e. in this case fur harvest, Voigt and Tinline, 1982) but also points to the weakness of the assumption that fox numbers are directly correlated with hunting tallies (and in turn with rabies incidence). The most common incarnation of this assumption is embodied in the HIPD (Hunting Indicator of Population Density— number of Red Foxes killed per km² per annum, Bogel *et al.*, 1974). Bogel and Moegle (1980) stressed that this measure is only valid for areas of over 2000 km² in extent. Bearing in mind the great heterogeneity of the European landscape and the probably even greater local variation in fox population parameters, 2000 km² units must encompass a multitude of epizootiological phenomena (see Bacon, Chapter 5, this volume). Indeed, in Ontario areas which might be thought of as epizootiological units in that they have distinct case incidence patterns, out of phase with neighbouring areas of comparable size, the units measure about 1000 km². Gessler and Spittler (1982) have argued that the class of fox killed may be just as important as the total numbers killed. They speculate that the absence of rabies from an area where the HIPD was high was due to selective hunting of sub-adult foxes. Wandeler (1980b) discussed the many factors that confuse the HIPD. Quite apart from difficulty of assessing vector numbers, epizootiological patterns may themselves partly reflect biases; Braunschweig (1980) estimated

that only 2–10% of Red Fox cases in Germany were reported, and Bacon (1981) has shown how that level of inadequate monitoring could disable various control plans. Similarly, the low incidence of wildlife rabies in developing countries may also reflect inadequate monitoring. Acha (1982) noted that improved control of dog rabies in some Latin American towns is now disclosing a previously unacknowledged reservoir among rats. Finally, differing topographies may affect chances of contacts (Adamovich, 1978), both among rabid vectors themselves and between people and rabid vectors. The latter will affect reported rates even within a jurisdiction.

Nobody knows the threshold population density below which contact rate falls to a level at which the disease dies out, and probably it varies between populations. Using the European epizootic as a model, Bacon and Macdonald (1980) estimated the critical contact rate at 1.2, and in another model (using different parameter values) David et al. (1982) concluded that the threshold population density was 1 fox/160 ha (0.63 foxes/km^2). However, these and similar estimates can be taken with caution since one can always argue with the choice of parameters in the absence of direct field corroboration.

IV. Vector Biology

A. THE RED FOX

1. Behavioural Ecology

The Red Fox is a medium-sized (5–6 kg) canid, whose opportunistic behaviour and omnivorous diet facilitate its survival in a wide variety of habitats. The Red Fox is so flexible in its habits that only the broadest generalisations survive much scrutiny. Adult foxes live in pairs or small family groups of one male and up to five females (vixens). The females are likely to be relatives. The home ranges of members of a social group overlap widely with each other and relatively little, or not at all, with those of neighbouring groups; that evidence, together with observations of encounters and scent marking, suggest that foxes are generally territorial, although there are habitats where that may not be so (e.g. Harris, 1980). The extent of overlap between neighbouring group ranges differs between populations in different habitats (and also varies greatly even in the same locality). Home range sizes vary among habitats, with extremes of 10 ha and over 2000 ha, and within a habitat type there is no obvious relationship between territory size and adult group size. Rather, those parameters seem to be independently affected by the dispersion and abundance of available food and by the pattern of mortality. The effect of different patterns of mortality on the social organisation of the survivors is particularly poorly understood. Macdonald

(1981) described local variation in the social organisation of foxes and Voigt and Macdonald (1985) compared two populations at opposite extremes of the spectrum of home range sizes (see also Sargeant, 1972; von Schantz, 1981; Lindstrom, 1982). Kruuk (1976) and Macdonald (1983) have reviewed the factors that may underlie variation in group and territory sizes within and between species of Carnivora.

In temperate zones foxes give birth in the spring. Mean vixen productivity varies greatly between areas and, where food availability moves in cycles with a several-year as well as seasonal periodicity, between years (Englund, 1970; Lindstrom, 1982). Two mechanisms affect mean vixen productivity: (1) variation in litter size and (2) variation in the percentage of vixens breeding. Part of this variation has a proximate ecological basis: mean litter sizes vary from 3.0 to 8.6 in a way that is probably a reflection of available food. Another part of the variation in average vixen productivity is the result of proximate social factors, such as the postponement of reproduction by subordinate (generally young) vixens (Macdonald, 1979, 1980a; Harris, 1979; Voigt and Macdonald, 1985). The highest proportion of non-breeding vixens (36%) was recorded in Sweden by Englund (1970). In Ontario, non-breeding vixens (5–15%) are largely yearlings (D. R. Voigt, unpublished data). However, over large areas of Europe, litter sizes averaged 4.3, with only 3.8% barren vixens, and there were no indications of age affecting reproductive performance (Artois *et al.*, 1982; see also Lloyd *et al.*, 1976).

In the autumn, young of the year begin to disperse. A variable proportion of sub-adult vixens and almost all of the sub-adult males leave their natal range. Mean dispersal distances vary greatly within and between habitats, but despite that the average dispersal distance of males is invariably further than that of females from the same habitat, even excluding those females who do not disperse at all (Storm *et al.*, 1976; Lloyd, 1975; Jensen, 1968, 1973). The mean male dispersal distance appears to increase with local mean home range size (Macdonald and Bacon, 1982; Newdick, 1983). A small proportion of sub-adults disperse over relatively enormous disances of 100 km or more (Storm *et al.*, 1976; Englund, 1980; Lindstrom, 1982). In Ontario, several young males distances greater than 150 km start-to-finish point distance, following zigzag routes of over 400 km (see also Ables, 1965). The autumn fox population is thus composed of resident and itinerant sections of fox society. The process of dispersal and the fate of the itinerants are even less understood than are some other aspects of fox society. However, it is certain that many of the travelling foxes die during the first winter. Although the idea that itinerant animals suffer higher mortality than residents (due to unfamiliarity with their surroundings and perhaps poorer physical condition) has intuitive appeal, data have not been forthcoming to support it.

The age structure of fox populations is difficult to assess since it is normally gauged from *post mortem* material which provides a sample of those dying, but is not necessarily representative of those that survive. However, it is indisputable that the age structures of Red Fox populations differ greatly, mainly due to the influence of man and of disease. In some populations, *post mortem* data suggest that few foxes survive 3 years, elsewhere animals of 5–6 years are not uncommon (e.g. Fairley, 1969; Storm *et al.*, 1976; Harris, 1979; Lloyd, 1980; Voigt and Macdonald, 1985).

General reviews of Red Fox biology, together with discussion of its implication for rabies control can be found in Lloyd (1980) and Macdonald (1980b).

2. The Fox as a Victim of Rabies

Red Foxes are very susceptible to rabies. They can succumb when challenged by a single mouse LD_{50} dose, a virus concentration of only $1/10,000$ the strength of that required to infect humans. Once infected, most foxes incubate the disease for 19–20 days before they become infective and begin to shed virus in their saliva. The virus in 1 ml of suspension of virulent fox salivary gland is, theoretically, sufficient to infect 34 million others! (Blancou *et al.*, 1979). They shed virus for up to 6 days. At that point symptoms may begin to appear after which the fox may survive 24 hours or more, but seldom more than 4 days. Symptoms may take several forms (1) the notorious (but less common) furious form which is typified by high, irregular mobility and attacks upon any object encountered (11% of artificially infected cases in captivity), (2) increasing paralysis, and (3) docile, apparently friendly, approaches to normally frightening stimuli such as children. Symptoms include aggressive attacks on other objects, including other foxes [as illustrated in George *et al.* (1980)]. All these "forms" may occur in the same fox. Bacon and Macdonald (1980) speculated that in terms of "game theory", combinations of these symptoms insure rabies virus transmission in a whole suit of vulpine circumstances. The fear that has beset biologists trying to understand rabies epizootiology has always been that the behaviour of rabid foxes might differ so greatly from that of healthy foxes as to invalidate any extrapolations from the latter. However, there are good grounds for seeking to analyse rabies epizootiology on the basis of studies of the behaviour of healthy foxes: (1) there is a long period after infection but prior to the onset of symptoms when the fox is not infective, (2) Andral *et al.* (1982) have radio-tracked three wild foxes artificially infected with rabies and found that they travelled approximately the same home range after the onset of symptoms, and (3) two radio-collared foxes in Ontario contracted the disease, and thereafter no difference in their movements was apparent until their death. Matters would be simplest if it transpired that rabid foxes generally behave like healthy ones (i.e. have the same movement patterns and frequency of social encounters) yet become more aggressive. In that case, the contact rate of the disease might approximate the frequency of social encounters (or a constant factor of it). The frequency of encounters is difficult, but possible, to measure.

In evolutionary terms, it is surprising that foxes have not developed resistance to rabies. Because the disease can cause a 10-fold or greater reduction in fox numbers, the selective pressure it exerts is immense. Steck (1982) reported HIPD falling from 1 to 6 per km^2 to 0.1 per km^2 due to rabies. Carey and McClean (1978) reported that in Virginia (United States), 2% of Red Foxes and 7% of Grey Foxes had rabies serum neutralising antibodies (i.e. implying that they had survived the disease and developed some immunity). Amongst the Grey Foxes, which were the principal vectors in that area, the portion of the same with SN antibodies reached 29% in some localities. Ramsden and Johnston (1975) also found rabies SNA in some foxes and skunks but at ower levels. The implications of these results are unclear (see discussion following Carey, 1982). The detection of rabies antibodies in the absence of challenge experiments does not constitute proof of immunity against rabies. Furthermore, the existence of strain differences and variation in 'test virus' complicate the virological picture. Nonetheless, some species such as Raccoons sometimes show a higher incidence of rabies antibody (McClean, 1975; Carey, this volume). It has generally been assumed that antibody levels develop after a low exposure to the virus. A carrier state in rabies (as distinct from natural immunity) has not been generally accepted despite reports (e.g. Yurkovsky, 1962) of people contracting the disease from dogs which showed no symptoms and survived.

Concerning the evolution of resistance to rabies, it is interesting that Lodmell (1983) has shown that resistance to intraperitoneally inoculated street rabies virus is under genetic control and that within resistant strains of mice females were more resistant than males.

In both the major fox rabies enzootic areas of Canada and Europe, there were low rates of antibody occurrence in non-rabid foxes. In Switzerland Steck (1982) found that less than 2% of 239 foxes survived and became immune after experimental infection (see Wandeler *et al.,* 1974). He concluded that naturally acquired immunity was not a major factor in the epizootiology of rabies. If this were not the case, then conventional control by culling could be counterproductive in increasing the proportion of susceptibles in the population [as Everard *et al.* (1976) argued regarding mongoose rabies; see Chapter 3, this volume].

B. THE SKUNK

Skunks are not nearly as widespread as foxes, but in North America, at least, they are just as commonly associated with rabies. Among the 13 recognised species of skunks, only one, the Striped Skunk is generally a major vector of rabies. The Spotted Skunk has been diagnosed rabid especially in the south-ernmost states (Johnson, 1959), but our discussion of skunk ecology and epi-zootiology will be based on the species most often diagnosed, rabid—the Striped Skunk (for a general review, see Verts, 1967). These skunks vary from 1 to 5.5 kg in weight, but most individuals are 1.3 to 2.7 kg. They are nocturnal and wander over homes ranges of up to 7 km^2 in a wide variety of habitats, ranging from urban centres, to open prairies, to heavily forested areas but are especially prevalent in agricultural areas. They are distributed throughout southern Canada and the contiguous United States. Litters, usually of 4–6 (range 2–10) are born in May after a 63-day gestation. The time of independent foraging of kits (young skunks) varies among families, but it occurs most often from July through September. Nonetheless, communal denning is well documented (Houseknecht, 1969; Allen and Shapton, 1942) and is most common during winter (from De-cember through March) when northern populations of skunks aestivate, under-taking only occasional foraging excursions on mild nights (Schowalter and Gun-son, 1982). Dens are commonly ground burrows or shelters under buildings, and several sites may be used by the same individual over the course of the winter (Storm, 1972). These burrows are shared by Woodchucks, Porcupines, Coyotes, Red Foxes, Grey Foxes, and Rabbits (*Sylvilagus floridanus*). Although simul-taneous occupancy by several species is not common, these burrows do provide high potential for disease exposure and transmission both interspecifically and intraspecifically. At other times of the year, male skunks are seldom associated with the female and offspring(s). Indeed, there is some evidence of intraspecific strife between adult males and females with kits (Sargeant *et al.*, 1982). The home ranges of several females may overlap, however, and groups of skunk recorded together included adult females and juveniles but rarely more than one male (Allen and Shapton, 1942). Thus denning behaviour and local activity of skunks provide a high potential for intraspecific spread of rabies.

Dispersal in skunks is even less understood than in foxes. Long-range move-ments (>10 km) of both adults and juveniles have been recorded (Bjorge *et al.*, 1981; Verts, 1967; Sargeant *et al.*, 1982; Andersen, 1981; Rosatte, 1984). However, it is not known whether such movements are commonplace, when they most often take place or what the sex and age distributions of dispersers are.

The fox–skunk–rabies interaction varies between areas. Several authors in the United States have suggested that areas with rabies among skunks were distinct from areas with rabies among foxes (Verts and Storm, 1966; Parker, 1961). Now that the rabies enzootic in Ontario is better understood, we recognise that large areas where both species are heavily involved with rabies also occur.

The following five reasons have been indentified, which alone or together lead to differences in the geographic distribution of fox–skunk rabies in North America:

1. Differences in the susceptibility of each species to rabies in different areas.

2. Differences in the infectivity (saliva virus concentration) of each species in different areas.

3. Difference in the social organisation and thus activity, movements and dispersal of each species in different areas, which is a primary determinant of contact rate.

4. Difference in the mortality by non-rabies factors and related to that, differences in density of each species.

5. Historical sequence of rabies and subsequent control efforts.

Areas where fox–skunk rabies is enzootic can be classed into three regions: (1) the central and southern plains of the United States, including the Canadian prairie extension (Parker, 1975), (2) the eastern woodlands of the United States (see Carey, Chapter 2, this volume), (3) southern Ontario (Webster et al., 1974; Johnston and Beauregard, 1969). The first region has little fox rabies, the second has few cases in skunks, and in the third, Ontario, both foxes and skunks are often diagnosed rabid.

There are no measures of fox to skunk (or vice versa) transmission rates. Foxes have been recorded carrying dead skunks, scent-marking them and rubbing and rolling on carcasses (D. R. Voigt and P. Bachmann, unpublished data). Houseknecht and Huempfner (1970) recorded encounters between live skunks and foxes, but the studies on oral infectivity of rabies by Ramsden and Johnston (1975) demonstrate that transmission from a corpse is possible. The invasion of rabies into Ontario clearly suggests that foxes can transmit rabies to skunks as prior to rabies in foxes, rabies in skunks (or any other wildlife) was unknown and as cases of skunk rabies appeared in Ontario 1–2 years after fox epizootics. Today a similar pattern occurs, although the lag may be only 3–6 months. The monthly distribution of rabies cases in skunks is similar to that among foxes, with a winter peak (Johnston and Beauregard, 1969). However, in the rabies outbreaks among skunks in the United States and western Canada where foxes are not implicated, the peaks occur in April through June (Webster et al., 1974; Rosatte, 1984). In many parts of Ontario, as in Europe, fox rabies occurs in 3-year cycles but incidence of skunk rabies do not show the same consistent pattern. Together with the persistence of rabies in skunks in some urban centres, this suggests that skunk rabies in Ontario might persist without fox rabies. Since skunks can incubate rabies for long periods (up to 10 months), it is tempting to speculate that skunks do play a role in the persistence of fox rabies in Ontario. Further, the studies of Sikes (1962) showed that skunks secreted more virus in their saliva than foxes and that foxes were suceptible to even small amounts of infective virus. Thus, transmission from skunks to foxes seems probable from a virological viewpoint but transmission from foxes to skunks was more obvious from epizootiological studies. Differences in the probability of those events could explain differences in rabies incidence in North America. Furthermore, evidence is accumulating of differences between strains of rabies virus in those hosts (see Wiktor *et al.*, 1980).

The anomalies in the skunk–fox rabies incidence have repercussions for rabies control and attempts at simulation modelling. Fox population control is invariably difficult and of questionable effectiveness. Skunks are easier than foxes to trap and gas, and, with their more limited movements, control operations could be expected to be longer-lasting. However, disease recurrence rates, productivity and rabies epizootics after depopulation suggest that skunk depopulation is also a difficult undertaking with inconclusive results (Sargeant *et al.*, 1982; R. J. Greenwood, personal communication; Rosatte, 1984; Gunson *et al.*, 1978). Control might be most effective before a rabies invasion by limiting contact rate. The simulation model by Voigt *et al.* described later in this volume (chapter 13) clearly shows that reintroduction need occur only at a very low rate to successfully initiate new outbreaks. Reintroduction to a population may be fundamental in maintaining rabies in a 'local' area.

C. EPIZOOTIOLOGICAL GENERALISATIONS

The foregoing account of vector biology provides possible explanations for the following features shared by the epizootics in central Europe and eastern Canada.

1. The relatively steady, slow advance of the epizootic front suggests that transmission is generally from one resident social unit to the next. Within any one area, and within any one social group, the majority of foxes probably contract the disease (see also Ball, 1981, and Chapter 8, this volume). Bogel and Moegle (1980) found that 93% of new cases in Germany were reported within 10 km of the previous month's front line. Assuming an interval of about a month between successive infections, and circular home range sizes of 500 ha, then the front could advance at a maximum of 1.6 km per month (i.e. one home range diameter) by interneighbour contact alone.

2. Outbreaks of the disease well ahead of the front were typical of the early invasion of Ontario and are known in Europe too. Those probably resulted from transmission via a dispersing animal.

3. The periodic recurrence of rabies in enzootic areas is a consequence of recovery from the devastating effects of this lethal disease on a population of highly susceptible vectors and, probably more importantly, of colonisation by vectors from neighbouring areas. Few foxes survive the epizootic, and it takes 2–4 years (longer if control is intensive) for their numbers to recover sufficiently for the contact rate to sustain a further enzootic. Dispersal provides one mechanism for "reintroduction" of rabies.

4. The seasonal peak during winter can be linked to dispersal, competition for territories and mating activity, all of which increase the chances of encounters. More foxes engage in more interactions and elevate the contact rate which is then mirrored in the seasonal pattern of rabies incidence. Johnston and Beauregard (1969) hypothesised that both dispersing juveniles, and pregnant vixens are stressed and therefore especially susceptible to infection. The population of susceptibles is renewed annually with the birth of cubs in spring. Such young foxes may not directly encounter non-family members until the late summer. Figures 6A and B show a steady increase in the percentage of fox cases each month from a minimum in June to the peak in March or April. Note that the incidence

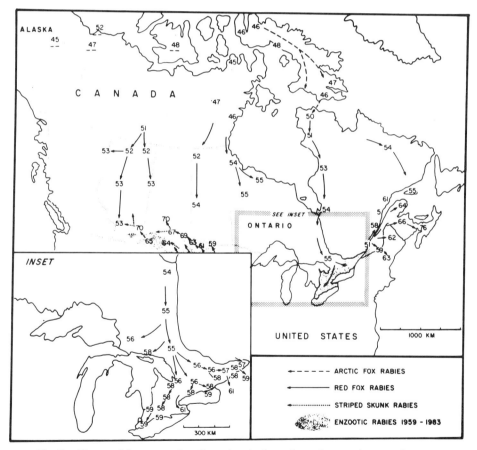

Fig. 7. History of the present Canadian epizootic. Inset shows the annual progression across Ontario. Redrawn from Tabel *et al.* (1974) and Tinline and Pond (1976).

pattern of rabies cases is likely to lag about 1 month behind the infection pattern due to the incubation period, i.e. if most foxes are found to be rabid in March, then most were bitten in February during the peak of mating.

5. Linked to (4), the low representation of youngsters in the summer rabies figures may reflect their lower involvement in certain classes of social interaction (such as territorial behaviour) and/or under-reporting. For example, although in summer over 70% of foxes may be the young of the year, it was found in Switzerland that they comprise only 15–40% of the sample dying of rabies (Steck, 1982). The subsequent increase in youngsters among the rabid sample may reflect the deaths of cubs who contracted the disease from their parents who were infected a month or so earlier. Dispersing animals (i.e largely sub-adults) in the autumn and winter are probably over represented in samples dying if they are more likely to be killed travelling through unfamiliar terrain. They may also be more prone to infection if they are especially subject to attack from residents (Wandeler et al., 1974). Alternatively, the age structure of the dying may genuinely reflect the extent of differential mortality due to rabies among age-classes. Thus Artois and Aubert (1982) argued that the lower ratio of young (5–13 months) to older foxes, ahead of the rabies front wave rather than behind it, indicates that, in comparison to adults, a smaller proportion of sub-adults contracted rabies. They concluded that this differential susceptibility to infection led to the observed lower age structure in rabies epizootic areas.

6. Variation in the incidence of rabies from one locality to the next may indicate any or all of (1) surveillance efficiency, (2) variation in fox numbers due to either resource availability or mortality (see Section V), and (3) variation in contact rate. The number of rabid foxes reported in an area does not necessarily indicate either the number dying of rabies or the size of the surviving population. Within a particulr area, however, reports of rabies can be used to indicate trends if surveillance efficiency is known or does not change.

7. In many regions, the tendency for the epizootic to follow topographical features may be partly due to the behaviour of some foxes, which tend to travel along such features (e.g. rivers, roads) when dispersing. However, except for very large rivers and motorways, it is more probably a consequence of topography correlating with fox numbers (e.g. valleys are more productive than mountain peaks, and roads and rivers often follow valleys and ecotones.).

There are differences in rabies epizootiology between central Europe and eastern Canada that can be partly explained as follows:

1. The incidence of the disease is lower in Canada than it is in Europe. This may be entirely due to a lower density of foxes in Canada, but unfortunately there are no conclusive field data which demonstrate that contact rate is proportional to, or a simple function of, density. Generally, where rabies occurs,

density of foxes and rabies incidence are correlated within an area. The apparent differences in rabies incidence between areas are probably real, despite the unquestionable local differences in reporting rate.

2. Rabies is enzootic in Canada at estimated fox densities that are below those at which it dies out in Europe. A more varied group of vectors, as in Ontario, may be the simplest answer to that anomaly. Skunks, for example, incubate the virus for longer than do foxes and may consequently act as reservoirs, initiating reintroduction of the disease to the fox population. Since rabies epizootics in large contiguous areas in Ontario are often not concurrent, the possibility of reinfection by rabid foxes from nearby areas is high. That possibility is perhaps less probable in the more broken countryside typical of much of Europe, where physical barriers between areas may effectively partition rabies into smaller, largely independent epizootiological units.

3. The rate of spread during the initial epizootic was high in Canada. There are two related explanations for that phenomenon. Territories of foxes (10 km^2) and dispersal distance (up to 150 km) are both larger in Canada. There is a correlation between size of fox territories and dispersal distances (Macdonald and Bacon, 1982). Greater dispersal distances explain a higher rate of disease spread, as could larger territories, if contact rate was independent of territory size. The latter relationship is unproven. Macdonald *et al.* (1980) and D. R. Voigt (unpublished data) found that foxes could meet their neighbours several times each night in both high and low density areas. However, those data were insufficient to resolve adequately the relationship between contact rate and territory size. It is probable that throughout much of the wide variation in Red Fox population densities, interaction frequency varies between limits at which *per capita* contact rate is always greater than 1.0.

The ability to explain the broad features of rabies epizootics in terms of vector biology may create an illusion of greater understanding than actually prevails. Fox densities vary at least 70-fold between habitats, and probably 40-fold within rabies endemic areas, and so specific extrapolations from one study area to another are unwarranted. It is clear that habitat types affect fox populations, at least to the extent that habitats mirror different levels of resource availability. Similarly, it is clear that contact rate between foxes and fox population density are related to rabies spread. However, fox density is notoriously difficult to measure, and the precise relationship between density and contact rate is unknown: for some purposes, such as evaluating control, this precise form is crucial, as shown by Mollison, Chapter 9, this volume. Accordingly, studying or predicting the course of rabies epizootics on the basis of foxes has often been thwarted by inadequate knowledge in the past. In the following section, we will discuss an alternative method, namely the study of the habitat–rabies epizootiology link.

V. Habitat Structure and Rabies Epizootiology

An ecologist's studies of epizootiology should be studies of factors affecting contact rate among vectors. It is widely, but only tacitly, assumed that contact rate amongst foxes is directly proportional to their population density and simple models may assume that it depends on density alone, regardless of carrying capacity (see Chapters 6 and 7, this volume, and as explained and criticised by Mollison in Chapter 9). There are no data to support or to refute this assumption, but revelations of the complexity of mammalian social behaviour make it, *a priori*, a questionable proposition. Although the relationship is clearly not simple, it is generally true that outbreaks of rabies have been more intense where foxes were more numerous. Bogel and Moegle (1980) reported a weak correlation between fox rabies incidence and HIPD; Voigt and Tinline (1982) showed strong correlations between rabies incidence and fox harvests within similar areas, but they also demonstrated much variation between years and different regions.

Local differences in numbers of foxes at least partly reflect variation in resource (prey) availability and mortality. Bacon and Macdonald (1980) and Macdonald *et al.* (1981) investigated the idea that fox populations might be estimated from habitat characteristics, to the extent that these are indicators of prey availability. Habitats appear to be easier to measure than fox numbers, and correlates of habitat might indicate not only fox numbers but the structure of fox society (cf. Macdonald, 1983). These in turn could be compared with independent estimates of both population density and contact rate (as reflected in rabies incidence).

At first sight this approach is promising. Common knowledge that fox density varies among habitats is reinforced by published studies (e.g. Macdonald, 1981; Voigt and Macdonald, 1985), and Macdonald *et al.* (1981) presented a method whereby fox densities over a wide area could be estimated from a knowledge of the habitat features that may effect their number locally. Similarly, other studies indicated that the spread of rabies was influenced by habitat types (e.g. Carey *et al.*, 1978). Three studies, all using fox rabies incidence data from France, have sought to quantify the role of habitat type. Ball (1981; Chapters 8 and 11, this volume) found a tendency for the velocity of the epizootic front wave to vary depending on landscape features. His analysis suggested that features (read from maps) such as altitude, the presence of fruit trees and vines and aspects of geology were important, as was the presence of railway lines. If the effect is real, then the impact of railway lines could be in either or both of two respects. First, railway lines may congregate in particular habitats, such as valleys, which for other reasons favour high fox contact rate. Second, foxes sometimes follow roads and railways while dispersing, so the front may move rapidly near such features because it is directed along them. Jackson (1979) examined fox rabies

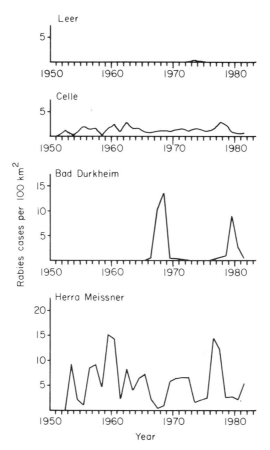

Fig. 8. Three of the patterns of rabies incidence noted by Jackson (1982) among counties in West Germany.

incidence data in France from 20 × 20 km quadrats, which were each allocated to given land classes. She found that a high incidence of rabies classes was associated with only some land classes. Ross (1981) produced quarterly contours, which delineated the progress of the epizootic across France. Superimposing the trajectory of the accumulated progression of contours on a geological map indicated a striking coincidence between the path of the epizootic and limestone bedrock. A plausible conclusion is that the bedrock underlies a habitat supporting a high density fox population with a high contact rate. In a second analysis, Ross examined the temporal pattern of fox rabies incidence in grid cells (20 × 20 km) categorised by the same indicator species analysis (ISA) procedure used by both Jackson and Ball. She found more than one distinct pattern. In mixed habitats, the epizootic was sudden and devastating, a dramatic peak in cases being swiftly followed by rapid decline to a low level. In more uniform habitats, the wave was less clearly defined, more protracted and, in some cases, slower to escalate. Mixed habitats are generally associated with numerous foxes. Jackson (1982) also noted different patterns of rabies incidence among counties in West Germany (although neighbouring counties often approximated the same pattern). Over the years that they were infected, the mean annual incidence of rabies in foxes for all counties was 1.8 cases per 100 km^2, with the maximum for any one county of 9.8 cases per 100 km^2. In general, high incidence counties were in the uplands of central and southern Germany, whereas low incidence was typical of lowlands to the north and west. Three of the patterns that Jackson described are shown in Fig. 8. The differences between the patterns are similar to differences generated in a computer model of rabies by alteration of the contact rate among foxes (cf. Bacon and Macdonald, 1980, and this volume).

Although this "habitat–fox–rabies" approach still holds promise, it is constrained by the facts that (1) habitat types do not invariably indicate prey availability, (2) patterns of mortality are not directly considered (although they can vary with habitat type, e.g., Gessler and Spittler, 1982), (3) on a wide scale the reliability of the case incidence data, even as an index, varies, and (4) suitable habitat may be occupied by a competitor (e.g. Voigt and Earle, 1983). It is important to recognise, however, that large areas are not homogeneous either from the viewpoint of fox ecology or rabies epizootiology.

VI. Discussion

Many of the broad features of rabies outbreaks can be explained in terms of fox behaviour, as can some of the differences between outbreaks in different areas. However, it is all too tempting to conjure up an average fox which rears two cubs before contracting rabies, infecting a couple of neighbours and dying. Such foxes can participate obligingly in mathematical models, which can generate patterns rather like those produced by the rabies virus. Probably the basic similarity between many real rabies outbreaks and model rabies outbreaks is indeed due to fundamental facts of fox life that drive them both. However, models are only helpful in so far as they tell us something that we did not already know. For instance, it is unknown why previous waves of rabies disappeared in Europe or in the boreal forests of northern Ontario. Indeed, although dog rabies was not uncommon in nineteenth century England, the disease appears not to have infected wildlife. Today, it is puzzling that bats in North America are involved in rabies (Fischman and Young, 1976), but those in Europe seldom are, and why should Uruguay be free of rabies while neighbouring countries are heavily infected. Similarly, why should Raccoon rabies be a feature of only parts of eastern United States and not be as widespread as is the Raccoon? Why are there areas with rabies commonly in skunks but rarely in foxes and vice versa? Perhaps some of the answers to these particular questions lie in the disease being more complicated than often assumed, perhaps being composed of regionally distinct strains of virus (*vide* the use of monoclonal antibodies, Wiktor *et al.*, 1980). Other answers may lie in vector behaviour. Why, for example, are city dwelling foxes more common in England than elsewhere (Harris, 1980; Macdonald and Newdick, 1982). Certainly the feature of foxes most likely to complicate the efforts of modellers is variation in their behaviour between populations.

In practice, models have emphasised the great sensitivity of rabies epizootiology to contact rate (Bacon and Macdonald, 1980; Anderson *et al.*, 1981; Macdonald and Bacon, 1982; see also this volume). Admittedly this finding leads biologists to glum reflection upon failed attempts to measure this variable, but it also holds future challenge. The details of vector social behaviour hold the key to understanding the disease and its management.

Acknowledgements

We are grateful to A. J. Crowley for helping to collate case incidence records and to Drs. M. Artois, H. Hofer, G. Kerby and M. Newdick for helpful suggestions on an earlier draft. The Rabies Research Unit staff at the Ontario Ministry of Natural Resources provided much assistance throughout the studies in Ontario, as did R. Tinline of Queen's University. The support of the Rabies Advisory Committee is gratefully acknowledged.

References

Ables, E. D. (1965). An exceptional fox movement. *J. Mammal.* **46**, 102.

Acha, P. N. (1966). Rabies in the Americas. *In* "Proceedings of the National Rabies Symposium," pp. 140–143. National Center for Disease Control, Atlanta, Georgia.

Acha, P. N. (1982). A review of rabies prevention and control in the Americas 1970–1980. C.N.E.R.–W.H.O. Science Meeting on Animal Rabies. Malzeville, France.

Adamovich, U. L. (1978). Landscape-ecological prerequisites for the existence of natural foci of rabies infection. *Zool. Zh.* **57**(2), 260–271.

Allen, D. L., and Shapton, W. W. (1942). An ecological study of winter dens, with special references to the eastern skunk. *Ecology* **23**, 59–68.

Andersen, P. (1981). Movements, activity patterns, and denning habits of the Striped Skunk in the mixed-grass prairie. M.Sc. Thesis, University of Calgary, Calgary.

Anderson, R. M., Jackson, H. C., May, R. M., and Smith, A. D. M. (1981). Population dynamics of fox rabies in Europe. *Nature (London)* **289**, 765–771.

Andral, L. (1982). *Rabies Bull. Eur.* **4**, 5.

Andral, L., Artois, M., Aubert, M. F. A., and Blancou, J. (1982). Radio-pistage de renards enrages. *Comp. Immunol. Microbiol. Infect. Dis.* **5**, 285–291.

Artois, M. (1976). Prophylaxie écologique de la rage vulpine. Thèse med-vet., Poulouse, France.

Artois, M., and Aubert, F. A. (1982). Structure des populations (age et sex) de renards en zones indemnes ou atteintes de rage. *Comp. Immunol. Microbiol. Infect. Dis.* **5**, 237–245.

Artois, M., Aubert, M. F. A., and Gerard, Y. (1982). Reproduction du renard roux (*Vulpes vulpes*) en France. Rythme saisonnier et fecondite des femelles. *Acta Oecol.* **3**, 205–216.

Bacon, P. J. (1981). The consequences of unreported fox rabies. *J. Environ. Manage.* **13**, 195–200.

Bacon, P. J., and Macdonald, D. W. (1980). To control rabies: Vaccinate foxes. *New Sci.* **87**, 640–645.

Baer, G. (1975). Bovine paralytic rabies in the vampire bat. *In* "The Natural History of Rabies" (G. M. Baer, ed.), Vol. 2, pp. 261–266. Academic Press, New York.

Bailey, N. T. J. (1975). "The Mathematical theory of infectious diseases," 2nd ed. Griffin, London.

Ball, F. (1981). Rabies spread and habitats in France. *In* "Habitat Classification, Fox Populations and Rabies Spread" (P. J. Bacon and D. W. Macdonald, eds.), Merlewood Res. and Dev. Pap. No. 81, pp. 24–25. Institute of Terrestrial Ecology, U.K.

Ballantyne, E. E., and O'Donoghue, S. G. (1954). Rabies control in Alberta. *J. Am. Vet. Med. Assoc.* **125**, 316–326.

Barnard, B. J. H. (1979). The role played by wildlife in the epizootiology of rabies in South Africa and South West Africa. *Onderstepoort J. Vet. Res.* **46**, 155–163.

Beran, G. W., Nocate, A. P., Elvina, O., Gregorio, S. B., Moreno, R. R., Nakas, J. C., Burchett, G. A., Lanizares, H. L., and Macasaet, F. F. (1972). Epidemiological and control studies on rabies in the Philippines. *Southeast Asian J. Trop. Med. Public Health* **3**, 433–445.

Bjorge, R. R., Gunson, J. R., and Samuel, W. M. (1981). Population dynamics of Striped Skunks in central Alberta. *Can. Field Nat.* **95**, 149–155.

Blancou, J., Aubert, M. F. A., Andral, L., and Artois, M. (1979). Rage expérimental du renard roux (*Vulpes vulpes*). *Rev. Med. Vet. (Toulouse)* **130**, 1001–1015.

Bogel, N., and Moegle, H. (1980). Characteristics of the spread of a wildlife rabies epidemic in Europe. *In* "The Red Fox, Behaviour and Ecology" (E. Zimen, ed.), pp. 251–258. Junk Publ., The Hague.

Bogel, K., Arata, A., Moegle, H., and Knorpp, F. (1974). Recovery of a reduced fox population under rabies control. *Zentralbl. Veterinaermed., Reihe B* **21**, 401–412.

Bogel, K., Moegle, H., Knorpp, F., Arata, A., Dietz, N., and Diethelm, P. (1976). Characteristics of the spread of a wildlife rabies epidemic in Europe. *Bull. W. H. O.* **54**, 433–447.

Braunschweig, A. (1980). Ein Modell fur die Fuchspopulationsdynamik in der Bundersrepublik Deutschland. *In* "The Red Fox, Behaviour and Ecology" (E. Zimen, ed.), pp. 97–106. Junk Publ., The Hague.

Carey, A. B. (1982). The ecology of red foxes, gray foxes, and rabies in the eastern United States. *Wildl. Soc. Bull.* **10**, 18–26.

Carey, A. B., and McClean, R. G. (1978). Rabies antibody prevalence and virus tissue tropism in wild carnivores in Virginia. *J. Wildl. Dis.* **14**, 487–491.

Carey, A. B., Giles, R. H., and McLean, R. G. (1978). The landscape epidemiology of rabies in Virginia. *Am. J. Trop. Med. Hyg.* **27**, 573–580.

Constantine, D. G. (1971). Bat rabies: Current knowledge and future research. *In* "Rabies" (Y. Nagano and F. M. Davenport, eds.), pp. 253–262. University Park Press, Baltimore, Maryland.

Cumming, D. H. M. (1982). A case history of the spread of rabies in an African country. *S. Afr. J. Sci.* **78**, 443–447.

David, J. M., Andral, L., and Artois, M. (1982). Computer simulation model of the epi-enzootic disease of vulpine rabies. *Ecol. Modell.* **15**, 107–125.

Englund, J. (1970). Some aspects of reproduction and mortality rates in Swedish foxes (*Vulpes vulpes*), 1961–63 and 1966–69. *Viltrevy* **8**, 1–82.

Englund, J. (1980). Yearly variations of recovery and dispersal rates of fox cubs tagged in Swedish coniferous forests. *In* "The Red Fox, Behaviour and Ecology" (E. Zimen, ed.), pp. 195–207. Junk Publ., The Hague.

Everard, C. O. R., Baer, G. M., and James, A. C. (1974). Epidemiology of mongoose rabies in Grenada. *J. Wildl. Dis.* **10,** 190–196.

Everard, C. O. R., Race, N. W., Price, J. L., and Baer, G. M. (1976). Recent epizootiological findings in wildlife rabies in Grenada. *Proc. Symp. Adv. Rabies Res., 1976,* p. 8.

Everard, C. O. R., James, A. C., and da Breo, S. (1979). Ten years of rabies surveillance in Grenada, 1968–1977. *Bull. Pan. Am. Health Organ.* **13,** 342–353.

Fairley, J. S. (1969). Survival of fox (*Vulpes vulpes*) cubs in Northern Ireland. *J. Zool.* **159,** 532–534.

Fischman, H. R., and Young, G. S. (1976). An association between the occurrence of fox rabies and the presence of caves. *Am. J. Epidemiol.* **104,** 593–601.

George, J. P., George, J., Blancou, J., and Aubert, M. F. A. (1980). Description clinique de la rage du renard: Etude Expérimentale. *Rev. Med. Vet. (Toulouse)* **131,** 153–160.

Gessler, M., and Spittler, H. (1982). Relations entre population de renards et limitatiin de la propogation de la rage en Rhenanie—Westphalie. *Comp. Immunol. Microbiol. Infect. Dis.* **5,** 293–302.

Gomez Orosco, A. (1981). Canine and bovine rabies in Colombia. *In* "Habitat Classification, Fox Populations and Rabies Spread" (P. J. Bacon and D. W. Macdonald, eds.), Merlewood Res. Dev. Pap. No. 81, pp. 47–55. Institute of Terrestrial Ecology, U.K.

Gunson, J. R., Dorward, W. J., and Schowalter, D. B. (1978). An evaluation of rabies control in skunks in Alberta. *Can. Vet. J.* **19,** 214–220.

Harris, S. (1979). Age-related fertility and productivity in red foxes, *Vulpes vulpes,* in suburban London. *J. Zool.* **187,** 195–199.

Harris, S. (1980). Home ranges and patterns of distribution of foxes (*Vulpes vulpes*) in an urban area, as revealed by radio tracking. *In* "A Handbook on Biotelemetry and Radiotracking" (C. J. Amlaner and D. W. Macdonald, eds.), pp. 685–690. Pergamon, Oxford.

Hassel, R. H. (1982). Incidence of rabies in kudu in South West Africa/Namibia. *S. Afr. J. Sci.* **78,** 418–421.

Houseknecht, C. R. (1969). Denning habits of the Striped Skunk and the exposure potential for disease. *Bull. Wildl. Dis. Assoc.,* No. 5, pp. 302–306.

Houseknecht, C. R., and Huempfner, R. A. (1970). A red fox–striped skunk encounter. *Am. Midl. Nat.* **83,** 304–306.

Jackson, H. C. (1979). A contribution to the study of fox rabies in relation to habitat in Europe. M.Sc. Thesis, Imperial College, University of London.

Jackson, H. C. (1982). Rabies in the Federal Republic of Germany. *Comp. Immunol. Microbiol. Infect. Dis.* **5,** 309–313.

Jensen, B. (1968). Preliminary results from the marking of foxes (*Vulpes vulpes* L.) in Denmark. *Dan. Rev. Game Biol.* **5,** 3–8.

Jensen, B. (1973). Movements of the red fox in Denmark investigated by marking and recovery. *Dan. Rev. Game Biol.* **8,** 1–20.

Johnson, H. N. (1959). The role of the spotted skunk in rabies. *In* "Proceedings of the 63rd Annual Meeting of the U.S. Livestock Sanitary Association," pp. 267–274. Minneapolis, Minnesota.

Johnston, D. H., and Beauregard, M. (1969). Rabies epidemiology in Ontario. *Bull. Wildl. Dis. Assoc.* **5,** 357–370.

Kruuk, H. (1976). Functional aspects of social hunting in carnivores. *In* "Function and Evolution in Behaviour" (G. Baerends, C. Beer, and A. Manning, eds.), pp. 119–141. Oxford Univ. Press, London and New York.

Lindstrom, E. (1982). Population ecology of the red fox (*Vulpes vulpes* L.) in relation to food supply. Ph.D. Thesis, Stockholm.

Lloyd, H. G. (1975). The red fox in Britain. *In* "The Wild Canids" (M. W. Fox, ed.), pp. 207–215. Van Nostrand-Reinhold, Princeton, New Jersey.

Lloyd, H. G. (1980). "The Red Fox." Batsford Press, London.

Lloyd, H. G., Jensen, B., van Haaften, J. L., Niewold, F. J., Wandeler, A., Bogel, K., and Arata, A. A. (1976). Annual turnover of fox populations in Europe. *Zentralbl. Veterinaermed., Reihe B* **23**, 580–589.

Lodmell, D. L. (1983). Genetic control of resistance to street rabies virus in mice. *J. Exp. Med.* **157**, 451–460.

McClean, R. G. (1975). Raccoon rabies. *In* "The Natural History of Rabies" (G. M. Baer, ed.), Vol. 2, pp. 53–76. Academic Press, New York.

Macdonald, D. W. (1979). Helpers in fox society. *Nature (London)* **282**, 69–71.

Macdonald, D. W. (1980a). Social factors affecting reproduction amongst red foxes (Vulpes vulpes L., 1758). *In* "The Red Fox, Behaviour and Ecology" (E. Zimen, ed.), pp. 123–175. Junk Publ., The Hague.

Macdonald, D. W. (1980b). "Rabies and Wildlife, A Biologist's Perspective." Oxford Univ. Press, London and New York.

Macdonald, D. W. (1981). Resource dispersion and the social organisation of the red fox (*Vulpes vulpes*). *In* "Worldwide Furbearer Conference Proceedings" (J. Chapman and D. Pursely, eds.), pp. 918–949. R. H. Donnelly & Sons, Falls Church, Virginia.

Macdonald, D. W. (1983). The ecology of carnivore and social behaviour. *Nature (London)* **301**, 379–384.

Macdonald, D. W., and Bacon, P. J. (1982). Fox society, contact rates, and rabies epizootiology. *J. Comp. Immunol. Microbiol. Infect. Dis.* **5**, 247–256.

Macdonald, D. W., and Newdick, M. T. (1982). The distribution and ecology of foxes, *Vulpes vulpes* (L) in urban areas. *In* "Urban Ecology" (R. Bornkamm, J. A. Lee, and M. R. Seeward, eds.), pp. 123–135. Blackwell, Oxford.

Macdonald, D. W., Ball, F., and Hough, N. G. (1980). The evaluation of home range size and configuration using radio tracking data. *In* "A Handbook on Biotelemetry and Radio Tracking" (C. J. Amlaner and D. W. Macdonald, eds.), pp. 405–424. Pergamon, Oxford.

Macdonald, D. W., Bunce, R. G. H., and Bacon, P. J. (1981). Fox populations, habitat characterisation, and rabies control. *J. Biogeogr.* **8**, 145–151.

May, R. M. (1983). Parasitic infections as regulators of animal populations. *Am. Sci.* **71**, 36–45.

Meredith, C. D. (1982). Wildlife rabies: Past and present in South Africa. *S. Afr. J. Sci.* **78**, 411–415.

Muller, J. (1971). The effect of fox reduction on the occurrence of rabies. Observations from two outbreaks of rabies in Denmark. *Bull. Off. Int. Epizoot.* **75**, 763–776.

Newdick, M. T. (1983). Behavioural ecology of urban foxes in Oxford. Ph. D. Thesis, University of Oxford.

Parker, R. L. (1961). Rabies in skunks in the North-central states. *In* "Proceedings of the 65th Annual Meeting of the U.S. Livestock Sanitary Association," pp. 273–280. Minneapolis, Minnesota.

Parker, R. L. (1975). Rabies in skunks. In "The Natural History of Rabies" (G. M. Baer, ed.), Vol. 2, pp. 41–51. Academic Press, New York.

Parker, R. L., and Wilsnack, R. E. (1966). Pathogenisis of skunk rabies virus: Quantitation in skunks and foxes. *Am. J. Vet. Res.* **27**, 33–38.

Ramsden, R. O., and Johnston, D. H. (1975). Studies of the oral infectivety of rabies virus in Carnivora. *J. Wildl. Dis.* **11**, 318–324.

Rosatte, R. C. (1984). Seasonal occurrence and habital preference of rabid skunks in southern Alberta. *Can. Vet. J.* **25**, 142–144.

Ross, J. (1981). Rabies spread and land classes in France. *In* "Habitat Classification, Fox Populations and Rabies Spread" (P. J. Bacon and D. W. Macdonald, eds.), Merlewood Res. Dev. Pap. No. 81, pp. 26–30 and supplement.

Sargeant, A. B. (1972). Red fox spatial characteristics in relation to waterfowl predation. *J. Wildl. Manage.* **36,** 225–236.

Sargeant, A. B., Greenwood, R. J., Piehl, J. L., and Bicknell, W. B. (1982). Recurrence, mortality and dispersal of prairie striped skunks, *Mephitis mephitis,* and implications to rabies epizootiology. *Can. Field Nat.* **96,** 312–316.

Schowalter, D. B. (1980). Characteristics of bat rabies in Alberta. *Can. J. Comp. Med.* **44,** 70–76.

Schowalter, D. B., and Gunson, J. R. (1982). Parameters of population and seasonal activity of Striped Skunks, *Mephitis mephitis* in Alberta and Saskatchewan. *Can. Field Nat.* **96,** 409–420.

Sikes, R. W. (1962). Pathogenesis of rabies in wildlife. Comparative effects of varying doses of rabies virus inoculated into foxes and skunks. *Am. J. Vet. Res.* **23,** 1041–1047.

Steck, F. (1982). Rabies in wildlife. *Symp. Zool. Soc. London* **50,** 57–75.

Steck, F., Wandeler, A., Bicksel, P., Capt, S., Hafliger, U., and Schneider, L. (1982). Oral immunization of foxes aginst rabies: Laboratory and field studies. *Comp. Immunol. Microbiol. Infect. Dis.* **5,** 165–171.

Steel, J. H. (1975). History of rabies. *In* ''The Natural History of Rabies'' (G. M. Baer, ed.), Vol. 1, pp. 1–29. Academic Press, New York.

Storm, G. L. (1972). Daytime retreats and movements of skunks in farmlands in Illinois. *J. Wildl. Manage.* **36,** 31–45.

Storm, G. L., and Verts, B. J. (1966). Movements of a Striped Skunk infected with rabies. *J. Mammal.* **47**(4), 705–708.

Storm, G. L., Andrews, R. D., Phillips, R. L., Bishop, R. A., Sineff, D. B., and Tester, J. R. (1976). Morphology, reproduction, dispersal and mortality of mid-western fox populations. *Wildl. Monogr.* **49,** 1–82.

Tabel, H., Corner, A. H., Webster, W. A., and Casey, C. A. (1974). History and epizootiology of rabies in Canada. *Can. Vet. J.* **15,** 271–281.

Tinline, R. R., and Pond, B. A. (1976). Rabies incidence in Ontario: A Grey County example. *''Queen's'' Geogr.* **3**(2), 1–18.

Tinline, R. R., Voigt, D. R., and Broekhoven, L. H. (1982). Evaluating tactics for the control of wildlife rabies in Ontario. *Int. Symp. Vet. Epidemiol. and Economics, 3rd, 1982,* 581–589.

Toma, B., and Andral, L. (1977). Epidemiology of fox rabies. *Adv. Virus Res.* **21,** 1–36.

Verts, B. J. (1967). ''The Biology of the Striped Skunk.'' Univ. of Illinois Press, Urbana.

Verts, B. J., and Storm, G. L. (1966). A local study of prevalence of rabies among foxes and striped skunks. *J. Wildl. Manage.* **30**(2), 419–421.

Voigt, D. R., and Earle, B. D. (1983). Avoidance of coyotes by red fox families. *J. Wildl. Manage.* **47,** 852–857.

Voigt, D. R., and Macdonald, D. W. (1985). Variation in the spatial and social behaviour of the red fox, *Vulpes vulpes. Acta Zool. Fenn.* **171,** 261–265.

Voigt, D. R., and Tinline, R. R. (1982). Fox rabies and trapping: A study of disease and fur harvest interaction. *In* ''43rd Midwest Wildlife Conference, Furbearer Symposium'' (G. C. Sanderson, ed.), pp. 139–156. Witchita, Kansas.

von Schantz, T. (1981). Female cooperation, male competition and dispersal in the red fox, *Vulpes vulpes. Oikos* **37,** 63–68.

Wachendorfer, G. (1977). The problem of rabies in the European region. Paper to 2nd European Conference on Surveillance and Control of Rabies, Frankfurt, November.

Wandeler, A. I. (1980a). Epidemiology of fox rabies. *In* ''The Red Fox, Behaviour and Ecology'' (E. Zimen, ed.), pp. 237–250. Junk Publ.. The Hague.

Wandeler, A. I. (1980b). Hunting indicators of fox numbers. *In* ''Habitat Classification, Fox Populations and Rabies Spread'' (P. J. Bacon and D. W. Macdonald, eds.), Merlewood Res. Dev. Pap. No. 81, pp. 38–39. Institute of Terrestrial Ecology, U. K.

Wandeler, A. I., Wachendorfer, G., Forster, U., Krekel, H., Schale, W., Muller, J., and Steck, F. (1974). Rabies in wild carnivores in Central Europe. III. Ecology and biology of the fox in relation to control operations. *Zentralbl. Veterinaermed., Reihe B* **21,** 765–773.

Webster, W. A., Casey, G. A., Tabel, A., and Corner, A. H. (1974). Skunk rabies in Ontario. *Can Vet. J.* **15,** 163–167.

Westergaard, J. M. (1982). Measures applied in Denmark to control the rabies epizootic in 1977–1980. *Comp. Immunol. Microbiol. Infect. Dis.* **5,** 383–387.

Wiktor, T. J., Flamand, A., and Koprowski, H. (1980). Use of monoclonal antibodies in diagnosis of rabies virus infection and differentiation of rabies and rabies-related viruses. *J. Virol. Methods* **1,** 33–46.

Yurkovsky, A. M. (1962). Hydrophobia following the bite of apparently healthy dogs. *J. Hyg., Epidemiol., Microbiol., Immunol.* **6,** 73–78.

Zumpt, I. F. (1976). The yellow mongoose (Cynictis penicillata) as a latent focus of rabies in South Africa. *J. S. Afr. Vet. Assoc.,* **47,** 211–213.

A Systems Analysis of Wildlife Rabies Epizootics

5

P. J. Bacon

Institute of Terrestrial Ecology,
Merlewood Research Station,
Grange-over-Sands, Cumbria, England

I. Introduction

The phrase systems analysis is in vogue at present, and it means many things to many people, generally conjuring up vague pictures of complex mathematical analyses. In the context of this chapter, I simply use it to imply "a systematic approach to investigating complex situations and 'solving' complex problems". The essence of the approach is to begin by clearly defining the topic to be considered and by obtaining a broad overview of the problem before commencing any detailed work. This approach may be contrasted with more subjective stances, which might decree that the problem lay predominantly in a particular scientific discipline and so should be carried out under the aegis of a specialist from that field. For example, the initial models of classical epidemiology assume that the population size, N, is constant, whereas, in practice, there is considerable dynamic interaction between the numbers of hosts and the disease 'level' for many diseases (e.g. Anderson and May, 1979). The results of the dynamic interaction can take many forms, but, with a disease of high lethality, such as rabies in European foxes, will be very likely to cause a drastic decrease in the population size of foxes in the short term. It is easy to think of other examples where the traditional approach of any one discipline might predispose a researcher to adopt an approach simply because it is familiar and convenient, and hence he will implicitly make a number of assumptions about the new situation without assessing them rigorously. Another reason for beginning a study by consulting with a body of specialists from different fields is to try and ensure the use of consistent terminology and definitions. In the present context, a simple example would be the phrase 'reproductive rate of a disease' from epidemiological literature. To a mathematician or physicist, the word rate implies 'some quantity per unit time', but, to an epidemiologist, the 'reproductive rate of a disease, r,' is a dimensionless ratio representing 'the (average) number of secondary infections resulting per any single initial infection'. Clearly, such differences in terminology, and more subtle differences in precise meaning and definitions of how particular parameters are defined for measuring, could cause serious problems of communication and understanding. There are indeed a number of computer-aided techniques designed by psychologists to help unravel the basic structure of concepts from the differing words and jargon that may be used to describe them. (Interactive elicitation of personal models, Shaw, 1980).

The purpose of this chapter is not to provide an exhaustive list of all the potential pitfalls to producing mathematical models of rabies epizootics, but rather, by indicating several major snags, and some of lesser importance, to encourage the reader to assess critically the content of the following chapters. Further, it should not be thought that the succeeding chapters are entirely free from conceptual errors or oversimplifications. Indeed, they were chosen to represent a broad spectrum of approaches and complexity; all have their different strengths and weaknesses. We would do well to remember when considering these, and other, models that a modeller may strive to incorporate into his representation of the real world differing degrees of three fundamental aspects: *generality, realism* and *precision*. The meanings of these words are such that a high degree of any two automatically excludes the possibility of a high degree of the third. In assessing any model, one should not use a yardstick of 'degree of perfection relative to the real world' but rather, having discerned its purpose and decided whether that purpose is worthwhile, judge the model on whether its assumptions and structure allow it to fulfil adequately the purpose for which it was designed. A predictive model may be highly accurate, but based on a mathematical formulation whose coefficients and parameters are quite uninterpretable in relation to the causal processes. Such obscurity would not matter if the model aimed only to predict; however, if on the basis of that prediction we may wish to modify the system to produce a more desirable outcome, such as fewer rabid foxes in 10 years' time, we must be careful. Our predictive model has been parameterised in one situation, with which we are about to interfere; it may be that our interference with the system will alter its internal interactions (which are glossed over by the predictive model) and appreciably alter the natural system in a way that the predictive model can not capture. It would, for example, be possible to perform a Fourier analysis of fox population density and rabid fox density with time and to use this analysis to predict fox densities at some future time: it would clearly be rather pointless to use this formula to predict how fox numbers and rabid fox numbers would behave after a cull (killing $P\%$ of all foxes), as the effects of a real cull could produce interactions outside the descriptive scope of the Fourier model (Fig. 1). In order to have any faith in a model of a situation that is to be perturbed (by human management of any other unusual factor) outside the conditions under which the model has formerly operated, we must have great confidence that our model *realistically* mimics the underlying processes of cause and effect. Experience has shown that failure to do this in environmental management can lead to grossly serious errors. Regrettably, accounting for causes and effects is difficult and, at best, very tenuous if the cause–effect relationships must be extrapolated, rather than interpolated, from one set of known conditions to a set outside previous experience (Holling, 1978).

II. What Are We Dealing With?

As we have seen from the previous chapters, rabies is a disease that effects many species in many different ways. How can we begin to simplify this com-

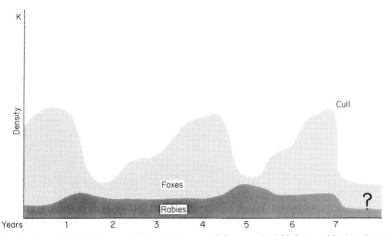

Fig. 1. Hypothetical diagram of the incidences of foxes and rabid foxes with time in years. Although the regular cycles could be *described* by a method such as Fourier analysis, such a description could not predict the outcomes of novel events, such as control by culling.

plex situation? A useful general structure is to simplify it in terms of fundamental *entities, attributes, processes* and *relationships*. Some of these significant to rabies are shown in Fig. 2.

An *entity* is basically a classificatory term, a name for a class of real objects that exist. Examples from everyday life might be ships, aeroplanes, cars, houses or hotels. In biology, species provide useful distinctions for entities (e.g. cats, dogs, foxes, rabies viruses). It is important to realise the distinction between an entity class, e.g. humans, and occurrences of particular examples of that class, e.g. John Smith, Mary Evans. Specific examples of entities will share a number of common features, some of which will be unvarying, such as sex, number of chromosomes, date of birth, while others will vary during the life of a particular individual, such as age, location in space, weight. Some of these features, or *attributes*, of particular examples of entities, or individuals, are of importance to

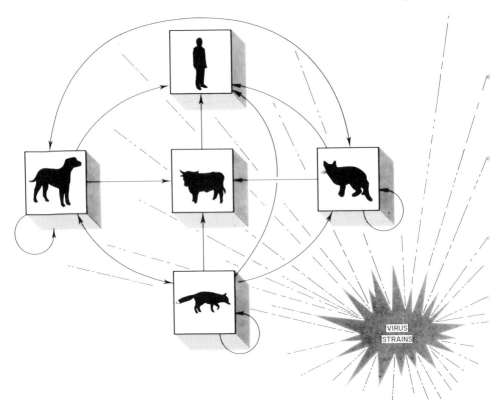

Fig. 2. Some entities and processes important in rabies epizootics. Host species represent one entity type, which are infected by rabies virus strains, a second entity type, by both intra- and inter-specific infection processes, indicated by the arrows.

our study of epidemiological processes and some are not. The fact that dogs, cats and foxes walk on four legs and have tails, whereas humans walk on two legs and are tail-less is irrelevant to us, whereas the fact that the European Red Fox rarely acquires immunity to rabies while the Vampire Bat, the Mongooses and the Grey Fox may often become immune is clearly important. We can perhaps envisage making a list of the attributes likely to be important in relation to rabies epidemiology and then considering whether we need to include them in our model for reasonable accuracy. For which species do we need to know the age distribution of a population in order to model the population's dynamics? Which species always live in monogamous pairs? Which species always live in small or large packs? Do some species sometimes live in pairs and sometimes in groups? Will these different life styles affect the epidemiology? In short, the more attributes we decide are important in determining what happens, the more complex our resulting model will be.

Processes represent changes in the system. Individuals become older with time; movement and dispersal redistribute individuals in space; births increase population size; deaths decrease population size. What factors determine the rates at which these processes take place, or the probability that a particular event will or will not occur? Age is clearly uniquely dependent upon time, while birth and death rates will depend on population density. Infection and acquisition of immunity (see Fig. 3) are clearly important processes in general epidemidogy, although, as we shall see later, we can make considerable progress in understanding the dynamics of natural wildlife rabies in European foxes by ignoring immunity, as it is acquired so rarely.

Relationships indicate especial associations between entities. One fox may be a parent of several others, a sister of two others and the mate of yet another; we would expect these relationships [*parent, sister* (or *sibling*) and *mate*] to imply different types of interactive behaviour if such individuals meet. Similarly, the relationship '*lives in*', referring to a home range or den site implies differing chances that particular foxes will meet depending upon whether they are members of a set, or group, who live in the same den or home range. Further, in spatial terms, the chances of two foxes meeting will depend on whether one is a *neighbour* of another, while any homeless *itinerant* fox will have much higher than normal chances of meeting many widely spaced foxes in a given time interval.

Such formal definitions may at first seem pedantic, but they can serve a useful function by clarifying our thoughts about complex interrelations. Assessing our concepts and ideas in relation to such a framework can help us distinguish between causes and effects, give guidance about what information is necessary, how it relates to the processes and what measurable attributes should be taken to elucidate the system's behaviour.

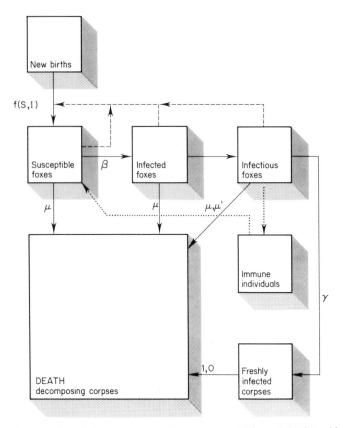

Fig. 3. The interactions between fox population processes (births and deaths) with disease infection processes. The continuous arrows represent the disease processes and indicate the paths individuals could follow around the epidemiological entity classes. Stippled arrows represent rare processes for fox rabies in Europe, which are here considered unimportant. The broken arrows represent feedback effects, such as fox density on fox birth rate.

Consider the diagramatic model of Fig. 2, which shows species interactions that comprise the chains of infection that are rabies epizootics. There are two main entity types: virus parasite and host species.

Within the entity *virus*, there are a number of different strains that have differing pathogenicities to different host species. However, our ability to identify these different strains was, until recently, very limited, and although we know different strains exist, we still know rather little about how they vary with respect of important properties such as infectivities and lethalities to different hosts. Serial passage of a strain of virus through one host species can alter the properties and the pathogenicity of the strain: the course of infection in a skunk bitten by a skunk is likely to be different from that in a skunk bitten by a fox, but we do not really know how different it will be.

Turning our attention to the entity *hosts,* the diagram is much more complex and reflects the more advanced state of our knowledge and ability to identify species of mammals as opposed to strains of virus. It is relatively simple to ascertain the species of a mammal corpse that has been diagnosed to have rabies, and even its sex and approximate age. (We might note in passing, however, that such data are rarely actually recorded, perhaps because the microbiologist technicians making the diagnoses do not have the relevant experience, do not know how important such information is, or more likely, do not have the time. Whatever the reason, lack of such data seriously militates against our chances of contrasting different models of rabies epizootics). The species figured in the diagram are by no means exhaustive, merely a selection of the more important ones. However, a number of interesting things are apparent. The arrows going to and from the entity boxes for the species represent the processes 'infection by' and 'infects'. It can be seen that some species such as humans, cattle and 'deer' become infected, but do not (at least only very rarely) pass the infection on: such 'dead end' species only become infected as a result of cross-infections from other species. Other species, such as fox, dog and Racoon Dog are not only infected by other species and frequently themselves infect other species but also maintain chains of infection among members of their own species (indicated by the closed-loop arrows in Fig. 2). It is interesting that social carnivores form a high proportion of species that appear to suffer rabies epizootics primarily because of intra-specific infections.

It is easy to think of attributes about individual foxes, dogs and cats that contain useful information about likelihood of rabies spread to, or by, the individual (age, sex, social status, home-range, local population density, etc.). Regrettably, it is very difficult to record a lot of these for a wild population. Conversely, it is extremely difficult to think of measurable attributes of rabies virus that could be recorded directly. Different strains can now be identified (Schneider, 1982), but their differing properties in different hosts remain largely unknown. Except in a living host or recent corpse, the virus is largely inviable (except in dark damp places, such as bat caves, for short periods); the measured concentration of virus in an animal may not be related closely to the chances that infection *has been* or *might be* passed on. In these circumstances, while the entity *virus* sub-divided into occurrences of different virus strains logically exists, it may often in practice be impossible to define it in terms other than 'an occurrence of host species S infected with an unknown strain V of rabies virus'. If we admit this limitation and recognise that, in the wild, we will not know from which species a particular rabid animal was initially infected, we must recognise that there are some aspects of wildlife rabies epizootics, which we can never hope to model. For example: in circumstances where infections between several species are common, and virus strains from one species produce different effects in others; in the spread of a primary epizootic, if the initial strain is modified by selection (as happened to myxomatosis virus in Australian rabbits, where continued exposure produced both higher resistance in the rabbits and lower virulence in the virus: see, e.g. Ross, 1982), then secondary outbreaks will not operate with the same parameters as determined the primary wave. The latter example may be pertinent to rabies, as data for primary waves are often more detailed and reliable.

Contrast Fig. 2 with the diagram of Fig. 3 which shows the various courses that infection could take within an individual. By implication Fig. 3 refers to infection processes within a single species, the entity being the *species* and occurrences of the entity individuals of the species (having attributes of age, sex, breeding condition). The epidemiological classes (susceptibles, infecteds, infectious, immune) refer to sub-sets of individuals. Visually, the diagram emphasises the epidemiological classes and the various progressive courses through these classes that an individual might follow between birth (starting class) and death (ending class). We may think of this diagram as indicating details of the types of processes summarised by the arrows of 'infectious processes' shown in Fig. 2, while suggesting that the attributes of individuals, which are nowhere indicated on the diagram, will not have important consequences for the outcome of the overall process. By default, the effects of different virus strains are also assumed to reduce to an 'average' value.

Figure 4 emphasises the details of the infection process between individuals, and the course of the disease within an infected host, indicating the likely environmental factors that will impinge on the rates of these detailed processes or the chances of their happening. The set of factors in the top left of the diagram are environmental parameters and biological concepts, which are known to be important in population dynamics. These will affect movement patterns of normal individuals and hence their chances of meeting other individuals, either normal or rabid, as indicated by the chain of processes at the bottom of the diagram. If virus is transmitted from one individual to another, then a number of factors determine whether an infection will result (i.e. does the virus reach the sanctuary of nerve tissue before it is eliminated by the host's antibody response?). If an infection does result, the infected animal may or may not die before it becomes infectious, and it will demonstrate *dumb* and *furious* rabies in differing degrees if it becomes rabid, which, in turn, affect the chances that the disease will be passed on.

The single box 'control' refers to a variety of measures that humans might impose on the system in attempts to modify the process. Note that the results of control, such as killing foxes, will affect fox population density, which is likely to alter population recruitment rate, breeding and dispersal. Hence, by its very nature, control killing is likely to affect the dynamics of these processes. If such

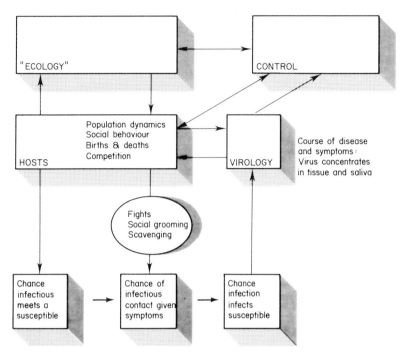

Fig. 4. The interplay between ecological conditions, especially the population ecology of the host species, and the chances that rabid hosts will successfully infect susceptible hosts. Any events that alter these conditions, such as control measures implemented by man but including natural deaths from rabies, will affect the subsequent course of events through feedback effects.

feedback effects are important, as they are likely to be, then models aimed at evaluating control strategies will need to be based on precise and realistic reflections of spatial population processes. These complex feedbacks of 'results of control method' on the 'future behaviour of the system' would not, however, be expected to result from control by oral immunisation of foxes, and so we could place more faith in the predictions of a fairly unrealistic model of fox population dynamics in reflecting the outcome of control by vaccination than in the ability of the same model to reflect the effects of control by killing.

Having considered some of the complexities of wildlife rabies epizootics, let us pause for a moment and consider the complexity of human society in terms of those people who have responsibilities for disease control and the various experts on whom they rely for information and recommendations. The main aspects are illustrated in Fig. 5; they can be seen to reflect five or so different professions or specialities: virology, ecology, pest and disease control, mathematics, politics. The previous section has highlighted some of the complex virological and ecological issues of wildlife rabies and equally tortuous details will plague the topics

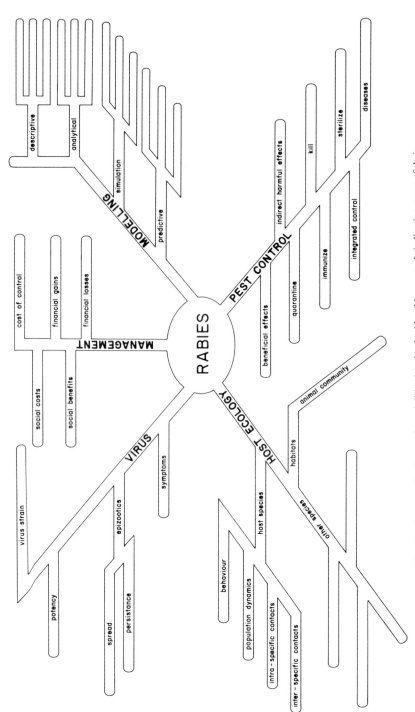

Fig. 5. Some professions and specialities involved with rabies control, indicating some of their main aspects of concern.

of politics, control methods and mathematical modelling. We cannot however expect the managers and politicians to immerse themselves in the complexities of ecology or the solution of partial differential equations, anymore than we could expect, or would wish, a mathematician to make the final decisions on the acceptability and economics of a particular control policy. The aim of systems analysis should be to produce an early dialogue between the different expert groups so that each profession understands the requirements, limitations and findings of the others. For example, the managers must understand broadly the types of questions that scientists can be expected to answer, at what cost, with what certainty and over how long a time scale, while the scientists must take pains to ensure their results are relevant, comprehensive and presented in such fashion that the findings and their likely accuracies are clear to non-experts.

At this stage, we might usefully expend some thought on how the merits of a particular control policy might be evaluated. First, let us make the point that it is impossible to evaluate any control policy in the absence of some model (however crude) of how the system would behave in the absence of control. Plagues and epidemics are, by definition, transitory phenomena, so that the disappearance of a disease coinciding with the use of one new control effort from a successive series of attempts should not necessarily be taken to indicate that the new control caused the decline. Indeed, if the burgermasters of Hamelin were mindful of the way lemmings apparently throw themselves into the sea during lemming 'plagues' and were sceptical of the reasons for the dancing rats, their final offer of 50 guilders to the Pied Piper might be thought generous, rather than niggardly! [though their suspicions would have been disproved by subsequent events (Browning, 1889)]. In similar vein, it is unreasonable for Medical Health officials to expect rigorous scientific proof that proposed new control measures will definitely be better than their current ones unless they already have a rigorous assessment of the efficiency of their present policy. Indeed, when this unreasonable demand was once put to me, the official concerned could not produce any firm evidence that present policy might not even be making matters slightly worse! (I do not imply that the policies were likely to have been impairing the situation, the anecdote is intended only to highlight sloppy thinking).

The assessment of control effectiveness should not only be safeguarded to ensure that the scientific requirements (such as vaccinating 60% of all foxes in a large area within a few weeks) can be met with the money and manpower available to the authorities, but should also consider the thorny problem of the time-scale over which any cost–benefit analysis should be applied. Clearly, it needs to be assessed over a time or geographic scale sufficient to iron out fluctuations caused by the cyclic nature of rabies outbreaks (every 3 to 5 years in the current European epizootic). On the other hand, an extremely expensive control procedure that is predicted to eradicate rabies (with very high confidence) could be made to look financially attractive by accounting its benefits for many decades into the future.

III. Dangers of Assumption

I have emphasised the complexity of biological systems, and fox–rabies interactions in particular, listing a number of important factors that might be expected to affect details, if not fundamental aspects, of the epizootiology. Before I go on to consider other aspects that are often assumed to be constants in models, but that we would expect evolution to alter, I would first sound a note of practical caution.

A. SIMULATION CONSTRAINTS

Let us assume we have decided that a spatial model is required to cope with stochastic variation of fox density in a spatially heterogeneous environment, plus the local movements of rabid foxes (giving rise to local concentrations of infection) and the dispersal of fox cubs. We wish to consider four categories of fox (rabid foxes, normal susceptibles, cubs and itinerant adults), incubation periods among the categories for the non-rabid groups, and carrying capacity. As rabies can have long incubation periods, up to 6 months, we might wish to record up to 6 different incubation periods in each category. We feel a model area based on a 100×100 grid would be adequate to study the spatial processes, while a 10×10 grid would not. If these figures seem reasonable, we should realise that they

TABLE I

Approximate Computer Core Storage Requirements for a Complex Spatial Model of Rabies

Grid size NG[a]	Incubator classes NI[b]	1 sex[c] NG² * (5 + 3 * NI)	2 sexes[d] NG² * (9 + 6 * NI)
10	6	2.3K	10K
30	6	21K	89K
50	6	57K	247K
80	6	147K	633K
100	6	230K	990K

[a] NG: numeric size of grid.

[b] NI: number of incubator classes.

[c] 5: carrying capacity; rabids; susceptible resident adults and juveniles; susceptible dispersers. $3 \times$ NI: incubator categories for the three susceptible classes.

[d] Two sexes for above classes.

imply the model stores between 2000 and 230,000 pieces of information for a uni-sex fox model and between 10,000 and 990,000 pieces of information for a model of sexual foxes! (See Table I.) Simulation packages might well require one word of store per piece of information (i.e. between 2 and 990k of core!); while such storage overheads could be reduced by coding the multiple information into one byte/word, this will either increase running time (already likely to be high) or require machine-code programming. Clearly, the computing overheads for such information-hungry models would be high, and we should realise that the above values would be modest in comparison with a rabies model refined to the level of group interactions within single fox territories. If the latter level of detail seems ridiculously precise, consider the implications of a (hypothetical) animal population in which individuals nearly always go around in pairs (or larger groups) and can, even at low population density, nearly always find a new partner within 1 week or so (see Fig. 6). Such a situation would clearly shatter the assumptions of density dependent contact rates, made by many simple 'mixing' models (for example, see Chapters 6 and 7, this volume) as every individual

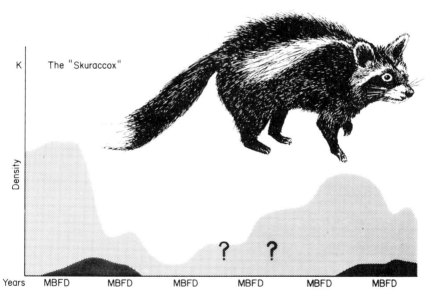

Fig. 6. Rabies incidence against time in a hypothetical host. It is fairly easy to understand the host population crash and its subsequent buildup, but the mechanisms allowing the presistance of rabies during the periods of very low host densities are poorly understood. The unrealistic assumptions of 'random host mixing', used in default of knowledge, can predict persistance in certain conditions, but the chances of disease persistance will be greatly enhanced by social behaviours, such as pairing, mating, births, family groups and cub dispersal. Such behaviours may keep individuals in groups of at least two animals in close contact for much of the year, thereby greatly increasing the chances of disease persistance. M, mating; B, births; F, families; D, cub dispersal.

would be almost continuously in contact with at least one other and the details of contacts would depend on complex social parameters.

B. IDENTICAL ORGANISMS?

It is fairly traditional in simple models of population dynamics to assume that all individuals in the population are identical, except perhaps for age and sex differences, despite the fact that the Darwinian (and neo-Darwinian) theories of evolution are based on individual differences between members of a population: the *implicit* assumption of identical individuals often pervades even sophisticated models of population processes. Population genetics has pointed to the consequences of genetically determined differences for over half a century (see, e.g. Gale, 1980). Some recent papers about population dynamics have returned to the theme of individual differences and demonstrate that the phenomenon of individual variations that affect survival, reproductive and breeding potential could be important mechanisms of populations regulation, even if these factors are not hereditary (Lomnicki, 1978; Bacon, 1982). As the lethality of rabies to foxes is very high, the selective advantages favouring foxes with increased resistance, decreased chances of contracting the disease, etc., would be very great, and we might expect quite rapid changes in the genetics of the fox population, increasing the frequency of these traits, if they were heritable. Such changes in the fox population would lead us to expect counteracting changes to affect the virus, leading to a new co-adaption between host and parasite, as was observed for rabbits and myxomatosis.

In this light, let us consider two aspects of rabies epidemiology, the variation of incubation periods and the 'abnormal' behaviour symptoms caused by the disease.

C. INCUBATION TIMES

The incubation time of rabies is extremely variable, from about 2 weeks to 6 months, with a mode around 3–4 weeks. Consider a virus type with short incubation periods. In a population of foxes where contacts are frequent, this virus type will spread rapidly and start to become commoner than a type with longer incubation periods. However, in a population of foxes where contacts are infrequent at low density, but population size is increasing, it will spread less rapidly, as its persistence will depend on the occurrence of several rare contacts per unit time at low density, whereas the persistence of a strain with longer incubation periods will depend on fewer such contacts. We could consider these interactions as a Game Theory Matrix, as shown in Fig. 7. Note that the mathematics of Game Theory does not permit quantitative solutions for cyclic phe-

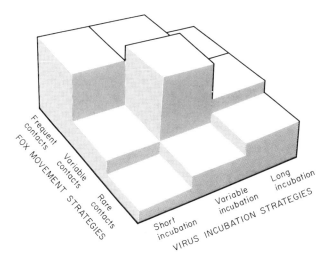

Fig. 7.   The possible interplay between different types of fox behaviour, in terms of movement strategies, and rabies virus properties, in terms of different durations of incubation. The strategies are arranged as a Game Theory matrix, with the heights of each block of the matrix representing likely 'payoffs of the game' to the viruses (i.e. relative numbers of infected hosts) for each combination of strategies and averaged over several cycles of rabies incidence.

nomena, but the qualitative principles are still illuminating. The long-term advantages to the virus are likely to be higher for the 'variable incubation' strategy. The long-term prospects for foxes are likely to be worst with frequent contacts and best with rare contacts between foxes. However, as foxes must meet to breed and defend their territories, the fox population is unlikely to be able to adopt the 'rare contacts' strategy—other constraints will force it to a 'more frequent contacts' style of existence and the actual frequency of contacts is likely to vary with both season of the year and suitability of habitats. As virus strains isolated from different species show different incubation times (when inoculated into a test host), it is likely that incubation times are alterable by natural selection on the virus genome. However, we do not know that short-term variations in virus 'incubation type' frequencies actually occur within the cycle period of natural epidemics; indeed, the observed variations of natural incubation times could be caused by variations in the site of the bite and the dose of virus inoculated by the bite. Models of rabies epidemiology generally assume the probability density function (PDF) of rabies incubation periods to be constant; the models 'select' appropriate periods at random from such a fixed distribution. We should note that the predictions of such models regarding the persistence of rabies at low fox contact frequencies would be biased if the form of the PDF changes during the course of the cycle.

D. FOX SOCIETY AND RABIES SYMPTOMS

The traditional view of rabies spread was that furiously rabid animals roamed
around over considerble distances attacking other animals and thereby spreading
the disease. Rabies has often been used as a classic demonstration of the power
of natural selection, as the symptoms produced promote its spread. These symptoms eventually progress to paralysis, coma and death. The rapid progression of
the disease to the paralytic (dumb) phase, with the aggressive phase sometimes
barely detectable would seem, at first sight, to give poorer prospects for disease
spread. We now know, however, that rabid individuals may become infective
before any symptoms appear, that there may be an initial 'friendly' period,
progressing through a period of wandering, irritable and aggressive behaviour, to
a paralytic phase (in which the animal can still snap and bite) to coma and death.
Many infected animals show all such symptoms, at least briefly, at some stage of
their illness. It seems, therefore, that evolution may have fashioned a more
sophisticated product. Considering the enormous range of abnormal behaviours
that brain malfunctions might be expected to produce (e.g. epilepsy, strokes and
various progressive nervous diseases), it is remarkable that, particularly among
social animals, nearly all the symptoms produced by rabies, not just aggression,
might be expected to promote the disease's spread. For example, photophobia
and paralysis might often result in an infective animal being confined to its den,
where it is likely to come into frequent contact with its mate and family; the
symptomless period will make it hard for foxes to evolve behavioural responses
for avoiding other foxes showing overt symptoms of rabies (note also that such a
behaviour could be exploited by 'cheating foxes' who "shammed furious
rabies" and that such cheats might thereby be able to poach food from the
territories of others!). Again, if we think of 'dumb' and 'furious' rabies as two
possible extremes of symptoms evinced by rabid foxes we may consider how
likely they are to spread in various fox societies in terms of a pay-off matrix, as
shown in Figure 8. We should again note that this is not a problem that could be
solved quantitatively by Game Theory, even if we could estimate the pay-offs
realistically: firstly, because it will refer to a cyclical epidemic in which the payoffs vary over the period of the cycle, and secondly because biological constraints will affect the 'Fox' strategy. The pay-off matrix of Fig. 8 would suggest
foxes should always play 'Solitary' to lose least to rabies, but, as foxes must
meet to raise cubs, it is clearly unrealistic for solitary to be a pure strategy (this
would exterminate foxes within one generation!). It does not matter very much in
this example whether 'dumb' or 'furious' depend on subtle differences in host
physiology, where the host was bitten, on the concentration of virus inoculated
into the host or even on rare mutations of the virus genome, the possibility for
evolution of fox behaviour to act on the total system is clearly there.

Before leaving the realm of Game Theory, we might usefully borrow its

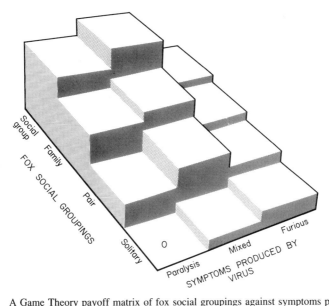

Fig. 8. A Game Theory payoff matrix of fox social groupings against symptoms produced by virus. As in Fig. 7, the block heights represent likely relative benefit payoffs to viruses, averaged over several cycles of rabies incidence.

concepts to think about the effects of control on the controlled population. Mammal pests are frequently controlled, to greater or lesser effectiveness, by the use of poisoned baits. Such controls are rarely completely effective, and the remaining populations often respond less readily to future controls, probably partly due to selection by the previous control for those animals less likely to take novel, even suspicious, food items. Consider a population of animals infected with rabies with individuals showing varying tendencies (which are probably heritable) to take novel food items. This population is presented with a variety of baits, which may or may not contain poison, vaccine or a temporary chemo-sterilant. Assume that the baits are perfectly prepared, so an animal finding a bait has no way of telling what type of bait it is. The possible outcomes are shown in Fig. 9. If the bait contains nothing, the animal gets a small gain from the food content for each bait it takes, so more frequent acceptors benefit more. However, if the bait contains poison frequent acceptors will die almost immediately and even rare acceptors are likely to suffer eventually the extreme penalty of death; hence the only safe strategy for 'Poison' is 'Never', implying poison would select very strongly against bait acceptors. Circumstances are dramatically different if the bait contains vaccine: animals never taking bait-with-vaccine are likely to die from rabies, whereas those taking the bait get both the food and immunity from rabies, and indeed, if this conferred immunity is temporary, more

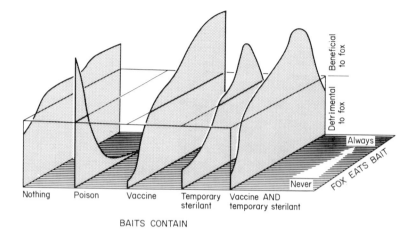

BAITS CONTAIN

Fig. 9. Game Theory considerations of the interplay between different methods of host population control and the responses of the target host population to that control. Control options are
discrete strategies of food baits containing the following: nothing, poison, vaccine, temporary sterilant, vaccine and temporary sterilant. The target population's strategy is a continuous variable, the
chances of an individual eating a novel food item such as a bait on any given encounter with such a
bait. The vertical axis represents likely payoffs to target hosts in terms of enhanced life expectation
and breeding potential: the overall shapes of the graphs relative to each other should be contrasted;
their details are not intended to be realistic.

frequent bait-acceptors will fare better. Thus, we have the possibility that, by
using an appropriate control technique (vaccination), natural selection can be
utilised to our benefit by tending to produce fox populations that are more likely
to respond to our control measures, in contrast to the well known effects of
control killing that often make the residual population harder and harder to kill.
This might not matter if, for example, control killing could readily reduce fox
populations below the 'threshold' level for rabies epidemics. Experience in
Europe suggests however that control killing can rarely achieve this on a wide
scale (even the intensively controlled Danish border area of Schleswick-Holstein
has been briefly invaded by rabies 3 times since 1940), so the prospects of having
the success of our control measures enhanced, rather than reduced, by natural
selection, are very attractive.

IV. Data Limitations

A. SCALE, RESOLUTION AND CHANCE

We have touched briefly on the likely biases in records of fox rabies and have
mentioned in passing that it is highly desirable that these biases should be

estimated by proper field survey. The main aim of this section is to point to a dilemma concerning necessary sample sizes for statistical treatment: subsequent chapters will present the pros and cons of temporal models (averaging events over a wide area) and spatio–temporal models (which consider time and space simultaneously).

Let us consider the scale of distances, in one dimension, that are of interest for different aspects of rabies epizootics and information collection, as illustrated in Fig. 10. The front wave of the epizootic moves 30 to 60 km a year; individual rabid foxes are thought to move mainly (>90% of cases) between 2 and 10 km (with very rare instances of up to 30 km, which probably represent dispersing individuals); the location of reported cases of rabies is sometimes very precise (e.g. 0.1 km), but often only to the nearest town, say 10 km or worse. Fox territories typically vary between 40 and 1300 ha (Macdonald, Chapter 4, this volume), or square territories of side 0.6–3.6 km. Habitat type can change dramatically over distances of a few hundred metres (0.1 km), or much less in environments modified by man, while, in mountainous regions, a horizontal displacement of 100 m could easily represent several hundred metres change in altitude with accompanying dramatic changes in habitat. There are some regions where vast tracts of land are essentially uniform habitat, such as the Dutch

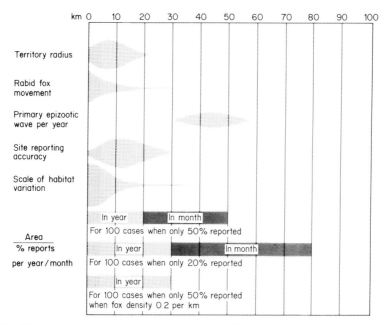

Fig. 10.   An illustration of the approximate different distances over which various parameters important to rabies epizootics are likely to vary significantly, expressed as kilometres (in one dimension). See text for details.

polders, the Polish steppes and forests, but, at least in much of Europe, such uniformity is rather uncommon.

Over how big an area do our reports of rabid foxes need to be collected before we can have fair confidence that they will provide reasonable epidemiological estimators of, say, disease prevalence? If we desire a sample size of 100 reports per year to give fair accuracy, assume 50% of rabid foxes are reported, assume 50% die from the disease, and consider an initial density of 1 fox/km² for the population (about the density at which European foxes reliably sustain rabies epizootics), then our sample represents some 250 km², or a 16 × 16 km² grid. However, as the incidence of rabies changes rapidly from month to month, we might decide we wanted 100 reports every one-tenth of a year, implying, by simple arithmetic, a sample drawn from an area of 2500 km² (50 × 50 km² grid). In practice, the calculation is over-simple, as 50% of the population would not die in a single month, but even if the mortality of 50% in a month were realistic, we are talking now of drawing our monthly sample from a grid so large that rabies would actually take a *year* to spread from one side to the other! We could perhaps make our sample area wide and shallow, say 5 × 500 km. But the habitats might not be similar all along this belt, and it might have to be bent about a bit to ensure that it represented the same temporal stage of the epidemic cycle all along its length. Without the sample *beforehand,* how do we decide where the "front" is? If we are prepared to accept 10 reports a year or 10 reports a month, we reduce our catchment area to 25 or 250 km², respectively (5 × 5 or 16 × 16 km). Hence the following dilemma: A small 'catchment' area for reports may be reasonably homogeneous as an environment, but it is unlikely to provide sufficient reports of rabid foxes for statistically accurate analysis, whereas an area large enough to provide a sample giving adequate accuracy is likely to be extremely heterogeneous. In geographic regions that are typically very heterogeneous, there may be no suitable 'quadrat' size for such gross data summarisation.

A possible way around such difficulties would be to choose a size of recording area that would be fairly homogeneous *as a habitat* and contain a fair number of foxes, and then use some multi-variate descriptive technique, or classificatory system, to describe a large number of such units over a wider contiguous region. A spatial model of rabies spread in a heterogeneous (model) environment could then be used to investigate likely patterns of spread for a defined mosaic of environments and then to assess whether patterns of spread were more similar than expected by chance for similar habitats. In this vein, Macdonald *et al.* (1981; see also Bunce *et al.,* 1981; Benefield and Bunce, 1982) investigated the feasibility of predicting potential carrying capacity densities of foxes from readily recordable landscape features and over a wide geographic area—the entire United Kingdom. A similar approach was used by Ball (1982, and Chapter 8, this volume) to investigate factors affecting rates of rabies spread in France. These investigations complement earlier works by Adamovich (1978) and Carey

(1982, and Chapter 2, this volume), which show associations between landscape types and epizootiological parameters.

B. CONTROL, VACUUM EFFECTS AND DISPERSAL

Intensive killing of animals in one area inherently produces a region that is favourable for their existence but presently contains very few. Consequently, any animals from surrounding areas (which may be over populated) that move into the cleared area are likely to remain there. These events are often referred to as *biological vacua*, as the cleared areas appear to 'suck-in' animals of the controlled species from surrounding regions. Clearly, such events will be important not only with regard to rabies control efforts, as too small a control region might promote both influx and conflict and, hence, increase the chances of disease spread even at a lower density, but also during the course of a natural wildlife epizootic as rabies itself may kill a sufficient proportion of its main host population to create a strong vacuum effect. Although we know that animals on the fringes of such vacua are likely to disperse into them, we know very little about when, why, how far they will move and how they decide to settle. Consequently, we are poorly placed to model the process. We do have data on how far particular individuals have dispersed from a natal home range to a new one, but these data often come from study populations near their carrying capacity densities and may not be relevant to the 'vacuum' situation. Is it realistic to observe how far dispersers move at high density and then to select a random distance from that frequency distribution and apply it to individuals who have an abundance of spare territories in their immediate neighbourhood? It seems unlikely, but it also seems unlikely that dispersers would settle in the first reasonably suitable area— if there is plenty of choice they might find an even better area nearby. Indeed, might we expect much of the surviving population to concentrate into the better areas?

As dispersing juveniles that are incubating rabies are thought to be responsible for the increased prevalence and spread of rabies in late autumn and winter, dispersal is clearly important for rabies epizootics even at normal population levels. Recent theoretical works on population processes (Lomnicki, 1978; Bacon, 1982) have even suggested that selective emigration could serve as a mechanism of population regulation and such possibilities emphasise that understanding dispersal processes could be crucial to rabies modelling.

V. Summary

This chapter aims to give an overview of the elements of rabies epizootics in terms to the entities, attributes, relationships and processes that comprise infectious diseases. First, it is hoped that this framework and the examples will allow the reader to clarify his thoughts and to aid his assessments, for particular objectives, of where he should stand in the dilemma between 'requiring too much data' and 'making too many unrealistic assumptions'. Second, it is hoped that the reader will take a similar stance of informed, constructive criticism in evaluating the merits of the models proposed in the remainder of the book as in the assessment of his own present thoughts.

References

Adamovich, V. L. (1978). Landscape-ecological foundations of the local foci of rabies infection. *Zool. Zh.* **57**(2), 260–271.

Anderson, R. M., and May, R. M. (1979). Population biology of infectious disease. Part 1. *Nature (London)* **280**, 361–367.

Bacon, P. J. (1982). "Population Dynamics: Models Based on Individual Growth, Resource Allocation and Competitive Ethology," Merlewood R&D Pap. No. 88. Institute of Terrestrial Ecology, Grange-over-Sands, Cumbria, England.

Ball, F. G. (1982). Some statistical problems in the epidemiology of fox rabies. Ph.D. Thesis, University of Oxford.

Benefield, C. B., and Bunce, R. G. H. (1982). "A Preliminary Visual Presentation of Land Classes in Britain," Merlewood R&D Pap. No. 91. Institute of Terrestrial Ecology, Grange-over-Sands, Cumbria, England.

Browning, R. (1889). "The Pied Piper of Hamelin." Warne, London.

Bunce, R. G. H., Barr, C. J., and Whittaker, H. A. (1981). "Land Classes in Great Britain. Preliminary Descriptions for Users of the Merlewood Method of Land Classification," Merlewood R&D Pap. No. 86. Institute of Terrestrial Ecology, Grange-over-Sands, Cumbria, England.

Carey, A. B. (1982). The ecology of Red Foxes, Grey Foxes and rabies in the Eastern United States. *Wildl. Soc. Bull.* **10**, 18–26.

Gale, J. S. (1980). "Population Genetics." Blackie, London.

Holling, C. S. (1978). Overview and conclusions. *In* "Adapture Environmental Assessment and Management" (C. S. Holling, ed.), pp. 1–21. Wiley, New York.

Lomnicki, A. (1978). Individual differences between animals and the natural regulation of their numbers. *J. Anim. Ecol.* **47**, 461–475.

Macdonald, D. W., Bunce, R. G. H., and Bacon, P. J. (1981). Fox populations, habitat characterisation and rabies control. *J. Biogeogr.* **8**, 145–151.

Ross, J. (1982). Myxomatosis: The natural evolution of the disease. *In* "Animal Disease in Relation to Animal Conservation" (M. A. Edwards and U. McDonnell, eds.), pp. 77–95. Academic Press, New York.

Schneider, L. G. (1982). Antigenic variants of rabies virus. *Comp. Immunol. Microbiol. Infect. Dis.* **5**, 101–107.

Shaw, M. L. G. (1980). "On Becoming A Personal Scientist: Interactive Computer Elicitation of Personal Models of the World." Academic Press, New York.

A Continuous Time Deterministic Model of Temporal Rabies

6

A. D. M. Smith[1]

Centre for Environmental Technology,
Imperial College,
London, England

I. Introduction

In exploring the dynamic relationship between rabies and foxes, the development of mathematical models can serve several functions. Models of a statistical nature can be used to *detect* or *describe* patterns in the distribution and abundance of cases in space and time. On the other hand, mechanistic models can be developed that also serve to *explain* such patterns in the dynamics of the interaction. Such models may range in complexity from simple analytical models involving a few variables and several equations to complex simulation models incorporating many variables and equations. These models generally require the use of a computer for their solution. Finally, both statistical and mechanistic

---

[1]Present address: Department of Zoology, University of Adelaide, Adelaide, South Australia, Australia 5001.

POPULATION DYNAMICS OF RABIES IN WILDLIFE

models may be used to *predict* the outcome of a variety of possible control measures that might be applied to reduce the incidence of rabies or even eradicate it altogether. Models used in this way form an important tool in many branches of applied ecology, in that the consequences of intervention can be, at least to some extent, judged prior to their actual implementation.

In this chapter we will examine the way in which a simple deterministic model of the interaction between foxes and rabies can be used both to explain certain features of the temporal dynamics of the disease and to explore the possible consequences of both fox culling and vaccination of wild foxes in efforts to control or eliminate rabies. The model described in this chapter was first developed by Anderson *et al.* (1981). The first section describes the rationale for development of this model and the assumptions on which the model is based. The second section describes the basic predictions of the model and compares them with observed patterns in the epidemiology of fox rabies, particularly in Europe. The third section explores various elaborations of the basic model, including the incorporation of control measures such as culling and vaccination. The final section concludes with an assessment of the success of this approach and an indication of possible lines for future work.

II. The Basic Model

The model for fox rabies developed by Anderson *et al.* (1981) differs from most previous models on this topic in that it ignores the spatial aspects of epidemic spread of rabies to concentrate on temporal aspects of the disease in a single fox population. This approach, which was also followed by Bacon and Macdonald (1980), simplifies considerably the resultant model, making it analytically more tractable and increasing its explanatory power, albeit at the expense of understanding the importance of spatial factors in disease transmission. Where such spatial factors have been modelled explicitly (Preston, 1973; Smart and Giles, 1973; Berger, 1976), the resulting model has been large and complex and only numerical solutions could be obtained. Numerical solutions were also obtained by Bacon and Macdonald, as described in the following chapter.

The basic model of Anderson *et al.* was developed by first assuming that, in the absence of rabies, fox population growth could be modelled using the logistic equation. If N represents fox density or population size, then this model describes the rate of change in density by the equation

$$dN/dt = rN (1 - N/K) \tag{1}$$

where r is the intrinsic growth rate of the population at low density and K is the carrying capacity of the environment, that is, the density of foxes that can be maintained in a given type of habitat. The parameter r can be written $r = a - b$, where a is the per capita birth rate of foxes and b is the per capita death rate in the absence of intraspecific competition. (Expressed another way, $1/b$ is the expected life-span of a fox not subject to density-dependent mortality.) Differential equations are widely used in population models in ecology (and elsewhere). They are used to represent the rate of change of magnitude of a variable as a function of time. In Equation (1), this is expressed as dN/dt. The right-hand part of Equation (1) represents the assumptions of the logistic model for population growth, that there is some basic rate of population growth rN (exponential growth), which will decrease as population density N increases (represented by the term $(1 - N/K)$). The ''equilibrium solution'' for this equation is found by setting $dN/dt = 0$, that is, finding the conditions under which the population is tending neither to increase nor decrease. Thus $rN(1 - N/K) = 0$ is ''solved'' for the variable N either when $N = 0$ or $N = K$. The logistic equation is used widely in ecology to model the growth of single populations (see, e.g., May, 1976). It is not particularly realistic so far as mammal population growth is concerned, especially where birth rates are seasonal as in foxes and where the age structure of the population may be important. It does, however, describe the tendency of populations to increase at low densities and to stabilize at some density characteristic of a particular habitat type, and for this reason it is widely used as a basis for describing single species population growth.

The dynamic effects of rabies on foxes is incorporated in the model by dividing the fox population into three epidemiological classes: (1) susceptible individuals, (2) those incubating the disease (that is, infected but not yet infectious), and (3) infectious or rabid individuals. The population densities of these three classes are denoted X, H and Y, respectively, and total fox density is thus $N = X + H + Y$. There seems to be no clear evidence for the development of immunity to rabies in foxes in Europe (Toma and Andral, 1977), perhaps surprisingly so, considering the strong selective force exerted by this disease on fox populations in infected areas. The inclusion of a fourth, immune class is therefore not considered, except in a later elaboration of the model to include artificial immunity due to vaccination. The subdivision of the fox population into epidemiological classes follows traditional lines established in modelling microparasitic human infections (Bailey, 1975), except that in this case the total population size N is a dynamic variable, rather than a constant, and free to vary under the influence both of the disease and of the birth and death processes occurring in the fox population itself.

The fox rabies model is now developed by considering the factors affecting the rate of change in density of each epidemiological class in turn. The rate of disease transmission (that is, the rate at which susceptible individuals become infected) is given by βXY where β is a transmission parameter, which will be proportional to the average period of contact between individuals in the population or, in the case of territorial animals, between individuals of different social units occupying different territories. The parameter β is almost impossible to measure directly but can be inferred by a method described in Section II. The rate of disease transmission is also directly proportional to the densities of susceptible and infectious individuals in the population. This follows conventional lines in modelling infectious diseases (Bailey, 1975) and assumes, in effect, a random encounter rate between individuals in the population.

Infected individuals in the population become infectious at a per capita rate σ, where $1/\sigma$ is the mean incubation period of rabies in foxes, about 30 days (Winkler, 1972). Infectious or rabid individuals have a mortality rate α due to the disease. This rate can be estimated from the reciprocal of the mean duration of infectiveness (equivalent to the mean life-span of a rabid individual once clinical symptoms of the disease develop), which is about 5 days in foxes (Toma and Andral, 1977). All rabid animals die.

The basic model is derived by putting together all these assumptions concerning the basic biology of the fox and the impact of rabies on a fox population to yield a set of three differential equations expressing the rates of change in X, H and Y, namely

$$dX/dt = aX - bX - \phi NX - \beta XY$$
$$dH/dt = \beta XY - bH - \phi NH - \sigma H \qquad (2)$$
$$dY/dt = \sigma H - bY - \phi NY - \alpha Y$$

where $\phi = r/K$ is a measure of density dependent mortality due to intraspecific competition (mostly for territories in foxes). Note that it is assumed that only susceptible individuals contribute to reproduction in the population.

The model is derived, then, from a basic set of assumptions about the interaction between foxes and rabies. All the parameters in the model have biologically interpretable meanings (Table I) and all, except β, can be estimated from data available in the literature.

III. Model Predictions

The basic model outlined in the previous section makes four sets of predictions concerning the impact of rabies on a fox population. These predictions are in broad agreement with observed aspects of the epidemiology of rabies in foxes.

A. THRESHOLD DENSITY

The model predicts a threshold fox density below which rabies will not persist in the population. This threshold density is given by the equation

$$K_T = (a + \sigma)(a + \alpha)/\beta\sigma \qquad (3)$$

Equation (3) is obtained by setting $dX/dt = dH/dt = dY/dt = 0$ in Equation (2) (that is, solving for the equilibrium in which there is no change in X, H or Y), and

TABLE I

The Variables, Parameters and Control Variables Used in the Models[a]

Symbol	Meaning	Value
Variables		
N	Fox population density	
X	Density of susceptible foxes	
H	Density of infected foxes	
Y	Density of rabid foxes	
Z	Density of immune foxes	
Parameters		
a	*Per capita* birth rate	1.0
b	*Per capita* death rate	0.5
r	Intrinsic rate of increase	0.5
K	Carrying capacity	Various
φ	Degree of density dependence	Various
β	Transmission parameter	199
σ	$1/\sigma$ is mean incubation period	13
α	Rate of disease induced mortality	73
Controls		
c	Culling rate	
v	Vaccination rate	
i	Potential immigration rate	

[a] The parameter values are those used to generate the results in Figs. 1–5.

subsequently solving for the condition in which the disease is just eliminated (that is, $H = Y = 0$). Since σ and α are much larger than a, K_T is approximately equal to α/β. High mortality rates for rabid animals will tend to increase K_T because individuals do not remain infectious for very long (they die very quickly thus reducing the probability of meeting a susceptible individual and so consequently reducing the rate of disease transmission). On the other hand, high rates of contact between individuals (high values of β) will tend to decrease the threshold fox density required for the persistence of rabies.

Such threshold densities for disease persistence have been widely observed for rabies in foxes (see, e.g. Lloyd, 1976). Fox density is difficult to measure directly and indirect measures such as the number of foxes killed per square kilometre are frequently used. In Europe, the threshold fox density for rabies persistence is reported to be about 0.4 foxes per km² (Steck and Wandeler, 1980). This allows an indirect estimation of the parameter β, since β is approximately equal to α/K_T.

B. FOX POPULATION DEPRESSION

Rabies acts as a very severe density dependent constraint limiting fox population growth. The model predicts that, provided $K > K_T$, the fox population

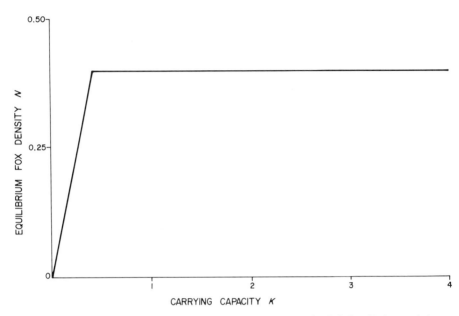

Fig. 1. Equilibrium fox density N as a function of carrying capacity K. Below K_T the population is unregulated by rabies.

density will be regulated to a level very close to K_T, independent of how large the population size would be in the absence of rabies (Fig. 1). This represents an increasing level of population depression by the disease as the carrying capacity of the environment, K, increases. Although good information on fox density is difficult to obtain, available data tend to confirm increasing population depression by rabies with increasing initial population density (Steck and Wandeler, 1980).

C. LOW PREVALENCE OF RABIES

The model predicts a low equilibrium prevalence of rabies, as measured by the proportion of the population, which is either rabid or is incubating the disease (Fig. 2). Even where the carrying capacity is high and the degree of depression of the fox population caused by the disease is also proportionately high, the prevalence of rabies is relatively low. This is explained by the relatively short durations of the incubation and infectious periods, causing high ''turnover'' rates in the population. Evidence from serological surveys in endemic areas of rabies support this prediction (Davis and Wood, 1959). Of course non-equilibrium prevalence of the disease may be very much higher, as in the case when rabies is initially introduced into a dense population not previously exposed to the disease.

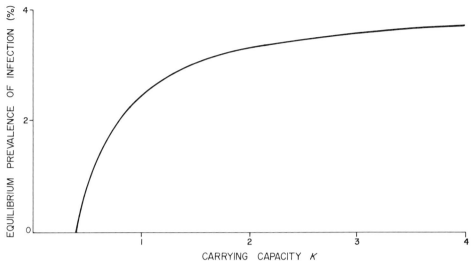

Fig. 2. Equilibrium prevalence of rabies [(H + Y)/N] expressed as a percentage, as a function of fox carrying capacity K.

D. CYCLES IN DISEASE INCIDENCE

The final major prediction of the basic model stems from an analysis of the stability properties of the model coupled with numerical integrations to predict the dynamic behaviour of the variables over time. In regions where rabies can persist in a population (i.e. $K > K_T$), the model predicts two possible patterns in the incidence of rabies over time (Anderson *et al.*, 1981). For $K_T < K < K_L$, the incidence of rabies will tend to oscillate after its initial introduction into a susceptible population, with the amplitude of the oscillations gradually decreasing until a steady equilibrium is achieved (Fig. 3a). Such cycles in incidence appear to be a common feature of the epidemiology of rabies in foxes. For the parameter values given in Table I, the value of K_L is about 3.4 foxes per km^2. Note also that the period of the cycles is about 3–4 years. For $K > K_L$, the oscillations in incidence do not damp out, but continue indefinitely (Fig. 3b). The period of the cycles is similar and is in broad agreement with values observed in a variety of studies (Lloyd, 1976; Toma and Andral, 1977; Kauker and Zettl, 1960). Moreover Johnston and Beauregard (1969) observed that the cycles were more pronounced in areas of good fox habitat.

The cause of the cycles is easily interpreted from the model. Rabies is acting as a very severe source of density-dependent mortality and as one which acts with a delay due at least in part to the incubation period of the disease. The other source of delay in response is the time required for the fox population to recover, having been reduced to a low level by rabies, to a density at which the disease

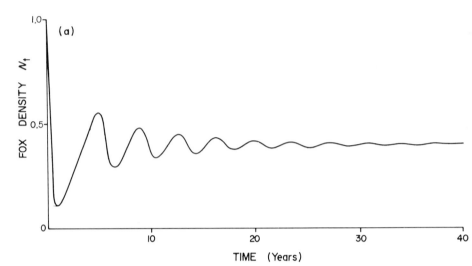

Fig. 3. Population density N_t as a function of time for two levels of fox carrying capacity: (a) K = 0.8 km^{-2} (b) K = 2.4 km^{-2}. Fluctuations in disease incidence follow fluctuations in fox density, but with a slight time lag.

can again spread through the population. It is well known that delays of this sort result in cyclic fluctuations in model behaviour for a wide range of ecological models (May, 1973).

IV. Model Extensions

Having determined that the basic model predicts certain broad features of the dynamics of rabies in foxes, one can use the structure of this model as a basis for investigating further features of the interaction between disease and host and of the effects of various control interventions on this interaction.

A. CONTROL BY CULLING

The most common method used in Europe in attempts to control fox rabies has been through efforts to reduce fox density by a variety of means including hunting, gassing, poisoning and trapping (Kaplan, 1977; Macdonald, 1980). These methods have not generally proved successful, but were motivated by the observed phenomenon of a threshold density below which rabies did not seem to persist in a fox population.

The potential effect of such measures can be explored theoretically by incorporating an additional mortality term in the model to represent fox culling. The

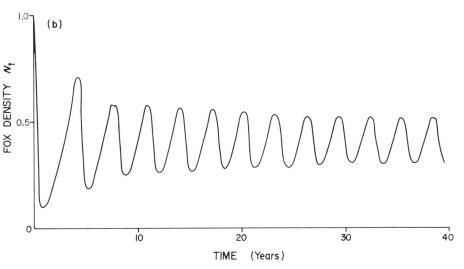

Fig. 3. (*Continued.*)

most appropriate way to incorporate this effect would seem to be via a constant per capita mortality rate c. This is analogous to a constant harvest effort widely used in fisheries models, and it might reflect a constant number of man hours spent in hunting or a constant number of traps set, and so on.

Incorporating this term in the model results in the set of equations

$$
\begin{aligned}
dX/dt &= aX - bX - \phi NX - \beta XY - cX \\
dH/dt &= \beta XY - bH - \phi NH - \sigma H - cH \\
dY/dt &= \sigma H - bY - \phi NY - \alpha Y - cY
\end{aligned}
\tag{4}
$$

The condition for disease eradication is that the culling rate c should exceed a fixed value, given by

$$
c > r (1 - K_T/K)
\tag{5}
$$

This expression is obtained, formally, by setting $dX/dt = dH/dt = dY/dt = 0$ in Equation (4) and subsequently determining the condition for which $H = Y = 0$. This involves a good deal of algebraic manipulation, but a more illuminating derivation can be obtained by examining the dynamics of culling in the absence of rabies. This is expressed as

$$
dN/dt = rN (1 - N/K) - cN
\tag{6}
$$

which can be solved by setting $dN/dt = 0$ to obtain

$$
N^* = K (1 - c/r)
\tag{7}
$$

To ensure that an outbreak of rabies cannot occur, the population density must be below the threshold density for disease eradication, i.e. $N^* < K_T$. Thus

$$K\,(1\,-\,c/r) < K_T \qquad (8)$$

from which Equation (5) is obtained by simple algebraic manipulation.

It is clear from Equation (5) that the culling rate for disease eradication must increase as K increases. In very good fox habitat prior to outbreak of rabies, the proportion of the fox population that must be removed to prevent an outbreak will approach 100%, and this effort must be maintained so long as rabies is endemic in the area. This explains, at least in part, why efforts at reducing fox density have not been generally effective in preventing the spread of rabies. Other aspects of the problem include the high reproductive potential of the fox and the tendency for immigration to rapidly repopulate areas in which fox densities have been reduced well below potential carrying capacity.

One interesting feature of culling predicted by the model is that, so long as rabies persists in the population, increased rates of culling have little effect on the equilibrium fox density N (Fig. 4). Culling simply acts to reduce the proportion

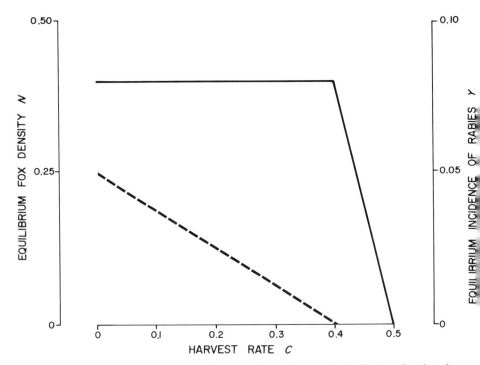

Fig. 4.   Population density N (solid line) and rabies incidence Y (broken line) as a function of c, the rate of removal of foxes.

of the population that is infected, up to the point at which rabies is finally eliminated. There appear to be no good data to verify whether, in fact, this happens. In any case, the results bear only on equilibrium densities, and actual densities may vary widely from these.

B. CONTROL BY VACCINATION

The basic model may be elaborated to include the effects of vaccinating wild foxes, a more recently developed control measure and one which appears to show some promise of success. The model must be extended to include an immune class, with density denoted Z, which will also contribute to reproduction. If the per capita rate of vaccination is v, and assuming no loss of immunity, the model becomes

$$
\begin{aligned}
dX/dt &= a(X + Z) - bX - \phi NX - \beta XY - vX \\
dH/dt &= \beta XY - bH - \phi NH - \sigma H \\
dY/dt &= \sigma H - bY - \phi NY - \alpha Y \\
dZ/dt &= vX - bZ - \phi NZ
\end{aligned}
\tag{9}
$$

where now $N = X + H + Y + Z$. Once again, the condition for disease eradication is the variable of interest. This condition can be expressed as

$$
v > a(K/K_T - 1)
\tag{10}
$$

which again will increase as K increases. Equation (10) can be derived, as in the case of culling, by examining the case in which rabies is not present in the population. Thus, only susceptible and immune individuals are present, and their dynamics are described by the equations

$$
\begin{aligned}
dX/dt &= a(X + Z) - bX - \phi NX - vX \\
dZ/dt &= vX - bZ - \phi NZ
\end{aligned}
\tag{11}
$$

where $N = X + Z$. Solving Equation (11) by setting $dX/dt = dZ/dt = 0$, the equilibrium density N^* is equal to the carrying capacity K, and

$$
\begin{aligned}
X^* &= aK/a + v \\
Z^* &= vK/a + v
\end{aligned}
\tag{12}
$$

Clearly if $v = 0$, $X^* = K$ and $Z^* = 0$, and as v increases Z^* increases and X^* decrease s. To ensure no outbreak of rabies, X^* must be decreased below the threshold density for disease persistence, i.e. we require $X^* < K_T$. This can be written as

$$
aK/a + v < K_T
\tag{13}
$$

from which Equation (10) follows directly. Another way of expressing both conditions (5) and (10) is that the proportion, p, of the population, which must be either culled or vaccinated to eradicate rabies, must fulfil the condition

$$p > 1 - K_T/K \qquad (14)$$

The effects of vaccinating foxes differ from those of fox culling in several important respects. One effect of an increasing vaccination rate is an increasing pool of immune individuals in the population and therefore an increasing overall density of foxes. Since the immune foxes contribute to reproduction, the net birth rate will increase, and hence the net rate of production of susceptible individuals since all foxes are born susceptible. The effect of this can be that for low rates of fox vaccination, the incidence of rabies can actually increase (Fig. 5). This would suggest that, as far as vaccination is concerned, some measure of control may not, in fact, be better than none. This stands at the moment as a theoretical possibility and remains to be validated in the field. Nevertheless it seems to warrant some attention. Although not predicted by the model used in Equation (4), it seems likely that some culling may also be detrimental, if it has the effect of increasing mixing rates in the population (e.g. mates of culled animals re-

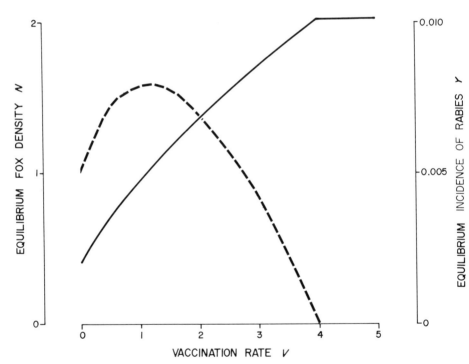

Fig. 5. Population density N (solid line) and rabies incidence Y (broken line) as a function of the vaccination rate v of wild foxes.

pairing, juveniles moving into vacated territories) thus increasing the contact rate β, and hence the disease incidence.

C. SPATIAL FACTORS

The basic model and the elaborations of it considered so far have focused on describing events in a single isolated fox population with implicit assumptions of homogeneity in factors such as the probability of contact between individuals in the population. The virtue of the lack of consideration of spatial factors has been the simplicity of formulation and solution of these models and the consequent ease of interpretation of the phenomena, which they (successfully) predict. In practice the idealized population considered in these models does not, of course, exist. This will be true of any mathematical formulation, no matter how complex, but there are reasons to believe that spatial factors may be important in determining some aspects of the dynamics of rabies in a population of foxes in any given location. This will be a consequence of, amongst other factors, the high mobility of the fox, and fine scale variations in habitat type influencing fox distribution and abundance.

One aspect in particular of the dynamic behaviour predicted by the basic model requires further consideration. This concerns the periodic fluctuations in the incidence of the disease, outlined in Fig. 3. It is evident that a consequence of the long period (3–4 years) of these fluctuations is that the incidence of rabies in a closed population will fall to very low levels over long periods of time (relative to the duration of the disease in any individual animal), and in a finite population the probability of stochastic extinction of the disease will be correspondingly high. The undoubted persistence of the disease over large areas may perhaps be a consequence of a reservoir in alternative hosts, but a more likely explanation is the high mobility of the fox coupled with asynchrony in the cycles of fox rabies incidence in neighbouring areas.

While periodic reinfection by rabid animals may be important in promoting persistence of the disease in any given area, immigration of susceptible individuals may also affect dynamic patterns in the association of rabies and foxes. The importance of such immigration was mentioned earlier with regard to the difficulty of maintaining fox densities below carrying capacity by culling in areas where rabies is not yet endemic. The effects of such immigration can be easily incorporated in the basic model, without expanding the model to a full spatial representation of adjacent populations. There is some advantage in retaining the structure of the basic model in that the effects of new assumptions can be assessed directly by comparing predictions with those made by the basic model.

It is assumed that there is a constant potential rate of immigration i of susceptible foxes from outside the population under consideration. This assumption will be most appropriate where rabies is entering the population for the first time, that is, at the front wave of the disease. The effective rate of immigration will depend on the density of foxes already present in the population, such that the full potential rate of immigration will be realized when this density is zero, and there will be no net immigration from outside the population when it is at its carrying capacity. This assumption leads to the new set of equations

$$dX/dt = aX - bX - \phi NX - \beta XY + i(1 - N/K)$$
$$dH/dt = \beta XY - bH - \phi NH - \sigma H \qquad\qquad (15)$$
$$dY/dt = \sigma H - bY - \phi NY - \alpha Y$$

Increasing levels of the immigration rate i tend to increase the prevalence of rabies, though not dramatically. The most notable effect of immigration is on the stability of the fox–rabies interaction. Increasing rates of immigration greatly reduce the amplitude of oscillations in incidence of rabies, as well as reducing the period of the cycles. This is due to the faster recovery of the population from low densities. Both these effects will thus tend to increase stability and decrease the likelihood of stochastic ''fadeout'' of the disease. This may be particularly important at the frontwave of the disease since the initial outbreak tends to be the most intense and produce the greatest depression in the fox population. Coupled with the effects of the immigration of occasional rabid individuals discussed earlier, the net effect of spatial movement in foxes seems to be to increase the stability of the association between rabies and foxes.

V. Discussion

Some general features of the approach used in developing the basic model outlined in Section II are worth outlining at this stage. Unlike most previous models of fox rabies, this model did not seek to address the problems of epidemic spread of rabies, but rather to focus on aspects of the endemic maintenance of the disease in a single population. This choice of focus has both advantages and limitations. One of the major advantages is the resulting simplicity of the model. The advantages of simplicity and analytical tractability are twofold. First, analysis of the full range of dynamic behaviour of the model is made possible. Second, the predictions of the model are more easily interpreted and this understanding can be used to interpret the dynamic behaviour of the real system (and of more complex models of it). The disadvantages stem from the greater level of abstraction required in the simple model. A more complex model can be made more realistic (though any model will always remain an abstraction). On the other hand, the more complex model will involve many more assumptions and will require a much more detailed *a priori* understanding of the system and better data on aspects such as fox behaviour and movement.

The choice of simple versus complex model may also depend on the particular questions about which answers or at least predictions are required. A detailed spatial model may be required to design a strategy to contain local outbreaks of rabies and prevent their spread. Such a model might address detailed tactical questions. On the other hand, the simple model may be more appropriate for addressing broad strategic questions concerning eradication of endemic rabies.

Stemming from the importance of simple models in the degree of insight they give to understanding at least their own predictions, they can prove useful in investigating the importance of individual processes or specific interventions by adding to or altering specific assumptions of the model whose basic structure is well understood. Thus simple models can be used as building blocks for more detailed and more realistic models, where any change in model behaviour at each step can be attributed to specific assumptions or factors.

Productive areas for future modelling of rabies lie in two areas. First, an investigation of the importance of spatial heterogeneity and fox mobility on the dynamics of rabies in foxes. Second, the importance of the development of naturally acquired immunity to rabies by foxes. Results from the model outlined in this chapter would tend to suggest that both spatial heterogeneity and natural immunity will tend to act as stabilizing influences on the association between rabies and foxes.

Acknowledgements

Much of the work reported here was done in collaboration with Roy Anderson to whom I am indebted for many stimulating ideas. The research was supported by a grant from the U.K. Department of the Environment on ''The stability and resilience of ecological systems and the implications for environmental management''.

References

Anderson, R. M., Jackson, H. C., May, R. M., and Smith, A. D. M. (1981). Population dynamics of fox rabies in Europe. *Nature, (London)* **289,** 765–771.

Bacon, P. J., and Macdonald, D. W. (1980). To control rabies: Vaccinate foxes. *New Sci.* **87,** 640–645.

Bailey, N. T. J. (1975). ''The Mathematical Theory of Infectious Diseases.'' Griffin, London.

Berger, J. (1976). Model of rabies control. *Lect. Notes Biomath.* **11,** 74–88.

Davis, D. E., and Wood, J. E. (1959). Ecology of foxes and rabies control. *Public Health Rep.* **72,** 115–118.

Johnston, D. H., and Beauregard, M. (1969). Rabies epidemiology in Ontario. *Bull. Wildl. Dis. Assoc.* **5,** 357–370.

Kaplan, C., ed. (1977). ''Rabies: The Facts.'' Oxford Univ. Press, London and New York.

Kauker, E., and Zettl, K. (1960). Die okologie der rotfuchses und ihre beziehung zur tollwut. *Dtsch. Tieraerztl. Wochenschr.* **67,** 463–467.

Lloyd, H. G. (1976). Wildlife rabies in Europe and the British situation. *Trans. R. Soc. Trop. Med. Hyg.* **70,** 179–187.

Macdonald, D. W. (1980). "Rabies and Wildlife. A Biologist's Perspective." Oxford Univ. Press, London and New York.

May, R. M. (1973). "Stability and Complexity in Model Ecosystems." Princeton Univ. Press, Princeton, New Jersey.

May, R. M. (1976). "Theoretical Ecology. Principles and Applications." Blackwell, Oxford.

Preston, E. M. (1973). Computer simulated dynamics of a rabies controlled fox population. *J. Wildl. Manage.* **11,** 318–324.

Smart, C. W., and Giles, R. H. (1973). A computer model of wildlife rabies epizootics and an analysis of incidence patterns. *Wildl. Dis.* **61,** 1–89.

Steck, F., and Wandeler, A. (1980). The epidemiology of fox rabies in Europe. *Epidemiol. Rev.* **2,** 71–96.

Toma, B., and Andral, L. (1977). Epidemiology of fox rabies. *Adv. Virus Res.* **21,** 1–26.

Winkler, W. G. (1972). Rabies in the United States 1951–1970. *J. Infect. Dis.* **125,** 674–675.

Discrete Time Temporal Models of Rabies

7

P. J. Bacon

Institute of Terrestrial Ecology,
Merlewood Research Station,
Grange-over-Sands,
Cumbria, England

147

I. Introduction—A Simple Model

A. BASIC MATHEMATICS

In the previous chapter, much of the background mathematics to epidemiology was described and attention was drawn to the importance of critical parameters that may underly the gross behaviour of the host–pathogen interaction. In 1979, I started working on rabies epizootics and was particularly struck by the fact that several highly complex simulation models had been developed but that, in general, their predictions had only been tested crudely against real data, to the extent that much simpler models were almost certain to 'fit' equally well. The model described in this chapter was developed as a self-teaching process, over the course of a few months, to investigate the complexity of behaviour that could be generated by a simple model.

The complexity of spatial processes, and especially the sparcity of accurate spatial–temporal data led me to concentrate initially on temporal models alone, and, indeed, as mentioned above, the adequacy of our knowledge is still rather poor for developing a realistic spatial model based on data for which we have adequate measures of the sub-processes illustrated in Figs 1 and 3. The striking aspects of the host–pathogen interactions of rabies, particularly in a host like the Red Fox, are as follows:

1. Rabies infections 'reoccur'–reproduce about once a month, on average.
2. Foxes only reproduce once a year.
3. Rabies is a lethal disease in foxes, and it may typically reduce the population to 20–40% of its former level.
4. As rabies is spread by contact, the density of fresh infections is likely to vary with the densities of both rabid and susceptible foxes.

Considering the above facts, we would expect, first, that, on a monthly time scale, no true steady state equilibrium can exist, as foxes are dying each month and are only born once a year, and, second, that, if rabies does affect between 40 and 70% of the fox population over a period of several months, it may take the fox population more than a single breeding season (i.e., more than a year) to make good those losses due to rabies.

We may develop this argument, starting with the logistic equation for population growth and the Lotka–Volterra prey–predator equations, with which many biologists will be familiar. The logistic equation gives the following:

Difference equation   Differential equation

$$N_{t+1} = N_t + rN_t(1 - N_t/K), \quad dN/dt = rN(1 - N/K) \qquad (1)$$

where N_t is the density of animals at time t; r is the (births − deaths) per capita; K is the carrying capacity density; t is the time in arbitrary units.

The Lotka–Volterra equations envisage additional prey deaths due to predation as specified by a constant contact rate C between prey and predators, and a predator sustenance term C' relating prey deaths to predator food needs, such that

$$N_{t+1} = N_t + rN_t(1 - N_t/K) - CP_tN_t \quad \text{or}$$
$$dN/dt = rN(1 - N/K) - CPN \quad (2)$$
$$P_{t+1} = P_t + C'N_tP_t - eP_t \quad or \quad (dP/dt) = C'NP - ep$$

where N is the prey density; P is the predator density; C is the proportion of the prey–predator contacts leading to prey death; C' is the ratio of prey–predator contacts sustaining a predator; e is the predator death and birth rate.

By analogy, if rabid foxes kill susceptible foxes by infecting them with rabies, we may write as follows:

$$N_{t+1} = N_t + rN_t(1 - N_t/K) - CN_tR_t \quad \text{or}$$
$$dN/dt = rN(1 - N/K) - CNR \quad (3)$$
$$R_{t+1} = R_t + C'N_tR_t - eR_t \quad or \quad dR/dt = C'NR - eR$$

where R is the rabid fox density; N is the normal–susceptible fox density; C and C' are contact ratios scaled per unit area.

Finally, by noting that rabid foxes cannot directly produce more rabid foxes and that by choosing a suitable time interval j such that all rabid foxes will die in such a period (1 month would be suitable for this), we may write as follows:

$$N_{t+}1 = N_t + r_{st}N_t(1 - N_t/K) - CN_tR_t$$
$$R_{t+1} = CN_tR_t \quad (4)$$

where $C = C'$ from Equation (3); r_{st} denotes seasonal reproduction of foxes.

It is well known that a time delay in linked difference equations (here the reproductive rate of foxes, r, is seasonal, which constitutes a time delay) can lead to oscilations (e.g. May, 1974; Bartlett, 1960). The incubation period provides a second time delay, which, in our first simple model but not the later model, is set equal to the model's time interval of 1 month.

B. A SIMPLE DIFFERENCE EQUATION MODEL

Figure 1A shows a diagram of the processes that we are trying to understand and relates the processes to Equations (4). These processes were translated into a computer program, illustrated in Fig. 1B and listed in Appendix 1.

The results of using this computer program and the parameters listed in Table I to model rabies are shown in Fig. 2. Figure 2A first demonstrates that the equations do produce a reasonable prediction of how the number of foxes in a

(A)

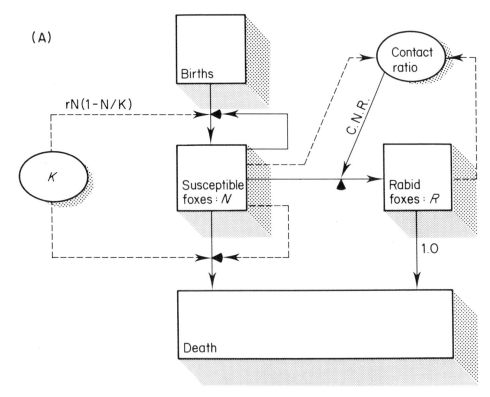

Fig. 1. (A) A simplified diagrammatic model of rabies in a fox population, showing the main entities (boxes), the major parameters affecting these (ovoids), the population and disease processes (open arrows) and the mathematical relationships used (formulae on line arrows). (B) A flow-diagram of the above simple model; the computer code implementing the flow diagram is given in Appendix 1.

population would vary over time in the absence of rabies: this is achieved by 'starting' the model population at low density (10% of carrying capacity) with a realistic per-capita birth rate and observing, in Fig. 2A, how the equations predict the population increasing in density and stabilizing at the carrying capacity level. If the population had been started above carrying capacity, the equations would show a stepwise drop to that level, but this prediction is not illustrated. We may take it, therefore, that the equations represent, albeit crudely, a reasonable set of population processes.

The remaining parts of Figure 2 (B–I) show model fox populations starting at carrying capacity and affected by rabies with differing contact parameters: in these figures, $K = 1000$, $N = 1000$, $R = 10$, fecundity $= 2.0$ and contact parameters vary between 0.00099 and 0.0028. The values of K, N and R here represent numbers per unspecified size area. (Note: with $N = 1000$, $R = 10$, $C = 0.001$, $C * N * R = 10 = R$, initially.) In Fig. 2B, the contact parameter is

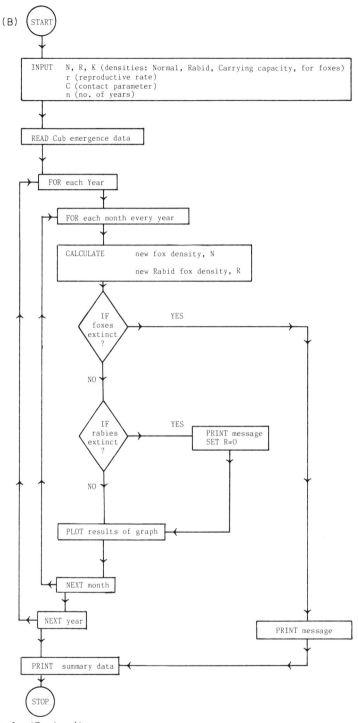

(B)

START

INPUT   N, R, K (densities: Normal, Rabid, Carrying capacity, for foxes)
        r (reproductive rate)
        C (contact parameter)
        n (no. of years)

READ Cub emergence data

FOR each Year

FOR each month every year

CALCULATE   new fox density, N

               new Rabid fox density, R

IF foxes extinct ?   YES

NO

IF rabies extinct ?   YES   PRINT message
                                    SET R=0

NO

PLOT results of graph

NEXT month

NEXT year

PRINT message

PRINT summary data

STOP

Fig. 1.   (*Continued.*)

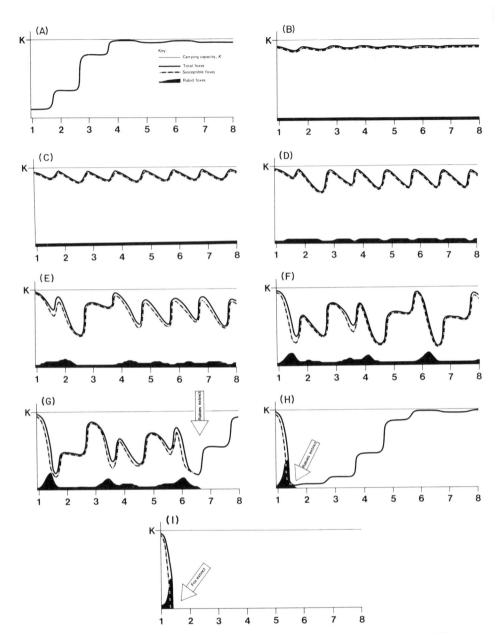

Fig. 2. (A–F). Results from the simple rabies model showing numbers of foxes, relative to carrying capacity K, against time in years since the disease started, for various levels of the contact ratio parameter. The thick solid line represents total fox density, both susceptible and rabid; the black shading represents rabid foxes; the dashed line shows the separate total of susceptible foxes when this can, on the graph, be distinguished from 'total foxes'.

Note that, as the value of the contact parameter increases through the graphs on Fig. 2B–I, that the level of the fox population is increasingly depressed below K with rising variability, leading eventually to oscillations and extinctions. See text for details. (B) $C = 0.0010$; (C) $C = 0.0011$; (D) $C = 0.0012$; (E) $C = 0.0014$; (F) $C = 0.0018$; (G) $C = 0.0020$; (H) $C = 0.0026$; (I) $C = 0.0028$.

TABLE I

Parameters Used in the Simple Model RABSHR.BAS

Factor	Value(s)												
Number of foxes at start	1000												
Number of rabid foxes at start	10												
Carrying capacity, K	1000												
Per capita fecundity	2	(1–3 reasonable)											
Contact ratio value	0.002												
	[0.001–0.003 : scaled relative to K (see text)]												
Month	J	F	M	A	M	J	J	A	S	O	N	D	
Proportion cubs emerging per month	0	0	0	0	0	0	0	0	0.2	0.6	0.2	0	
Number years to simulate	15	(5–100)											

0.0010, and rabies remains at a low level throughout the simulation; eventually, rabies become extinct ($R < 1$) in year 12. In Fig. 2C, the contact parameter is 0.0011, and rabies persists for at least 12 years, causing minor fluctuations in fox population density from K, of around 5% of the magnitude of K. In Fig. 2D, the contact parameter is 0.0012; rabies persists for at least 12 years and now shows annual fluctuations in numbers of rabid animals, whose frequencies rise on occasion to 2% of K. The amplitude of the annual variation in fox numbers is now around 30% of K and is still regular. Apart from an initial fluctuation in the first 2 years, the pattern of Fig. 2D is repeated with wider fluctuations in Fig. 2E, with the contact parameter of 0.0014. However, in Figure 2F, a bi-annual cycle becomes apparent when the contact parameter is 0.0018: the population crashes as rabies rises rapidly, regains its level slightly in the second year as rabies becomes less common, but, as the level rises a second time at the end of year 2, another rabies outbreak is triggered, and the 2-year cycle recommences.

In Fig. 2G, with the contact parameter of 0.0020, a high amplitude 2- to 3-year cycle starts, but, part way through the second repeat of this cycle, the numbers of rabid foxes drop so low that rabies becomes extinct ($R < 1$) in year 6. In Fig. 2H, with the contact parameter of 0.0026, the initial outbreak is so severe that rabies becomes extinct in the first year. Finally, in Fig. 2I, with the contact parameter of 0.0028, the initial outbreak is so severe that both foxes and rabies become extinct (both N and $R < 1$) in the first few months.

These overall outcomes are summarised in Table II for two different fecundity levels—1.0 and 2.0 per capita—the latter value being that used in Fig. 2A–I. The overall outcome agrees broadly with a simple, continuous time deterministic model of rabies [Anderson et al. (1981); see Smith, Chapter 6, this volume]. When the contact parameter is, (1) below threshold, rabies dies out; (2) when just

TABLE II

Summary of Results from RABSHR.BAS Model

Extinction of		Values of contact parameter when		Outcome
Rabies	Foxes	Fecundity = 1.0	Fecundity = 2.0	
Yes	No	$C < 0.00100$	$C \leq 0.00100$	Slight initial decrease in N followed by extinction of R
No	No	$0.0011 < C < 0.0013$	$0.0011 < C < 0.0016$	N decreases to about 70% of K and both N and R fluctuate annually
No	No	$0.0014 < C < 0.0015$	$0.0016 < C < 0.0019$	decreases of N to less than 70% of K with 2–3 year cycles of N and R
Yes	No	$0.0015 < C < 0.0027$	$0.0019 < C < 0.0028$	Rapid initial drop in N, eventual extinction of R N then recovers
Yes	Yes	$C > 0.0027$	$C > 0.0028$	Catastropic drop in N; both N and R become extinct.

above threshold, both rabies and foxes persist, with small annual fluctuations. As the contact parameter rises well above threshold, the amplitudes of these fluctuations increase, eventually leading to (3) multiannual cycles; (4) extinction of rabies, and (5) extinction of both foxes and rabies.

These latter regions (4 and 5) were not specifically predicted by Anderson *et al.* (1981), simply because they did not include extinction thresholds, but they did indicate that such extinctions, particularly of rabies, were likely: their model also predicts damped oscillations, which can also be seen in Fig. 2, and they subsequently showed that seasonal factors would lengthen the dampening period (Anderson, 1982).

II. A More Complex Model

A. ELABORATION OF THE SIMPLE MODEL

The difference equation model just described is clearly over-simple, but its form, particularly as a computer program, can be readily expanded to investigate more complex aspects of the host–pathogen dynamics (such an expansion is described later). The overall form of the following model has been unchanged since early 1979, and some results from it reported elsewhere (Bacon and Macdonald, 1980; Macdonald and Bacon, 1982). However, the present program, listed in Appendix 2, has been simplified extensively from the original version (which developed piecemeal), and I am most grateful to Andreas Aigner for undertaking most of this revision, and, simultaneously, for providing a thorough check on my original logic and mathematics.

The structure of the model is shown in Fig. 3A, and a simplified flow diagram in Fig. 3B. The main differences from the foregoing model are as follows:

1. Addition of natural mortality, which may vary seasonally.
2. Variable distributions of incubation periods.
3. Seasonal variability in the contact-ratio parameter.
4. The inclusion of 'control' sub-routines to assess, in the model, the efficacy of various strategies for eliminating rabies, such as (1) killing foxes (2) temporarily sterilising foxes and (3) vaccinating foxes.

It should also be noted that the model has been made 'dimensionless' by scaling fox densities and rabid fox densities (N and R) relative to the carrying-capacity threshold, K. This scaling has been done for simplicity and convenience. As it is known that, in a dimensional model (e.g. Smith, Chapter 6, this volume), the parameter values are plausible, but as we are in practice unable to measure K, K' threshold or C with reasonable certainty, it is a useful and fair simplification to initially drop this dimension K from the model, but see Mollinson, Chapter 9, this volume, for some consequences of this approximation: the dynamic behaviour will be unaltered by the dimension chosen, (i.e. for any dimensioned value of K a value of C could be found to mimic that behaviour if K were expressed in any other unit). In addition, the procedure of scaling N relative to $K = 1.0$ has the attractive result of making the contact-ratio parameter, C, dimensionless and per capita, so that the values of C used in the model represent average susceptibles infected per rabid during its infectious stage.

B. MODEL FEATURES AND FORMULAE

These will be described first for the fox–rabies section of the model only; consideration of the control sections is deferred until later.

1. 'Births' or Cubs Emerging from the Den

'Births' have been made seasonal and density-dependent. It has been assumed that cubs do not contribute significantly to the disease until they emerge from their dens [this assumption could be wrong, but there is no clear evidence suggesting otherwise (Steck, 1982)], hence the births are scheduled for autumn. As fox numbers vary seasonally and during the course of a rabies outbreak, we

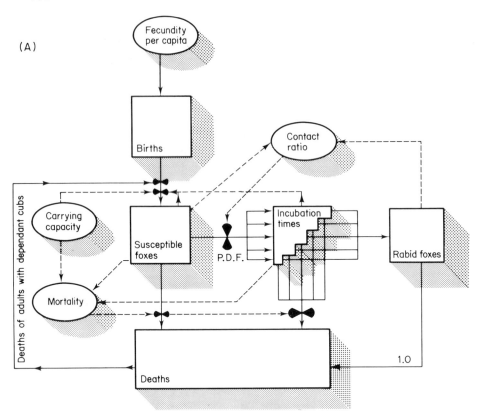

Fig. 3. (A) A diagrammatic model of a more complex description of fox rabies (RAB-BK1.BAS), incorporating variable incubation times. The time delay of rabies incubation now varies according to the Probability Density Function (PDF) of incubation times. Compare with Fig. 1A. (B) Flow diagram for the more complex rabies model, which also incorporates 'fox control' options. The diagram refers to equations in the text [e.g. Equation (*n*)] and line numbers of the computer program (e.g. 1250) listed in Appendix 2.

need to recognise that the maximum numbers of cubs 'born' will depend on the numbers conceived in spring, and the numbers surviving to emerge will depend on their parents' survival to feed them until they are independent. Thus, the equation for 'Births' is as follows:

$$\text{BORN} = \text{SPRD} * \text{FECUND} * \text{FEC(MTH)} * (1\text{-SPRD/KCAP}) * \\ (\text{AUTD/SPRD}) \tag{5}$$

where SPRD is the spring density; AUTD is the autumn density; FECUND is the per capita fecundity; FEC(MTH) is the proportion emerging *this* month; KCAP is the carrying capacity density (*K*).

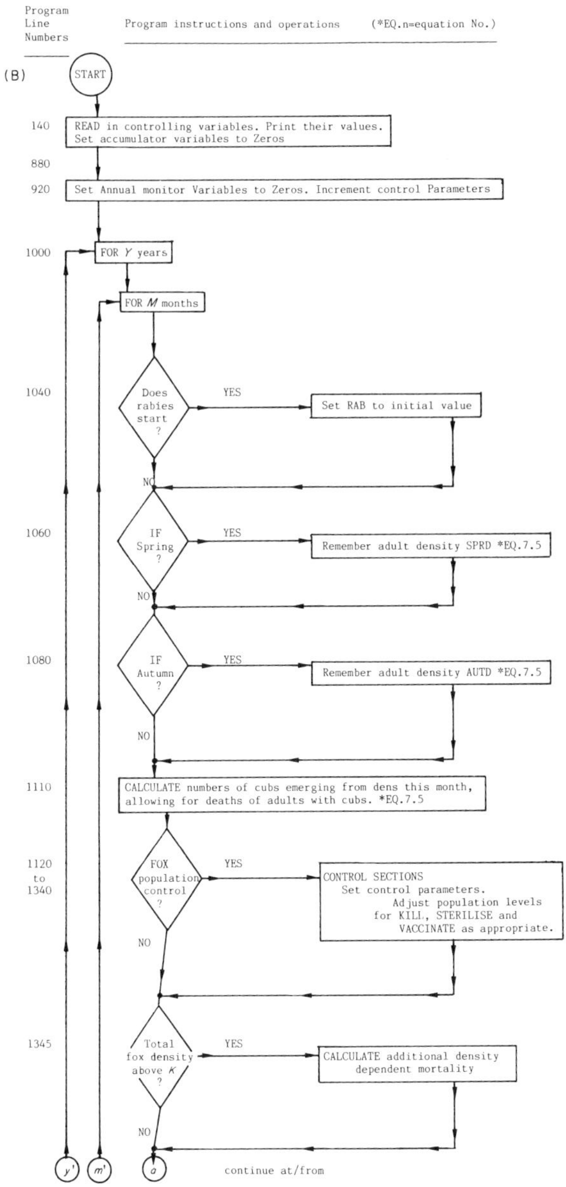

Program Line Numbers
Program instructions and operations (*EQ.n=equation No.)
(B)
START
140
READ in controlling variables. Print their values. Set accumulator variables to Zeros
880
920
Set Annual monitor Variables to Zeros. Increment control Parameters
1000
FOR Y years
FOR M months
1040
Does rabies start ?
YES
Set RAB to initial value
NO
1060
IF Spring ?
YES
Remember adult density SPRD *EQ.7.5
NO
1080
IF Autumn ?
YES
Remember adult density AUTD *EQ.7.5
NO
1110
CALCULATE numbers of cubs emerging from dens this month, allowing for deaths of adults with cubs. *EQ.7.5
1120 to 1340
FOX population control ?
YES
CONTROL SECTIONS Set control parameters. Adjust population levels for KILL, STERILISE and VACCINATE as appropriate.
NO
1345
Total fox density above K ?
YES
CALCULATE additional density dependent mortality
NO
y'
m'
a
continue at/from

Fig. 3. (*Continued.*)

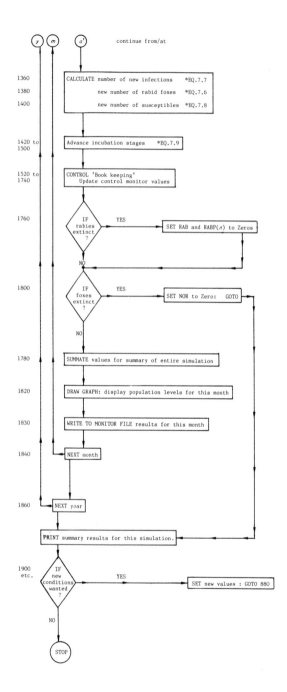

Fig. 3B. (*Continued.*)

2. Mortality

In a *seasonal* discrete-time model, it is no longer sufficient to calculate the net change in numbers (N − deaths + births), as deaths can occur in any month, but births occur only at certain seasons. Approximate estimates of seasonal mortality patterns are available (D. W. Macdonald, personal communication; see Table III), but it is not clear to what extent these mortalities are density dependent. Density dependence is included in the 'Birth' term of this model, and, as mortality and the disease will, for parameter values of interest to us, usually result in numbers being below carrying capacity ($N < K$), seasonal mortalities, which are density independent, would seem reasonable. However, at high densities ($N \gg K$), appreciable extra density-dependent mortality is clearly likely, and it is possible, with the birth Equation (5), for N to overshoot K considerably for some parameter values. If this happens ($N \gg K$), the present model uses a factor to simulate additional mortality, which is density dependent according to the following formula:

TABLE III

Parameters for the More Complex Rabies Model

Factor	Value
Carrying capacity, K	1.00000
Initial density of healthy foxes	0.99990
Initial density of rabid foxes	0.00010
Extinction limits	
Fox and Rabid fox limits	0.00001
Per capita births per year	2 (0.5–4)
Contact ratio parameter	2 (0.5–4)
Annual mortality, approximately	25%

Month	J	F	M[a]	A	M	J	J	A[a]	S	O	N	D
Breeding cycle												
Proportion cubs emerging per month	0	0	−1	0	0	0	0	−2	0.2	0.6	0.2	0
Percentage mortalities by month	3	3	1.5	0.5	0.5	0.5	0.5	0.5	3	3	3	3
Contact ratio adjustments per month												
Scenarios 1 and 2	1	1	1	1	1	1	1	1	1	1	1	1
Scenario 3	1	3	1	1	1	1	1	1	1	2	2	1

Incubation times: durations							
months of incubation	1	2	3	4	5	6	7
Percentage incubating N months:							
Scenario 1	100						
Scenarios 2 and 3	42	25	12	8	6	4	3

[a] Control codes; in the Cubs-emerging-per-month vector of values. The value −1 signifies spring conceptions, so RD is set. The value −2 signifies cubs are independent, so AUTD is set.

$$DDEC = 1.0 - [MORTAL * MORT(MTH)]$$
$$* [(NOR + RABT)/KCAP] \qquad (6)$$

where DDEC is the density dependent survival adjustment factor; MORTAL is the severity adjustment factor, usually 1.0; MORT(MTH) is the density independent mortality for this month; NORM is the fox density; RABT is the total of rabid and incubating fox densities; KCAP is the carrying capacity.

Equation (6) should be interpreted in relation to Equations (7)–(9). Experience of the model shows that, for most parameter values of interest to us, $N < K$ so frequently that the stabilising effects of Equation (6) are rarely utilised (see Section III,A).

3. New Infections

As before, contacts between rabids and susceptibles are assumed to be density dependent according to the formula,

$$RAB1 = NOR * RAB * CONTRATE * CONT(MTH) \qquad (7)$$

where RAB1 is the fresh infections this month; NOR is the density of susceptibles this month; RAB is the density of infectious rabids, this month; CONTRATE is the contact–ratio parameter; CONT(MTH) is the seasonal contact modifying factor, usually 1.0.

4. Infectious Rabids

This density is calculated from the surviving incubators with 1 month incubation remaining, modified by mortality: mortalities are the same for all classes of fox (susceptible, immune, incubating,):

$$RAB = RABN(1) * (1.0 - mortality) \qquad (8)$$

Susceptible foxes remaining are as follows:

$$NOR = [NOR - RAB1 + BORN] * (1.0 - mortality) \qquad (9)$$

5. Incubation Periods

The probability density function for incubation periods is stored in a matrix RABP (i), containing the proportions of infections having incubation periods of $1, 2, 3, \ldots, n$ months. The array RABN(i) is initially set to zeros and running totals subsequently held in it for the different incubation periods, which are updated each month according to the following formula.

$$RABN(i) = [RABN(i + 1) + RAB1 * RABP(i)]$$
$$* (1.0 - mortality) \qquad (10)$$

where i varies from 1 to (maximum incubation period $- 1$) and RABN(max $+ 1$) = zero.

Any reader requiring further details of the calculations is referred to the program listing in Appendix 2, but is recommended to read the description of the 'control option' variables (given in Section III) before studying the program in detail. The parameter values normally used in the model are given in Table III.

III. Results from the Model

A. FOX POPULATION DYNAMICS

The equations given above for the dynamics of the fox population are fairly complicated and slightly unconventional, so we should first satisfy ourselves that they are a reasonable description of a fox population without rabies. This test can be accomplished by observing the behaviour of the model in the absence of rabies. Figure 4 illustrates such results, starting with low fox density in year 1 (N = 0.10) and showing how the population builds up towards carrying capacity over 8 years, with per capita fecundities varying from 0.5 to 5.0 (equivalent to 1.0–8.0 cubs per litter emerging at independence). With the lowest fecundity (0.5 per caput), the overall births only just counterbalance overall deaths, and there is hardly any net increase; with a fecundity of 1.0, the population only

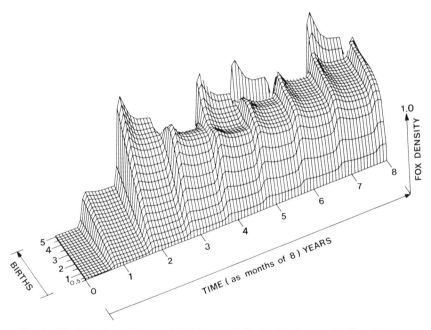

Fig. 4. The behaviour of the modelled fox population in the absence of rabies, for the more complex model. The density of the fox population, relative to $K = 1.0$, is plotted, Z axis, from low-starting densities against (1) time in years, X axis and (2) per capita birth rates, r, Y axis. The model behaviour can be seen to be reasonable for the likely range of per capita births ($r = 0.5–4.0$).

reaches 80% of carrying capacity after 8 years; with a fecundity of 2.0, the population reaches carrying capacity in year 4, and it is thereafter maintained just below it; with fecundity at 2.5, carrying capacity is slightly exceeded after cub emergence in year 3, and extra (density-dependent) mortality, of ~0.3% for a single month, is invoked by the model for the first time; this extra mortality is invoked about 2 times a year, for fecundities from 3.0 to 4.0, and keeps the population in check. However, with a fecundity of 4.5–5.0 or above, the system becomes unstable, in that births outweigh deaths to such an extent that, even with the extra mortality allowing for additional density dependent losses, the population stays above carrying capacity for long periods. When this happens, the birth term becomes negative, implying unrealistic catastrophic deaths on cub emergence, and the model population is thereby thrown into severe oscillations (indeed, if fecundity is increased to around 5.5–6.0, these oscillations become so extreme that the model population becomes extinct. However, such unrealistically high fecundities are not subsequently used, and the extra mortality is only very rarely invoked in the model runs reported throughout this chapter).

In Fig. 4 the fecundity was deliberately varied up to a maximum of 5.0 to illustrate the unrealistic behaviour of the model equations in the birth parameter range above 4. However, for litter sizes from 1.0–8.0 (fecundity 0.5–4.0 per caput), which adequately span the likely range of values of mean population litter sizes at cub independence, the model behaviour is good. Accordingly, it seems fair to assume that the model equations are satisfactory for our present purpose, that the model will produce tolerable behaviour for all likely values of fecundity (e.g. 0.5–4.0), and that a realistic fecundity value of 2.0 (litter size of approximately 4 at emergence in the absence of density-dependence) will achieve this satisfactory behaviour, in general, without even invoking our slightly novel method of accounting for density-dependent mortality.

B. FOX–RABIES DYNAMICS

The present model clearly contains too many parameters for it to be feasible, much less useful, to illustrate all possible outcomes for the whole range of likely parameters. Accordingly, we will first examine the effects of two major factors—fecundity and contact rate—in three different scenarios of other factors, and then we will proceed to a simple sensitivity analysis of the third scenario, which we argue is the more realistic. The two main factors we shall examine as different scenarios are as follows:

1. The distribution of incubation time periods.

2. Seasonal variations in the contact ratio. These will be presented as three scenarios, as shown in Table IV.

These scenarios correspond to differing assumptions that might be built into simpler models, and it is our purpose to illustrate what the effects of these

TABLE IV

Values of Fecundity and Contact Ratio in Three Scenarios

Scenario	Incubation period	Contact ratios
1	1 month only	Uniform (not seasonal)
2	Variable	Uniform
3	Variable	Vary with season

assumptions would be. For each scenario, we will present (1) a three-dimensional time series graph showing the effect of rabies on the fox population, similar to Fig. 4, but starting with the fox population at K, and illustrating only the final situation as represented by the last few years of a 100-year simulation, with fecundity constant at 2.0 and the contact ratio varying from 0.8 to 4.0 (Figs 5, 6 and 7, respectively); (2) time-series graphs, similar to those of Fig. 2, showing levels of foxes and rabid foxes for specified contact ratio and fecundities, illustrating both the initial 5 years and the final 5 years of a 100-year simulation (Figs 8, 9 and 10, respectively); (3) three-dimensional graphs illustrating the effects of varying, simultaneously, fecundity and contact ratio on the overall outcome as illustrated by (a) average fox density, (b) average rabid density (c) variation in fox density (Figs 11, 12 and 13A–C, respectively; all averaged over a 100-year simulation).

C. SCENARIO 1

The results are illustrated in the time-series graph of Fig. 5 for the last 5 years. As the contact ratio varies from 0.8 to 4.0, outcomes broadly similar to those of the simpler model for Fig. 2 are evident. Below a contact ratio of about 1.2, rabies dies out, and it also dies out above a contact ratio of about 3.0 (following a crash in fox numbers). In both cases, the *outcome,* as shown in Fig. 5, is the same, resulting in plateau fox populations once rabies has died out. If the contact ratio goes above 3.4, both foxes and rabies suffer early catastrophic extinction, so that no results can be illustrated for years 95–100. In the intervening range of the contact parameter (1.5–3.0), we move from depressed fox population with annual fluctuations to a 3- to 4-year cycle in fox abundance. We should note that the seasonality of both fox births and fox mortality are alone sufficient to synchronise the system on an annual basis: note that the ridges and troughs of the fox numbers are continually perpendicular to the time axis [confirmed when the three-dimensional graphs of Figs 5, 6 and 7 are viewed from this aspect (not illustrated)].

Turning now to the graph of Fig. 8, we may confirm our interpretations of Fig. 5 and note more clearly the form of the epidemic and the level and pattern of

Figs 5, 6 and 7. The modelled variations of
fox densities with time, at the end of 100-year
simulations, for varying values of the contact
ratio parameter. The different figures (5, 6, 7)
correspond to different scenarios of other parameters (scenarios 1,2,3 respectively, see text).
Note: Within each figure, how the nature of fluctuations in fox densities vary with the contact
ratio and, between the figures, how they change
for the same values of contact ratio depending on
the scenario (see text for details). Further details
are shown by Figs 8,9,10A–C, which correspond to 'sections' through these three-dimensional graphs, with additional information.

(5)

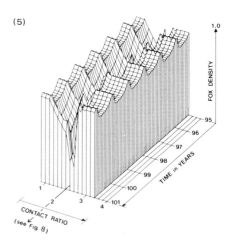

Figs 8, 9 and 10. Modelled variations in
densities, relative to K, of the following: total
foxes, susceptible foxes, rabid foxes and foxes
incubating rabies plotted against time, at both
the beginnings and ends of 100-year simulations. The figures (8,9,10) refer to scenarios
1,2,3, respectively. See text and Figs. 5,6, and 7
for further details.

Note the different outcomes between the scenarios when contact ratio = 2.0 (Figs 8,9,10B)
and the differences in outcomes of scenario 3
(Figs 10A–C) for contact ratios 1.5, 2.0, 2.5,
respectively. Similar graphs, not illustrated,
show that for many combinations of parameters
the patterns of fluctuations established in the early simulated years persist throughout the 100-
simulated years (e.g. Figs 8,9,10A and C),
while other parameter combinations may start
with multi-annual cycles which dampen and reg-
ularise over simulated time (e.g. Fig 10B).

(6)

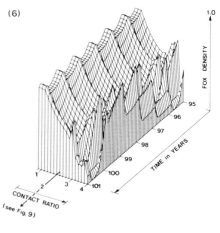

(7)

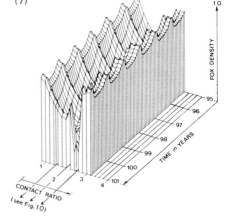

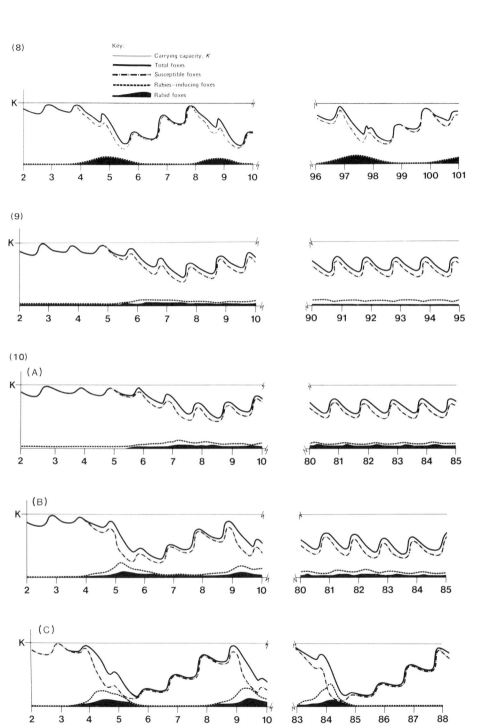

occurrence of rabies: a contact ratio of 2.0 gives 3- to 4-year cycles with a fairly high and long drawn-out incidence of rabies during the epidemic phase. The three-dimensional graphs of Fig. 11 illustrate the outcomes for the whole of the likely realistic ranges of contact ratio and fecundity. Figure 11A confirms the existence of two rabies extinction plateaus on either side of an endemic–epidemic valley in the response surface. It is interesting to note the projections into this epidemic valley of ridges of the second rabies extinction plateau (for contact ratios of about 2.2); these presumably arise from the interactions between the epidemic period and the seasonal emergence of fox cubs. Further illustrated as the top right-hand corner of Fig. 11A is a catastrophic dual extinction region, caused by both high fecundity and high contact ratio, representing the early extinction of both foxes and rabies. These interpretations are borne out by Figs 11B and C, which illustrate the average density of rabies and the standard deviation of fox numbers, respectively, over the whole 100-year simulation period.

D. SCENARIO 2

With variable incubation times (see Table III), the results are strikingly different from those of Scenario 1. In Fig. 6, we see that the region of oscilellatory, cyclic behaviour has been extended into a higher range of the contact parameter: extreme cycles now occur in the range $3 < C < 4$, whereas, previously, this happened in the range $2 < C < 3$, with the system becoming unstable when $C > 3.4$. Figure 9, again, shows a time-series section through Fig. 6 when $C = 2.0$: this section starts with annual variations in fox numbers, which, although variable, are closely similar and which, by years 95–100, have settled into a regular *annual* pattern.

The dramatic change in overall outcome is most clearly shown by contrasting Fig. 12A with Fig. 11A: Figure 12A shows only a single rabies extinction plateau at low contact ratios. The second rabies extinction plateau of Fig. 11A ($2.8 < C < 3.6$) has been smoothed out completely, and we may confirm, from Fig. 12B and C, respectively, that the whole parameter space above $C = 2$ results in relatively high averages of rabid foxes, and high to extreme variation in fox numbers between months and years. The inclusion of longer incubation periods [which also increase the mean incubation period relative to the typical (model) value of a month] clearly helps perpetuate the disease by promoting the persistence of rabies through the periods of low population densities.

E. SCENARIO 3

In addition to variable incubation times, the contact-ratio parameter is now increased in spring and autumn (see Table III) and produces a further profound effect on the overall outcome of the model. We may see from Fig. 7 that, at the end of 100 year simulations, the incorporation of seasonally increased contacts has 'reverted' to an outcome more similar to Scenario 1 than to Scenario 2. The extreme cyclic patterns are again confined to around $1.8 < C < 2.6$, there is a narrow rabies extinction plateau ($2.8 < C < 3.2$) and a catastrophic extinction plane for both foxes and rabies (when $C > 3.2$). Figure 10 shows time-series sections for three values of contact ratio for this scenario. Figure 10A ($C = 1.5$) goes quickly into annual cycles of regular magnitude; with $C = 2.0$, in Fig. 10B, the system starts with a 3- to 4-year cycle, but the magnitude of the 3- to 4-year fluctuation decreases and, by the end of the simulation (years 80 onwards), it has been damped to a regular annual oscillation. With $C = 2.5$, in Fig. 10C, we start with a 4–5 year cycle, which is maintained throughout the whole 100 years of the simulation. Figures 13A–C confirm these deductions: Fig. 13A shows a narrow rabies extinction plateau when $3.0 < C < 3.4$, followed by a catastrophic double extinction plane when $C > 3.4$. Figure 13B shows that numbers of rabid foxes are now high over much of the parameter space and Fig. 13C shows that the long-term fluctuations in fox numbers (i.e. 3- to 5-year cycles) are occurring at higher contact ratios ($2.4 < C < 2.8$ as compared to $1.8 < C < 2.2$ in Fig. 11C).

F. ASSESSMENT

Starting with a very simple difference equation model (Figs 1 and 2), we developed a more realistic and complex model (Figs 3–13), which is capable of generating the whole range of expected outcomes within reasonable parameter limits. Before going on to a sensitivity analysis of this model, we should re-member that the simulations illustrated so far show that considerable differences in overall behaviour can be generated by parameter changes, which are small compared with the accuracy with which we can estimate them from field data. We should further remember that the simulation results are as follows: (1) deter-ministic, (2) for a closed–isolated fox population with no spatial heterogeneity nor even spatial mixing, (3) averaged over a very long time period compared with field data. Accordingly, while the overall outcome of a simulation may show 3- to 5-year cycles damping to regular annual cycles after a few decades, we should remember that, in practice, stochastic extinction of rabies in local *spatial* pockets is much more likely than this model implies and would lead to more rapid recovery of local fox density. Because spatially adjacent habitat areas are unlikely to cycle in synchrony, it is quite likely that cycles could be perpetu-ated by a stochastic mechanism causing rapid local recovery of foxes (after local extinction of rabies) followed by a repeat epidemic caused by re-infection from an adjacent area. It would be fairly straightforward to set up a two-compartment theoretical system to demonstrate such an effect, but, yet again, rather hard to get data sufficient to validate such a model. In short, when considering the following sensitivity analysis, we should remember that it analyses the sensitivity of the

Figs 11, 12 and 13. The average outcomes, over 100-year simulations, of modelled fox rabies depending on the simultaneous varying of two driving parameters: (1) per capita fecundity, X axis, (2) contact ratio, Y axis. The vertical scales represent the responses of three output variables: figure (rows) A: average fox density, figure (rows) B: average rabid fox density (Note: different scale) and figure (rows) C: standard deviation of fox population density. The figure numbers (11,12, and 13; arranged as columns) represent results from Scenarios 1,2,3, respectively. For each response (rows A,B,C) contrast the widely differing shapes of response surface between the scenarios (columns). See text for details.

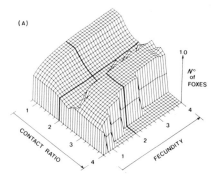

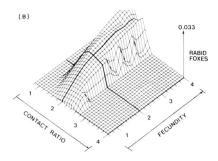

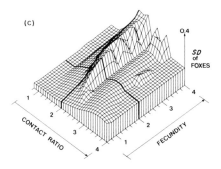

Fig. 11

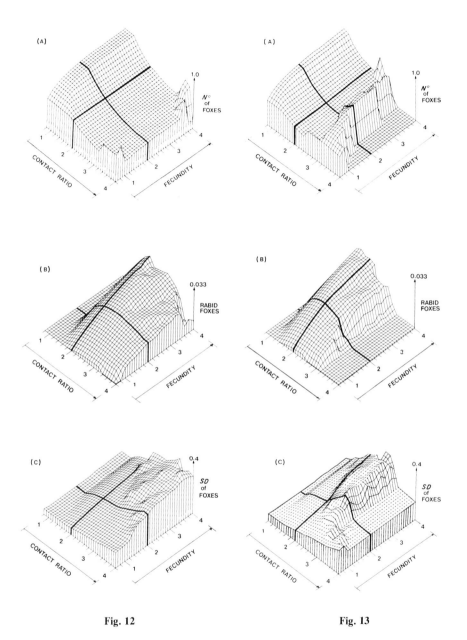

Fig. 12   Fig. 13

169

model, and, if the model is unrealistic, its sensitivity to changes of the model parameters may be a poor guide to the likely effects of these factors in reality.

IV. Sensitivity Analysis of the Model

A. METHOD OF SENSITIVITY ANALYSIS

As a rough guide to the behaviour of this model, we can consider designing an experiment, using the model, where we investigate the effects of making minor changes to the values of a list of driving parameters. Such an experiment can conveniently be set up as a Factorial Analysis of Variance (FACT ANOVA) design.

Consider the six factors shown in Table V: We could choose likely values for these, and vary them all by 5%. This procedure will give us two levels, or values, for each factor, so there will be $2^6 = 64$ different possible combinations of the factors; this number of runs of the model, 64, will allow us to assess, in the near neighbourhood of these chosen values, the relative importances of the model's parameters and also the interactions between them. A full description of such sensitivity testings and their limitations can be found in Dent and Blackie (1979) and Kleijnen (1972). Ideally, more than two levels of each factor should be used to permit clearer interpretation, but the realism of the present model is not sufficient to warrant such rigour. As the model is deterministic, it would be pointless to replicate each run, as there can be no stochastic 'error': this means we will have to use the sums of squares (SSQS) of the higher-order interaction effects to estimate the error variance when testing the main effects and first-order interactions. The simulation program can be readily modified to perform the 64 simulations by adding six nested loops to vary the values of the six choosen variables. The data used start as those given in Table III and are then increased by 5%.

TABLE V

Six Driving Parameters of Model Used in Sensitivity Analysis

Driving parameter in model	Term used in text
A Fox fecundity	Fecundity
B Contact ratio	Contact ratio
C Fox mortality	Mortality
D Mean of incubation period for rabies	Incubation mean
E SD of incubation period for rabies	Incubation SD
F Relative magnitude of seasonal variation in contact ratio	Seasonality

B. FIRST RUN OF SENSITIVITY ANALYSIS

In the first instance, the values shown in Table III were all increased by 5%, the 64 simulations each were run for 100 years, and summaries of (1) average fox density, (2) fox population SD (3) average rabid fox density, (4) fox extinction year and (5) rabies extinction year printed. Perhaps the most important result was that the model rabies became extinct in 6 of the 64 simulations: in each of these six cases, the magnitude of the seasonality of contact ratios (Factor 6) was always 5% high. This outcome is crucial both to our previous understanding and to our interpretation of any other sensitivity tests. Figures 11, 12 and 13, which demonstrated the effects of simultaneously altering fecundity and contact ratio, suggested that minor alterations of either of these two control variables, in the region Fec = 2, Cont = 2, would not greatly affect the outcome. However, we have just seen that similar minor alteration of control variables previously held constant can alter the outcome drastically, causing extinction of rabies in regions which otherwise showed long-lasting cycles. Accordingly, if we wished to obtain a full understanding of this model, we would need to investigate its threshold behaviours in respect of all likely values, and the combinations thereof, for each driving variable. As the model is not sufficiently realistic to justify such a large effort, we will proceed by investigating its (approximate) *local sensitivity only,* close to the region specified by the parameter values listed in Table III, and recognising that even minor changes could greatly affect the outcome.

C. SECOND RUN OF SENSITIVITY ANALYSIS

The controlling data were kept predominately as listed in Table III: 'second level' parameters were increased by 5% of these values for factors A–E, but factor F (magnitude of seasonal contact-changed) was *decreased* by 5%. With this set of control parameters, all 64 simulations modelled for 100 years without leading to extinction of either foxes or rabies, so a reasonable analysis could be undertaken.

D. SENSITIVITY OF WHICH OUTPUT VARIABLES?

The model output produced 64 average values of (1) fox density, (2) fox population SD and (3) rabid density: a fox ecologist might be interested in the sensitivity of (1), a conservationist in (1) and (2), and a health official in (3). There is no reason to believe that each factor would be similarly affected by all the changed parameters: Do we then need to investigate three different sensitivities? This difficulty can be simplified by performing some simple multivariate analyses on these three output data types.

Table VI lists the means, over the 64 runs, of each output parameter, and

TABLE VI

Output Variables Produced by Model for Sensitivity Analysis

Output variable	Mean level	CV (%)[a]
Fox population mean/month	0.45	1.6
Fox population SD/month	0.24	9.5
Rabid fox mean/year	0.19	7.5

[a] CV% = coefficient of variation = (SD/Mean)*100.

indicates by how much they vary: Table VII presents a correlation matrix of these three output variables, showing that two—fox SD and average rabids, are highly correlated. This relation makes good sense, because foxes die from rabies, which would be likely to increase the population's seasonal variance. Principal component analysis of the correlation matrix of Table VII is summarised in Tables VIII and IX and shows that the model's outputs can be reduced from the three dimensions to two dimensions because of the high intercorrelation of the fox SD and average rabids. The main dimension of the output derives from a contrast between the average number of rabids and the fox population SD, and explains two-thirds of the total output variance. The second dimension, explaining most of the remaining one-third of the variance, is the average magnitude of the fox population density. The residual 4% of variation in the final axis is unlikely to be important. This analysis suggests that the essential changes in the model output can be summarised in a two-dimensional diagram, as will be illustrated later (Fig. 14).

TABLE VII

Correlation Half Matrix of Output Parameters

Correlation coefficients	Correlated variables		
Correlated variables	Fox population (mean)	Fox population (SD)	Rabids/year (mean)
Fox population (mean)	1	—	—
Fox population (SD)	0.089	1	—
Rabids/year (mean)	0.34	−0.884[a]	1

[a] $P < 0.001$

TABLE VIII

Principal Component Analysis (PCA) of Model Output Values

Output factor	Eigen value	% variance	
		Component	Cumulative
Axis 1	1.88	62.8	62.8
Axis 2	1.01	33.6	96.4
Axis 3	0.11	3.6	100.0

E. FACTORIAL ANALYSES OF VARIANCE

On the basis of the above PCA analysis, factorial analysis of variance was carried out to investigate the sensitivity of (1) Fox numbers and (2) Rabid fox numbers to variations of the six driving parameter values: Because of the high intercorrelation of fox population SD with average rabids, the former can be considered sensitive to the same parameters.

As mentioned above, the error sum of squares had to be approximated by high-order interaction terms: the highest-order interaction, 5th order, has only 1 degree of freedom in a 2^6th design, and this number of degrees of freedom is too few for any test of significance with reasonable sensitivity; the 4th order interactions have 6 df, giving a total of 7 df for 5th- and 4th-order interactions, a number of degrees of freedom that is adequate but low; the 3rd-order interactions have 15 df, giving 22 df for sum of the 3d-, 4th- and 5th-order interactions; while 22 df would be preferable to 7 df, it is possible that some 3d order interactions could represent real effects, thereby unduly inflating the (approximated) error sum of squares and hence suggesting differences are less significant than they really are.

The sum of squares for the 5th-order interaction was first used as an estimate

TABLE IX

Eigen Vectors Scaled to Maximum of 1.0

Order of PCA axes	Axis represents	Fox population (mean)	Fox population (SD)	Rabid foxes/year (mean)	Main factors on axis
Axis 1	Contrast	0.062	1.000	−0.996	Fox SD contrasted with density of rabids
Axis 2	Magnitude	1.000	0.038	0.101	Fox mean
Axis 3	NS[a]	(−0.138)	(1.000)	(0.996)	NS[a]

[a] NS, not significant.

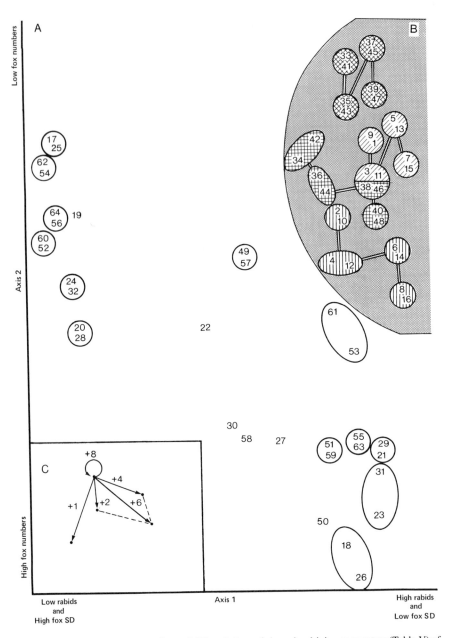

Fig. 14. Illustration of the effects of 5% variations of six major driving parameters (Table V) of the complex rabies model. The outcomes of combinations of the parameters are shown in two-dimensional Canonical Space, as defined by Principal Components Analysis (see Table VII and text). The numbers on Fig. 14A and B are simulation iteration sequence numbers (see Table XI): some pairs of iteration sequence numbers separated by 8 tend to cluster closely and are shown ringed (see text). A portion of the response plane of Fig. 14A is shown shaded in Fig. 14B; within this region

of the error variance, and the 4th-order interactions tested against this sum of squares; none of the 4th-order interactions were approaching a significant effect to this criterion. When the 4th- and 5th-order interaction SSQSs were pooled as a new estimate of the error and when the 3d-order interactions were tested, one of these 15 interactions approached significance ($p < 0.10$). As this particular interaction was later found to combine the effects of four factors, which had significant 1st-order interactions, it was concluded that some 3d-order interaction terms probably represented real effects and should not therefore be included in the estimate of the error sum of squares. Accordingly, the error sum of squares was taken to be estimated by the pooled 4th- and 5th-order interaction sum of squares with 7 *df*.

The sensitivity of the model outputs, for both fox numbers and rabid numbers values, were tested against this estimated error sum of squares, looking for the effects of the six main factors, A–F, (listed in Table V) and their 15 pairwise (1st order) interactions. [Again, these two outputs were chosen because they vary independently of each other, while the third output factor, fox SD, is highly correlated with rabid numbers (see Table VII): accordingly, these two output variables give an adequate picture of the sensitivity of all three output variables to the changes in the model's parameters (Table V)]. The significant effects detected accounted for about two-thirds of the variance of each data set (fox numbers and rabid fox numbers), but with some interesting differences between the two. The results are summarised in Table X. Within the parameter ranges of this analysis, all factors except fox mortality have significant influences on the outcomes, either directly as main effects or indirectly as interactions. By far the most influential factor is the contact ratio, which explains 40% of the variance of each data set. The next most influential factor is the magnitude of seasonal variation of the contact ratio: this is a significant main factor only for the rabid fox density data set (10% of variance), but, in this data set and the fox density data set, it participates in three significant 1st-order interactions, which contribute a total of 15% of explained variance between them. For each data set, the seasonality of contact ratio interacts with (1) actual contact ratio, (2) standard deviation of incubation time and (3) mean incubation time, each interaction explaining about 5% of variation in each data set. Finally, fox fecundity is significant as a main factor in each data set, but explains only about 3% of the variations.

These results make good sense. Previous analysis has shown contact ratio to be important, as has the work of Anderson. *et al.* (see Chapter 6, this volume).

---

fairly consistent changes in relative position are produced by certain changes in iteration sequence numbers. The vectors representing these changes are shown in Fig. 14C, and the relationships between the changes in iteration sequence numbers and the effects of the corresponding driving parameters are explained in the text.

TABLE X

Sensitivity Analysis of the Fox–Rabies Model by FACT-ANOVA, Showing the Percentages of Variance of Variance of Model Outcomes Explained by the Significant Driving Variables,[a] Both Alone and As First-order Interactions with Each Other

	Factor(s)		Fox density		Rabid fox density	
Effect	Main factor	Interacts with:	Average importance	% variance	Average importance	% variance
Main	Contact ratio		1st	40	1st	43
Main	Seasonality of contact ratio		—	—	2nd	10
Interaction	Seasonality of contact ratio	Contact ratio	2nd	7	3rd	5
Interaction	Seasonality of contact ratio	Incubation time SD	3rd	6	4th	4
Interaction	Seasonality of contact ratio	Incubation time mean	4th	5	5th	3
Main	Fecundity		5th	4	6th	3
Total variance explained				62		68
Estimated error variance as a percentage of total variance				0.7		0.4

[a] See Table V for list of driving parameters.

The seasonality of contact ratio, as defined in this model, temporarily elevates the usual contact ratio, so would be expected to have some effect, while its temporary nature means that such an effect is unlikely to be simply additive (and the two factors do interact significantly). Another effect of the Seasonality parameter is to introduce pulses of extra rabid and incubating foxes. The size and time lags between these pulses will affect the chances of the disease persisting, and, as the mean and variance of the incubation times will clearly affect the die-off rates of these pulses, these factors would also be expected to affect the outcome; their significant interactions show clearly that they do. In fact, we would also expect fox mortality, acting on incubating foxes to affect the die-off rates of these 'pulses', but the analysis shows its effect is small and non-significant compared to the other effects. Finally, it is interesting to note that fox fecundity, while clearly important to the overall dynamics of the fox–rabies cycle has less effect, at least on the local behaviour here analysed, than the separate interactions of the other factors.

F. WHAT ARE THE EFFECTS OF THE CONTROLLING FACTORS?

Having discovered from the above factorial analysis of variance that five factors have significant effects on the outcomes of the model, it is pertinent to ask what those effects are. They are illustrated in Fig. 14, especially the shaded part which comprises the two-dimensional plot of the PCA axes referred to above. The vertical axis represents the average fox population density, and the horizontal axis is the contrast between rabid density and fox SD, as indicated. The positions of each of the 64 model runs are shown in these two dimensions, indicated by a serial number, 1–64. The first run, 1, had the lowest of all six values; the second run, 2, kept the first five factors low, but used the 5% higher value of factor F = seasonality of contacts; the third run reverted to the low value for factor F, but increased that for factor E (i.e.: A, B, C, D and F were low; E was high); and so on. Thus, the levels of the factors are changed by nested loops, with factor F changing most rapidly; factor A, fecundity, is hence low for the first 32 runs, and then 5% higher for the last 32 runs; factor B, contact ratio, is low for runs 1–16 and for 33–48 and 5% higher for runs 17–32 and 49–64; and so on, as shown in Table XI.

Now let us look at Fig. 14B, which is the shaded portion in the top right-hand corner of Fig. 14A. Notice that rings have been drawn around spatially close neighbouring pairs of sequence numbers and that these close pairs are consistently separated by 8. This implies that variation in the level of the factor that alters at periods of 8 has negligable effect on the outcomes of the model as, if the other parameters are similar, the outcome is nearly the same. Which factor is this? The period repetition differences are: 1 = seasonality, 2 = incubation SD,

TABLE XI

Levels of Factors A–F in the 64 Iterations of the Sensitivity Analysis[a]

Iteration number	A	B	C	D	E	F	Iteration number	A	B	C	D	E	F
1	L	L	L	L	L	L	33	H	L	L	L	L	L
2	L	L	L	L	L	H	34	H	L	L	L	L	H
3	L	L	L	L	H	L	35	H	L	L	L	H	L
4	L	L	L	L	H	H	36	H	L	L	L	H	H
5	L	L	L	H	L	L	37	H	L	L	H	L	L
6	L	L	L	H	L	H	38	H	L	L	H	L	H
7	L	L	L	H	H	L	39	H	L	L	H	H	L
8	L	L	L	H	H	H	40	H	L	L	H	H	H
9	L	L	H	L	L	L	41	H	L	H	L	L	L
10	L	L	H	L	L	H	42	H	L	H	L	L	H
11	L	L	H	L	H	L	43	H	L	H	L	H	L
12	L	L	H	L	H	H	44	H	L	H	L	H	H
13	L	L	H	H	L	L	45	H	L	H	H	L	L
14	L	L	H	H	L	H	46	H	L	H	H	L	H
15	L	L	H	H	H	L	47	H	L	H	H	H	L
16	L	L	H	H	H	H	48	H	L	H	H	H	H
17	L	H	L	L	L	L	49	H	H	L	L	L	L
18	L	H	L	L	L	H	50	H	H	L	L	L	H
19	L	H	L	L	H	L	51	H	H	L	L	H	L
20	L	H	L	L	H	H	52	H	H	L	L	H	H
21	L	H	L	H	L	L	53	H	H	L	H	L	L
22	L	H	L	H	L	H	54	H	H	L	H	L	H
23	L	H	L	H	H	L	55	H	H	L	H	H	L
24	L	H	L	H	H	H	56	H	H	L	H	H	H
25	L	H	H	L	L	L	57	H	H	H	L	L	L
26	L	H	H	L	L	H	58	H	H	H	L	L	H
27	L	H	H	L	H	L	59	H	H	H	L	H	L
28	L	H	H	L	H	H	60	H	H	H	L	H	H
29	L	H	H	H	L	L	61	H	H	H	H	L	L
30	L	H	H	H	L	H	62	H	H	H	H	L	H
31	L	H	H	H	H	L	63	H	H	H	H	H	L
32	L	H	H	H	H	H	64	H	H	H	H	H	H

[a] Note that, within blocks of 16 iterations (1–16; 17–32; 33–48; 49–64), any pair of iterations separated by 8 (e.g. 1,9) differ in levels (L,H) only at factor C (fox mortality). It is precisely these 'pairs' of iterations that cluster closely in Fig. 14. Other pairwise combinations differing by 8 iterations can readily be found (e.g. 15,23; 32,40; 47,55), which differ in other factors *as well as* C but these do not cluster closely in Fig. 14. (L, low; H, high; see Table III for actual low levels.)

4 = incubation mean, 8 = mortality, 16 = contact ratio, 32 = fecundity, so the trival factor with period 8 is fox mortality, precisely that factor which the factorial analysis of variance showed to be non-significant. Now concentrate on the top right-hand corner of Fig. 14. Look at the pair (33,41); moving down the page, we find (35,43), which are two larger; from here, move up and right (37,45), two larger again; move down from here (39,47). Note that this approximate pattern is repeated within Figure 14B for the quartets of pairs starting (34,42), (1,9) and (2,10).

Now find the pair (1,9) and, using a pencil or ruler, find the distance and direction of this pair from the pair (2,10) (this distance and direction represents a vector translation). Now translate (or move) one end of this vector around the points (1,9), (3,11), (5,13) and (7,15) and confirm that the other end of your vector pointer tracks close to the points (2,10), (4,12), (6,14) and (8,16); check that this result also holds reasonably true for the quartets of pairs starting (33,41) and (34,42) as well. Remembering from above that the factor changing with period 1 = seasonality of contact, the vector we have just discerned represents the effect of increasing seasonality of contact by 5% *in this region of the response plane.* Such a vector, representing a fair 'downward' movement and a slight 'leftward shift' along the axes of Fig. 14 hence represents (1) a decrease in average fox population (vertical axis) with (2) a reduction in numbers of rabids and an elevation of the fox population SD (horizontal axis). In other words, the effect of increased seasonality of contact ratio is to reduce the average fox population density and increase the fox population SD while lowering the average numbers of rabid foxes. If this vector translation were always precise, it would suggest that no other factors interacted with this one; it is not precise, which suggests, as we know from the analysis of variance, that they do interact. Within the confines of Fig. 14B's parameter space, other vectors can be found for periods of 2,4, (6 = 2 + 4), 8 and 32, as illustrated in Fig. 14C, and these can be interpreted using the reasoning given above. The fact that 'period 6' translation ≏ 'period 2' + 'period 4' suggests that these two factors interact very little. Note that, as explained in the legend of Table XI, these iteration changes are only relevant for iteration changes in phase with the actual parameter level changes implemented by the nested loops of the program.

When we turn to the broader canvas of Fig. 14A, representing the larger parameter space of the entire sensitivity analysis, we can see that the intriguing geometric patterns of Fig. 14B (see top right-hand corner) are elsewhere severely disrupted. Ineeed, at first sight they are quite inconspicuous. Note, however, that repetitions separated by 8 still cluster closely and that the (49,57), (51,59) (61,53) (55,63) quartet of pairs resembles the former pattern. Clearly, contact ratio (repetition period = 16) has a major influence on the outcomes, and the lack of any consistent vector to represent its effect illustrates its profound interactions with other factors. Finally, note the symbols in Fig. 14 representing 'near identical outcomes' by several different iterations (e.g. 3,11,38,46). These occurrences clearly show that different combinations of parameter levels can produce effectively the same outcome, at least, in so far as Fig. 14 represents our description of that outcome. In other words, given an outcome as described in Fig. 14, we can not expect to find a unique set of parameters that could give such a result (i.e. the inverse mapping Outcome → Driving parameters is not unique).

G. SUMMARY

Within the localised parameter space investigated (5% variation above 'likely' values for the six controlling parameters of Table IV), the sensitivity analysis shows that all but one (fox mortality) have significant effects on the model's outcomes, either directly, or indirectly. It is interesting that the interactions of factors not usually considered can, in this parameter space, outweigh the effects of fox fecundity. (Note: If one compares the results of this model with that of Anderson *et al.* (1981; see Smith, Chapter 6, this volume), that their model assumes fox fecundity to be density independent, which is almost certain to result in greater effect being attached to the fecundity parameter in their model than in this one). The model is clearly sensitive to these other parameters (which are not considered in simpler models as dynamic interactions): varying these factors by 5% produces changes in the model outputs, expressed as C.V. %, of only 2% for fox density, but as 9% and as 7% for fox population S.D. and rabid fox density respectively (see Table IV). These factors and their interactions clearly have major effects on the model's outcomes. Finally, we should remember that this is a deterministic model, and it is possible that some of the effects discerned by the foregoing analysis would be blurred by random error in a stochastic version of the model, and perhaps even obliterated if the errors were large compared to the changes in the driving variables.

V. Simulated Control Strategies

A. TYPES OF CONTROL AND THEIR INCLUSION IN THE MODEL

The second, more complex, simulation program (Appendix 2) contains some simple coding to allow us to investigate the likely effects of various control strategies. These strategies envisage three forms of manipulation: (1) killing, which is assumed to reduce equally the numbers of both rabid and susceptible foxes, (2) the use of temporary sterilants to depress breeding success and (3) oral vaccination of foxes. These simulation routines are most realistic if we envisage a control system that presents foxes with baits containing poison, sterilant or vaccine respectively, and that a known fraction of the population eats these baits and succumbs to the control. We further assume that bait acceptance is random or that a fox that did not eat a bait in a previous control is not always less likely to eat one. These assumptions may be slightly unrealistic, as it is possible that some foxes are suspicious of novel foods, or that some areas are harder to bait reliably.

Data in the program specify if, when, and for how long control operations are to be modelled for each option, and also how often within this time span the control is repeated. The proportion of foxes affected is also given (always 0.60 in these examples) and, for sterility and immunity, the duration of their effects on individual foxes. Because of adverse effects on other wildlife, it is assumed sterilants would be temporary, lasting a few months (5 is chosen). Vaccine is assumed to give long-lasting protection for several years (4 years chosen).

The computer code contains sections (line: 1120–1180; 1200–1260; 1280–1340), which determine whether, in a particular model month, controls are due to operate. If they are due to operate, then control variables are set to values supplied in the data (e.g. Kill 60%) for this month only, otherwise 'no effect' parameter values are used.

Killing. Killing is incorporated into the mortality formulae in lines 1360, 1400, 1460 and 1680, and it alters the values of variables holding densities of rabid, susceptible foxes, incubating and immune foxes. It is an instantaneous control, and no other records of its effects are needed.

Sterility. Sterility acts on the numbers of foxes born by reducing the density of fertile foxes (lines 1060, 1100 and 1140). As sterility only lasts a few months, and if we assume it is always started in late winter, we may assume all foxes, including juveniles from the previous year, would be sterile, and hence calculate only the cumulative proportion sterilised (lines 1520–1620) as opposed to the numbers sterilised and surviving.

Immunity. The model assumes juvenile foxes do not acquire immunity either from their mother's milk or from 'baits' obtained before they emerge into the adult population. Because of this assumption, all cubs are susceptible, and, as immunity is long-lasting, we hence need to record densities of immune foxes (lines 1640–1740); this density (zero if no vaccine control) is subtracted from the density of susceptible foxes in the formula for fresh infections (line 1380). (*Note:* Anyone intending to use this model is advised that these control routines could be mis-used to produce very unrealistic results—they are not foolproof—so study the coding carefully before providing parameter values.)

B. EFFECTS OF THE DIFFERENT CONTROLS

Killing.   Killing reduces the numbers of rabid, incubating, susceptible and immune foxes. It will hence decrease contacts and infections by decreasing densities. However, density dependent births will counter its effects quite quickly for foxes. In practice, it severely disrupts the fox society, and it may promote movement, strife, and hence contacts in a manner which we cannot here model.

Sterilisation.   Sterilisation reduces birth rate, and hence keeps numbers low for longer after any drop in population, whether the initial drop was caused by control killing, rabies or natural mortality.

Vaccination.   Vaccination reduces the proportion of susceptibles without altering the population density, and hence decreases contacts and future infections. As unvaccinated foxes may die from rabies, their mortality will be higher, and the percentage that is immune will rise slightly from the initial level achieved, until new foxes are born (all of whom will be susceptible) at which time the immunity will fall much more. Accordingly, repeated applications of vaccine will be necessary to maintain a high level of immunity.

C. MODEL BEHAVIOURS

The effects of the different control strategies are illustrated in Figure 15A–H and should be interpreted with some caution. Detailed examination of model results not illustrated here show clearly, as would be expected, that controls reduce the density of rabid foxes to low levels. In such circumstances, a stochastic formulation would be more appropriate. This is perhaps particularly true for vaccination, for which a single application of vaccine can maintain low levels of rabid foxes for long periods. For example, a single spring and autumn application of vaccine to 60% of foxes reduces rabid density to so low a level that less than one rabid fox would be expected to survive per 1000, or less than one in 500 km² in good fox habitat; this result seems to be borne out in practice by field trials in Switzerland for a vaccinated area of 500 km² (see Figure 3 of Steck, 1982). However, to reduce rabid fox densities below 10^{-5} (the extinction limit used in this model) requires repeated spring–autumn vaccinations in the following 2 years.

For consistency with previous examples, the graphs of Fig. 15 have been constructed using an extinction threshold of 1×10^{-5} [<1 fox per 5000 km² good habitat (roughly a 70 × 70 km square)], which is probably over-rigorous for many practical purposes. These graphs should be taken to illustrate the sorts of outcomes that different controls might produce. More realistic assessments

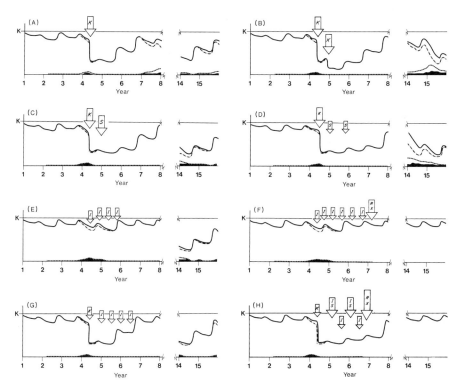

Fig. 15. The effects of different options of fox population control strategies (such as killing, temporary sterilisation, oral vaccination and combinations thereof) on the outcomes of modelled rabies epizootics. The first 7 and last 2 years of 15-year simulations are illustrated. Model rabies is started on the 1st of April of the second simulated year in every case, and the timings and natures of controls are indicated by labelled arrows. In the absence of controls, outcomes would be as shown in Fig. 10B. Note: The criterion for 'successful' control is probably over rigorous, see text. (A) Single Kill: reduces fox and rabid fox densities but disease persists. Control 'FAILS'. (B) Double Kill: foxes and rabid foxes kept lower for longer, but the disease still persists. Control 'FAILS'. (C) Single kill followed by single use of sterilant: foxes and rabid foxes reduced and kept low by effects of sterilisation. Disease persists, control 'FAILS'. (D) Single kill and sterilants used in 2 successive years: relative to C, densities are kept lower for longer, but disease still persists and control 'FAILS'. (E) Oral vaccination (spring and autumn) in 2 successive years: fox densities remain high while rabid fox densities are kept very low for a long time, but disease persists and control 'FAILS'. (F) Oral vaccination (spring and autumn) in 3 successive years: fox densities remain high, but rabid fox densities are kept very, low and the modelled disease becomes extinct (in year 7). Control 'SUC-CEEDS'. (G) Single kill followed by oral vaccination in 2 years: fox and rabid fox densities reduced by the kill, and rabid fox densities reduced to low levels for a long period (kill and vaccination), but disease persists and control 'FAILS'. (H) Single kill followed by both oral vaccination and sterilisation in 2 successive years: fox numbers reduced by kill and kept low by sterilisation; rabid fox numbers reduced by kill and kept low by low fox densities and vaccination. Model rabies becomes extinct in year 6, control 'SUCCEEDS'.

Key to arrow labels:

K, kill; S, sterilisation; I, immunise with vaccine; RX, rabies becomes extinct. Key to lines: same as for Figs 8, 9 and 10.

would require spatial stochastic models (see Chapters 12 and 13, this volume) parameterised with real data.

VI. Conclusions

Starting with some well-known equations for population dynamics and prey–predator interactions, we have developed a simple simulation model of fox rabies, which shows both annual and multiannual cycles. This model was subsequently elaborated to a more complex version. The effects of two major controlling parameters (fecundity and contact ratio) are illustrated for the more complex model, using three scenarios incorporating variations of other parameter values that correspond to differing degrees of simplifying assumptions that are often used in simple models. The levels of both fecundity and contact ratio factors and all the 'assumptions' mimicked by the three scenarios have profound effects on the model's outcomes. The model seems particularly sensitive to changes in contact ratio: Even if we knew which set of other parameters was appropriate, variations in the value of the contact-ratio parameter within (at present) the likely accuracy of its estimation could probably give rise to all extremes of outcome.

It is emphasised that this model lacks both spatial and stochastic elements, and should therefore only be interpreted as illustrating the likely effects of the modelled processes and *not* as realistically mimicking the behaviour of actual rabies outbreaks. Granting this lack of realism of the model, factorial analysis is used to investigate further the local effects of six parameters as driving variables on the model's outcomes. Three output variables are monitored, two of which are highly correlated but independent of the third one. Five of the six parameters have significant effects on both of the two independent output variables that were monitored: three of the significant parameters show their effects as mutual interactions, and these interactions produce greater effects on the outcomes than the direct effect of the parameter for fox fecundity. As fecundity is identified as an important driving variable in simpler models which ignore dynamic interactions between such other parameters, interpretations of such over-simple models should be treated with some caution.

The model incorporates routines to mimic, albeit crudely, the likely effects of different possible techniques for rabies control, such as killing, sterilisation and vaccination. Possible effects of different implementations of such controls are illustrated using the model. Assessment of the relative merits of different control strategies is difficult with a non-spatial deterministic model (particularly for control killing, which would promote violation of the model's assumptions). However, it is tentatively suggested that control by vaccination is preferable and that vaccination strategies, which are already considered safe and technically feasible, should succeed within 2–3 years. This suggestion is supported by one recent field trial of control by vaccination.

Appendix 1. Computer Program of Simple Model, RABSHR

This appendix is given in two parts. Part A is the computer program
which carries out the simulation calculations and Part B is a set of
three simple sub-routines which allow the results to be plotted as a
graph on a printer or VDU. NOTE THAT these identical graph plotting
routines (Annex 1.b) are also used in the more complex rabies model
RABBK1.BAS and are omitted from the listing of that program in
Appendix 2 for the sake of brevity.

The programs are written in BASIC PLUS for a PDP 11/34 computer
with a RSTS/E operating system.

```
      APPENDIX 1.a.
      *************

5     !      New version of QUIKRB.BAS for rabies book chapter,
      !  to fit in with formats of RABAAP.BAS, RABBK1.BAS, etc.

      P.J. BACON              RABSHR.BAS              28.6.82

10    EXTEND
20    DIM FEC(12), PR$(63)
30    GOSUB 5000                      ! set up plotting control
40    INPUT "Total number of FOXES at start < 1000 >  ", NORO
50    INPUT "Total number of RABIDS at start < 10 >  ", RABO
60    INPUT "Per captita birth for foxes < 1 - 3 >  ", FECUND
70    PRINT "Proportion of cubs born emerging in each month "
      FOR I%=1 TO 12 \ READ FEC(I%) \ PRINT FEC(I%) ; \ NEXT I%
/     PRINT \ PRINT
80    DATA 0, 0, 0, 0, 0, 0, .2, .6, .2, 0
      INPUT "Carrying Capacity   < 1000 >  ", KCAP
/     PRINT
//    PRINT "When giving CONTACT-RATIO remember the formula "
//    PRINT "Next_Rabid_numbers = Contact-ratio * RABIDS_NOW * Susceptibles_now"
//    PRINT
/     INPUT "Contact-ratio                            ", CONTR
/     !
100   INPUT "Number of years to print simulation  ", YRS%
140   GOSUB 6000                      ! plot AXIS for graph
145   NOR = NORO - RABO
```

(continued)

Appendix 1. (*Continued*)

```
/           RAB = RABO
/           PR$(63%)=""
/:
150         FOR YR% = 1 TO YRS%
200           FOR MTH% = 1 TO 12
220             RAB1 = CONTR * RAB * NOR
230             NOR1 = NOR - RAB1 + FECUND * ( FEC(MTH%) * (NOR+RAB) * (1.0 - (NOR+RAB)/KCAP ) )
280             IF NOR1 < 1.0 THEN 520
290             NOR = NOR1
                RAB = RAB1
295             IF RAB1 < 1.0  AND  RAB<> 0.0  THEN PR$(63%)="RABIES has DIED OUT !!"
300             IF RAB1 < 1.0  THEN RAB = 0.0
310             GOSUB 8000                        ; plot a line of GRAPH
320           NEXT MTH%
340         NEXT YR%
400         PRINT \ PRINT \ PRINT "Simulation ends OK" \ PRINT \ PRINT
500         STOP
520         PRINT \ PRINT \ PRINT "FOX population EXTINCT !! " \ PRINT \ PRINT
            STOP
/:


APPENDIX 1.b.   GRAPH-plotting routines for RABSHR.BAS and RABBK1.BAS
****************

5000        REM    Subroutine prints Graph Y axis
5020        PLMAX = 1.2
/           PRINT
/           PRINT "Max. value for Plotting is "; PLMAX ;" * Carrying_capacity"
/           PRINT
            MONTH$ = "#J- F M A M J J A S O N D "
5080        RETURN
/:

6000        REM    Subroutine sets up Graph Axis
6020        PRINT "SCALE-factor = ";
/           SCF = (60.0 / PLMAX / KCAP )
```

```
      PRINT SCF
      PRINT
      PRINT
      PRINT "        +++";
            FOR I%=1 TO 30
            PRINT "--";
            NEXT I%
      PRINT "+++++++++"
6080  RETURN

8000  REM    Subroutine prints a line of graph
8020  RMOD = INT( RAB ** SCF + 0.99999 )
      NMOD = INT( NOR ** SCF + 0.99999 )
      TMOD = INT( (NOR+RAB) * SCF + 0.99999 )
8040        FOR I%=1 TO 62
            PR$(I%) = " "
            NEXT I%
8060  IF RMOD > 60.0 THEN RMOD = 61
8080  IF TMOD > 60.0 THEN TMOD = 61
8100  IF NMOD > 60.0 THEN NMOD = 61
8120  PR$(RMOD) = "R"
8140  IF RMOD=NMOD THEN PR$(NMOD)="*"   ELSE PR$(NMOD)="N"
8160  IF TMOD=RMOD THEN PR$(TMOD)="r"   ELSE PR$(TMOD)="T"
8180  IF TMOD=NMOD THEN PR$(TMOD)="n"
8200  IF MTH% <> 1 THEN PRINT " ";   ELSE PRINT USING "### ", YR% ;
8210  PRINT MID$( MONTH$, 3*MTH%-2, 3 ) ;
8220  PRLINE$=""
            FOR I%=1 TO 63
            PRLINE$ = PRLINE$ + PR$(I%)
            NEXT I%
      PRINT CVT$$( PRLINE$, 128% )
8240  PR$(63%)=""
      RETURN

9999  END
Ready
```

Appendix 2. Computer Program of More Complex Model, RABBK1

This version of the program allows several output monitor files to be created, for example those needed to set up the data for plotting the 3-D graphs of Figures 5,7,8,10,11,13. Such sections could be omitted if not needed, but do not add greatly to the program's length, much of which is input/output routines. NOTE THAT the printer/VDU graph plotting routines for this program have been previously listed in Appendix 1.b.

The program is written in BASIC PLUS for a PDP 11/34 computer with a RSTS/E operating system.

```
5        Phil's THIRD 'Tweak-UP' of Andreas Aigner's
      version of CONRBC.BAS
            Var. INCT removed as redundent
            Breeding section modified
            Density dependent mortality if N+R>KCAP returned
            Mortality of Rabids modified. ( )ed terms
            Plot Out-put modified to give RABIDS and Incubators
            Immunity sub-section improved
            Summary output files included


      P.J.BACON/A.AIGNER            RABBK1.BAS            28.4.83


10     EXTEND
19PRINT                    ! gap between Output blocks
20     INPUT "Name for Output file for SUFRACE-2 ", SUR2$
/!     IF SUR2$<>"" THEN OPEN SUR2$ FOR OUTPUT AS FILE #5%
/!
25     INPUT "Name for file of summary statistics per run ", SUMSTAT$
/!     IF SUMSTAT$<>"" THEN OPEN SUMSTAT$ FOR OUTPUT AS FILE #6%
/!
30     INPUT "do you want to plot Individual graphs <Y or N> ", PLOTINDG$
/!     PLOTINDG$=CVT$$(LEFT(PLOTINDG$,1%),32%)
/!
100    GOSUB 5000
120    DIM MORT(12), FEC(12), CONTR(12), STER(20), IMMU(100), PR$(63)
```

```
140    PRINT "Monthly Mortality Factors"
           FOR I%=1 TO 12
           READ MORT(I%)
           PRINT MORT(I%) ;
           NEXT I%
180    PRINT / PRINT
       PRINT "Monthly Fecundity Factors"
           FOR I%=1 TO 12
           READ FEC(I%)
           PRINT FEC(I%) ;
           NEXT I%
220    PRINT / PRINT
       PRINT "Monthly Factors for Contact-rate/ratio"
           FOR I%=1 TO 12
           READ CONTR(I%)
           PRINT CONTR(I%) ;
           NEXT I%
260    PRINT / PRINT
       PRINT "Incubation time probabilty PDF"
           FOR I%=1 TO 10
           READ RABP(I%)
           PRINT RABP(I%) ;
           NEXT I%
300    PRINT / PRINT
       READ KCAP, NORO, RABO, MORTAL
       PRINT
       PRINT "Carrying capacity         = "; KCAP
       PRINT "Initial Density Normals = "; NORO
       PRINT "Initial Density Rabids   = "; RABO
       PRINT
       PRINT "Overall Mortality         = "; MORTAL
       READ LASTYR, PRON1Y, PROFF1Y, PRON2Y, PROFF2Y
       READ FECINIT, FECINCR, FECMAX
       READ CONTINIT, CONTINCR, CONTMAX
       READ FOXEXL, RABEXL
       PRINT
       PRINT "Fox extinction limit    "; FOXEXL
       PRINT "Rabies extinction limit "; RABEXL
       PRINT
520    READ RINFY, RINFM
```

(continued)

189

Appendix 2. (*Continued*)

```
        PRINT "Rabies infestation starts YEAR "; RINFY ;" in month "; RINFM
        PRINT
        PRINT
        PRINT "Control    Year  Month  Duration"
        PRINT
        READ KILLY, KILLM, KILLD
        READ STERY, STERM, STERD
        READ IMMUY, IMMUM, IMMUD
        PRINT "KILL";TAB(11); KILLY; TAB(17); KILLM; TAB(24); KILLD
        PRINT "Sterilise"; TAB(11); STERY; TAB(17); STERM; TAB(24); STERD
        PRINT "Immunise "; TAB(11); IMMUY; TAB(17); IMMUM; TAB(24); IMMUD
        PRINT
        READ KILLP, KILLIN
        PRINT "Kill proportion "; KILLP ;" every "; KILLIN ; "months"
        PRINT
740     READ STERP, STERMT, STERIN
        PRINT "Proportion "; STERP ;" sterilised. Sterility lasts for ";
        PRINT STERMT;"Months"
        PRINT "Sterilisation repeated every "; STERIN ;" "months of program"
        PRINT
800     READ IMMUP, IMMUMT, IMMUIN
        PRINT "Proportion "; IMMUP; "immunised.    Immuntiy lasts for ";
        PRINT IMMUMT;"Months"
        PRINT "immunisation repeated every "; IMMUIN; "Months of program"
        PRINT
        PRINT
        PRINT
'----    data input ends. SIMULATION STARTS
860     '
'----
870     IF PLOTINDG$<>"Y"  THEN EXECUTE=FNWRITE.DATA(1%)
'-
880     FOR FECUND=FECINIT TO FECMAX STEP FECINCR
'-
885     IF PLOTINDG$<>"Y"  THEN 900
890     PRINT "Fecundity per Fox "; FECUND
        PRINT
900     FOR CONTRATE = CONTINIT TO CONTMAX STEP CONTINCR
'-
905     IF PLOTINDG$<>"Y"  THEN 920
910     PRINT "Contact rate/ratio = "; CONTRATE
        PRINT
        PRINT
```

```
920    FOR I%=1 TO 10 \ RABN(I%)=0.0 \ NEXT I%
/      FOR I%=1 TO 20 \ STER(I%)=0.0 \ NEXT I%
/      FOR I%=1 TO 100 \ IMMU(I%)=0.0 \ NEXT I%
940    KILLC=0.0
/      STERC=0.0
/      STERT=0.0
/      IMMUT=0.0
/      RABT =0.0
/      SUMN =0.0
/      SUMN2=0.0
/      SUMR =0.0
/      IMMUC=0.0
/      NOR =NORO
/      RABEXY=0.0
/      FOXEXY=0.0
960    GOSUB 6000
980

       Yearly and Monthly Loops start here

1000   FOR YR% = 1 TO LASTYR
1020   FOR MTH% = 1 TO 12
1030 :           does raies start ?

1040 : IF YR% = RINFY AND MTH%=RINFM  THEN  RABN(1)=RABO  \  PR$(63)="RABIES"
1050 :           Fecundity; calculate foxes 'born'

1060   IF FEC(MTH%)= -1   THEN SPRD=NOR+RABT  \ ADJ=1.0 - STERT
1080   IF FEC(MTH%)= -2   THEN AUTD=NOR+RABT
1100   IF FEC(MTH%) > 0.0 THEN BORN = ADJ * (SPRD*FECUND*FEC(MTH%)*(1.0-SPRD/KCAP) ) * (
AUTD/SPRD)
                     ELSE BORN = 0.0
1110 : IF BORN < 0.0 THEN PR$(63)=PR$(63)+"-VE births! BORN= "+NUM$(BORN)
1117   KPER = 0.0
1120   IF YR%=KILLY AND MTH%=KILLM THEN PR$(63)=PR$(63)+"Killing Starts"
1130   IF ABS(12.0*YR%+MTH% - 12.0*KILLY-KILLM-KILLD/2.0 ) > KILLD/2.0  THEN  1200
1140   KILLC = KILLC + 1.0
1160   IF KILLC = KILLIN + 1.0  THEN KILLC = 1.0
/      IF KILLC = 1.0 THEN KPER = KILLP
1180 :
1200   SPER = 0.0
```

191

(continued)

Appendix 2. *(Continued)*

```
1210    IF YR% = STERY  AND MTH% = STERM  THEN PR$(63)=PR$(63)+"Steril. starts"
1220    IF ABS( 12.0*YR%+MTH% - 12.0*STERY-STERM-STERD/2.0 ) > STERD/2.0   THEN 1280
1240    STERC=STERC + 1.0
\       IF STERC=STERIN + 1 THEN STERC = 1
1260    IF STERC=1 THEN SPER = STERP
1270    !    immunise ??

1280    IPER = 0.0
1290    IF YR%=IMMUY  AND MTH%=IMMUM  THEN PR$(63)=PR$(63)+"Immun. starts"
1300    IF ABS(12.0*YR%+MTH% - 12.0*IMMUY-IMMUM-IMMUD/2.0) > IMMUD/2.0   THEN 1345
1320    IMMUC=IMMUC +1.0
\       IF IMMUC = IMMUIN + 1  THEN IMMUC = 1
1340    IF IMMUC = 1 THEN IPER = IMMUP
1341    !

                    Density-dependent mortality ?

1345    IF NOR+RABT > KCAP  THEN 1350     ELSE 1354
1350    DDEC=(1.0-( MORTAL*MORT(MTH%) * ((NOR+RABT)/KCAP) ) )
\       IF DDEC < 1.0  THEN PR$(63)=PR$(63)+"D.D.Mort.= "+NUM$(DDEC)
1351    GOTO 1360
1354    DDEC = 1.0
1359    !

                    work out new FOX and Rabids totals

1360    RAB  = RABN(1) * (1.0-KPER) * (1.0-MORTAL*MORT(MTH%))*DDEC
1380    RAB1 = ( NOR - IMMUT ) * RAB * CONTRATE * CONTR(MTH%)
1400    NOR  = ( NOR - RAB1 + BORN ) * ( 1.0-KPER ) * ( 1.0-MORTAL*MORT(MTH%))*DDEC
1420    RABT = 0.0
1440        FOR I%=1 TO 9
1460        RABN(I%) = ( RABN(I%+1) + RAB1*RABP(I%)  ) * (1.0-KPER) * (1.0-MORTAL*M
ORT(MTH%)) *
1480        RABT = RABT + RABN(I%)
1500        NEXT I%
1520    STERT = SPER
1540        FOR I%=1 TO STERMT - 1.0          ! altered
1560        STER(I%) = STER(I%+1) * (1.0 - SPER)        ! proportion
1580        STERT = STERT + STER(I%)
1600        NEXT I%
1620    STER(STERMT) = SPER
1640    IMMUT = IPER * NOR
1660        FOR I%=1 TO IMMUMT - 1.0
1680        IMMU(I%) = IMMU(I%+1) * (1.0-IPER) * (1.0-KPER)*(1.0-MORTAL*MORT(MTH%)) *
```

```
DDEC
1700              IMMUT=IMMUT+IMMU(IZ)
1720            NEXT IZ
1740          IMMU(IMMUMT) = IPER * NOR
1741          IF IMMUT > NOR THEN PRINT "Fatal error " \ STOP
1750        :
\:

1760      ? extinction of Rabies or Foxes
ELSE 1780
1770      IF RABT < RABEXL AND 12.0*YRZ+MTHZ > 12.0*RINFY+RINFM AND RABEXY=0.0    THEN 1770

          PR$(63)=PR$(63)+"RABIES EXTINCT"
          RABEXY = YRZ
          FOR IZ=1 TO 10 \ RABN(IZ)=0.0 \ NEXT IZ
1780      RAB = 0.0
          SUMN = SUMN + NOR
          SUMN2=SUMN2 + NOR*NOR
          SUMR = SUMR + RAB
          IF NOR < FOXEXL   THEN 1810  ELSE 1820
1800      PR$(63)=PR$(63)+ "Foxes extinct"
1810      FOXEXY=YRZ
          NOR = 0.0
          GOSUB 8000
          GOTO 1880
///
1820      IF (YRZ >= PRON1Y  AND  YRZ <= PROFF1Y )   OR   ( YRZ >= PRON2Y   AND   YRZ <= PRO
FF2Y )   THEN GOSUB 8000
1830      IF SUR2%<>"" AND   YRZ>=PRON2Y AND YRZ<=PROFF2Y THEN PRINT #5%, USING "####.####
###.#####  ###.####"; CONTRATE, (12
%*(YRZ-1Z)+MTHZ)-(12Z*(PRON2Y-1Z)), NOR : SURFACE-2 file
1840      PR$(63)=""
          NEXT MTHZ
//:
1850      IF YRZ+1 = PRON2Y  AND  PLOTINDG$="Y"   THEN PRINT "ZXX!!!"   FOR IZ=1 TO 15
1860      NEXT YRZ
1880      IF PLOTINDG$="Y" THEN EXECUTE = FNWRITE.DATA(2Z)
                           ELSE EXECUTE = FNWRITE.DATA(3Z)
1920      NEXT CONTRATE
1930      PRINT            ! gap to make BLOCKS of Output
1940      NEXT FECUND
:         end of loops
```

(continued)

Appendix 2. (*Continued*)

```
1980    PRINT
        CLOSE #6%
        PRINT "Data files closed", SUR2$, SUMSTAT$
        PRINT
        PRINT "Program ends OK"
        PRINT
        PRINT
        STOP
2000
3000    DATA 1.2
3020    DATA .03, .03, .015, .005, .005, .005, .03, .03, .03,.03
3040    DATA 0, 0, -1, 0, 0, 0, -2, 0.2, 0.6, 0.2, 0
3060    DATA 1,3,1,1,1,1,1,1,2,2,1
3080    DATA 0.00, 0.42, 0.25, 0.12, 0.08, 0.06, 0.04, 0.03, 0.00, 0.00
3100    DATA 1.0, 0.9999, 0.0001, 1.0
3121    DATA 15,0,15,99,100
3140    DATA 2, 0.5, 2.1
3160    DATA 2.0, 0.1, 2.05
3180    DATA 0.00001, 0.00001
3200    DATA 2, 4
3220    DATA 0, 0, 0
3240    DATA 0, 0, 0
3260    DATA 0, 0, 0
3280    DATA 0.6, 6
3300    DATA 0.6, 5, 12
3320    DATA 0.6, 48,6
4999    :
.
. :
5000    REM          Subroutine sets plot control         ) GRAPH PLOTTING
. :
. :
6000    REM          Subroutine prints Y axis of Graph     ) CODE GIVEN IN
. :
. : :
8000    REM          Subroutine prints a Line of Graph     ) APPENDIX 1.b.
. :
. :
9000 DEF FNWRITE.DATA(DJP%)                  ! Function prints Summary data for each run
9010    ON DJP% GOTO 9020, 9020, 9020, 9020, 9100
9020    PRINT \ PRINT \ PRINT                AVERAGE   AVERAGE   AVERAGE   ST. DEV. OF"
9040    PRINT"RAB. FOX FEC. CONT.            RABIDS    RABIDS    NORMALS   NORMALS"
        PRINT"EX. EX. PER RATE
```

194

```
          PRINT"YR.         YR.   FOX              MONTH        YEAR"
9050      ON DJP% GOTO 9175, 9100
9100      IF RABEXY <> 0 THEN PRINT RABEXY ;
9120      IF FOXEXY <> 0 THEN PRINT TAB(7); FOXEXY ;
9140      PRINT TAB(12); FECUND ; TAB(18); CONTRATE ; TAB(25) ; SUMR / LASTYR / 12.0 ;
9160      PRINT TAB(37) ; SUMR / LASTYR ; TAB(49); SUMN / 12.0 / LASTYR;
9165      NORMM = SUMN / 12.0 / LASTYR
/         NORSD = SUMN2 - ((SUMN*SUMN)/12.0/LASTYR)
/         NORSD = SQR( NORSD / (12.0*LASTYR-1.0) )
/         PRINT TAB(60%); NORSD
          IF SUMSTAT$<>"" THEN PRINT #6%, USING "###.##### ###.##### ###.#####", FECUND, CONTRATE,
NORMM
/!
9168      ON DJP%  GOTO 9175, 9170, 9180
9170      FOR I%=1 TO 8 \ PRINT \ NEXT I%
9175      PRINT
          PRINT
9180 FNEND
/!
9999      END

Ready
```

References

Anderson, R. M. (1982). Fox rabies. *In* "Population Dynamics of Infectious Diseases: Theory and Applications" (R. M. Anderson, ed.), pp. 242–261. Chapman & Hall, London.

Anderson, R. M., Jackson, H. C., May, R. M., and Smith, A. M. (1981). Population dynamics of fox rabies in Europe. *Nature (London)* **289,** 765–771.

Bacon, P. J., and Macdonald, D. W. (1980). To control rabies: Vaccinate foxes. *New Sci.* **87,** 640–645.

Bartlett, M. S. (1960). "Stochastic Population Models." Methuen, London.

Dent, J. B., and Blackie, M. J. (1979). "Systems Simulation in Agriculture." Appl. Sci. Publ., London.

Kleijnen, J. P. C. (1972). The statistical design and analysis of digital simulation: A summary. *Manage. Inf.,* **1**(2), 57–66.

Macdonald, D. W., and Bacon, P. J. (1982). Fox society, contact rate and rabies epizootiology. *Comp. Immunol. Microbiol. Infect. Dis.* **5**(1–3), 247–256.

May, R. M. (1974). "Stability and Complexity in Model Ecosystems, 2nd ed." Princeton Univ. Press, Princeton, New Jersey.

Steck, F. (1982). Rabies in wildlife. *In* "Animal Disease in Relation to Animal Conservation" (M. A. Edwards and U. McDonnell, eds.), pp. 57–75. Academic Press, New York.

Spatial Models for the Spread and Control of Rabies Incorporating Group Size

8

Frank G. Ball[1]

Department of Biomathematics,
University of Oxford,
Oxford, England

I. Introduction

The main purpose in constructing a mathematical model of the spread of rabies is to use that model to suggest and evaluate the efficacy of various control

[1]Present address: Department of Mathematics, University of Nottingham, University Park, Nottingham, NG7 2RD, England.

197

strategies. In this chapter we shall draw upon our knowledge of the behaviour of the Red Fox, in particular that obtained by David Macdonald (1977) from field studies spanning several years, to enable us to build such a model and then use our model to estimate the probabilities of success of control policies that reduce the fox population density in a region surrounding an initial case. Our model will differ in two important ways from the models presented in the previous two chapters, in that it will include both a spatial and a chance element.

A. SPATIAL ASPECTS

The models of Chapters 6 and 7, this volume, have all assumed that the population of foxes, amongst which rabies is spreading, is homogeneously mixing in that a given rabid fox is equally likely to infect *any* of the susceptible foxes in the population. This assumption is reasonable for small populations, such as a group of foxes sharing the same territory, but it is clearly invalid for large populations since a rabid fox is considerably more likely to encounter a fox from its own vicinity than one from afar off. In practice when using a homogeneously mixing model, one uses an average infection rate taken over the population as a whole. This is not entirely satisfactory since the resulting homogeneously mixing model will still behave quantitatively quite differently from the spatial model from which it was derived.

Apart from the theoretical deficiencies of homogeneously mixing models, there is also the practical problem in that when fox control is advocated or applied we require to know not only how intensive it should be but also where it should be applied. For example, a homogeneously mixing model will not be able to discriminate between the relative merits of a high intensity control over a small region and a low intensity control over a correspondingly larger region. Indeed, for a homogeneously mixing model to have any chance of predicting the success of a control policy, the control must be applied uniformly *throughout* the population.

B. STOCHASTIC EFFECTS

The previous models have also been deterministic in that given the mathematical mechanics of the model the spread of rabies was completely determined by the initial values of the parameters, thus there was no probability element. The main justification for using a deterministic formulation instead of a more realistic stochastic model, apart from the possible gain in mathematical tractability, is that for large populations we would expect the chance elements to average themselves out, and, thus, the deterministic epizootic should give a reasonable approximation to the more realistic stochastic one. However, for a deterministic formulation to reasonably approximate a spatial model, we shall require that the population is not only globally large but also *locally* large, which is often untrue. We shall construct below a model for the spread of rabies amongst foxes who live in groups, such groups rarely exceeding five foxes. Thus, we shall require a stochastic formulation, as five is not a very large number! Another reason for using a stochastic model is that the results are more readily interpreted than those of a deterministic model. With a deterministic model a control policy will either be successful or not successful but in real life the effects of rabies control will not be so clear cut: the same control policy will sometimes work and sometimes will not. Using a stochastic model we can calculate the probability that a given control policy is successful, or more likely estimate it from repeated simulations of the model, and it is precisely this probability that the disease control authorities should be most interested in.

Having described the advantages of a spatial stochastic model of fox rabies, we must now specify its details.

C. COMPLEXITY VERSUS SIMPLICITY

Any mathematical model must be sufficiently complex to be biologically realistic and at the same time sufficiently simple to be mathematically tractable; the art of modelling is to correctly adjust the balance. Even the simplest stochastic spatial epidemic models are notoriously difficult to analyse mathematically, and consequently, we shall resort to computer simulations for this model. However, the above balance must still be struck as introducing too many parameters into our model makes the results increasingly difficult to interpret, indeed it may become impossible to tell which parameter is doing what. Further, for the same computing time we shall obtain less simulations of the more complex model, with a corresponding drop of confidence in our results. In choosing a model, we should also bear in mind the purpose for which we intend to use our model, since this will obviously have an important bearing upon the final details.

D. DETAILS OF FOX ECOLOGY AND BEHAVIOUR

Radio tracking of foxes has revealed that, at least in some habitats, foxes live in groups, each group sharing a single territory with little overlap between neighbouring territories. This suggests that a model in which normal foxes live in groups, one group being located at each square of a lattice grid, would be appropriate. However, to build such a model, we have to decide upon the infection mechanism of rabid foxes.

There are two forms of fox rabies, namely furious and paralytic rabies, though the distinction between the two types is probably not as marked as once thought. In both forms the rabid foxes eventually became paralysed, but in the furious form, this is commonly thought to be preceded by a period of eratic behaviour.

However, there has been very little positive research into the movements of rabid foxes, and many biologists now believe that during most of its active infectious period, a rabid fox behaves not too dissimilarily from a normal fox. We thus assume that a rabid fox can only infect foxes within its own and immediately neighbouring groups, which leads to a nearest-neighbour model of epidemic spread.

E. POINT SOURCE VERSUS FRONT-WAVE EPIDEMICS

The most likely means of entry of rabies into the British fox population is via a smuggled pet that is incubating the disease, yielding the problem of controlling an epidemic that is spreading away from a point source. This contrasts sharply with the continental situation, where they are attempting to halt an advancing wave of rabies. The British government's contingency plans in the event of rabies entering Britain includes the killing of foxes within a region surrounding the initial reported case, and we shall use our model to examine the efficiency of such control measures under defined conditions. Experience of rabies control on the continent suggests that if rabies is not eradicated fairly quickly, then it is likely to remain enzootic for some time, in spite of quite widespread control measures. In this chapter we accordingly concentrate on the short-term behaviour, and, consequently, we will not incorporate natural changes in the fox population, due to births, deaths and migration, in our model as such parameters will not have time to play an important role. However, caution is required if rabies breaks out during either the breeding or dispersal season, since in the former case the group size will be higher than here assumed, whilst in the latter the fox population will have greater mobility than usual. However, in both cases we can make some appropriate adjustments to our control model.

II. The Basic Model

A. DESCRIPTION

We assume that foxes live in groups, one group being located at each square of a 49×49 square lattice. All uninfected foxes are susceptible and remain so until they are infected by a rabid fox. We assume that the latent period is constant and that the infectious period is reduced to a single point in time. This yields a discrete time epidemic with cases occurring at equal time intervals, the length of which is equal to the length of the latent period. These assumptions concerning the latent and infectious periods should be fairly reasonable for a model of fox rabies since the latent period is quite long, about 30 days, and the infectious period relatively short, about 4 days. Moreover, during the initial stages of an outbreak, there will be little difference between our discrete time model and a more realistic continuous time model, as the infectious periods are short compared to the latent periods.

At its point of infection, a rabid fox can infect any fox within its own group and its four nearest neighbouring groups. The probability that it infects a given fox in its own group is P_W (W, within a group) and that for infecting a given fox in a neighbouring group is P_B (B, between a group), all infections being independent of each other.

B. DYNAMICS OF THE MODEL

Suppose that at time t there are X_t susceptible foxes and Y_t rabid foxes in a given grid square. Suppose also that there are a total of Y_t' rabid foxes in the four neighbouring grid squares. Consider a given susceptible in this central grid square. To avoid infection it must avoid infection from foxes in its own and neighbouring groups. Thus, the probability that it avoids infection at time $t + 1$ is given by

P(it avoids infection at time $t + 1$) = P(it avoids infection from its own group). P(it avoids infection from neighbouring groups)

$$= (1 - P_W)^{Y_t} \cdot (1 - P_B)^{Y_t'}$$

as infections are independent.

$\therefore P$(it is infected at time $t + 1$) = $1 - (1 - P_W)^{Y_t} (1 - P_B)^{Y_t'}$. Thus, the number of rabid foxes in this grid square at time $t + 1$, Y_{t+1}, has a binominal distribution, $B(n,p)$, with parameters

$$n = X_t \qquad p = 1 - (1 - P_W)^{Y_t}(1 - P_B)^{Y_t'}$$

The number of susceptible foxes in this square at time $t + 1$ is clearly given by

$$X_{t+1} = X_t - Y_{t+1}$$

This model seems mathematically quite intractable and thus we resort to computer simulations, but before describing them we discuss some aspects of our model that have a bearing on whether rabies epizootics will 'take off' and spread or 'peter out' and vanish.

C. THE PROBABILITY THAT ONE FOX GROUP
INFECTS ANOTHER

The probability that one fox group, if infected, infects a given neighbouring group plays an important role in determining whether a rabies epizootic takes off, as intuitively the greater this probability is, the greater the probability of a true epizootic. To obtain a very close approximation to the above group infection probability, we consider two neighbouring fox groups of sizes N_1 and N_2, respectively. Suppose that one fox in the first group becomes rabid. What is the probability, P_G say, that at least one fox in the second group is infected by a fox from the first group, ignoring the part played by any other fox groups?

To calculate the group infection probability, P_G, we consider the size of an epidemic in the first group, ignoring any part the second group might play. Thus, if a total of N_R foxes become infected in group 1, the probability that group 2 avoids infection is $(1 - P_B)^{N_R N_2}$ since each of the N_2 foxes in group 2 must avoid infection from N_R rabid foxes in group 1 and consequently $N_R N_2$ independent possible infections must fail. Hence the probability that group 2 is infected is $1 - (1 - P_B)^{N_R N_2}$. Now N_R is a random variable and to find the unconditional probability that group 2 is infected, we must average over the distribution of N_R to yield

$$\begin{aligned}
P_G &= 1 - E_{N_R}[(1 - P_B)^{N_2 N_R}] \\
&= 1 - f((1 - P_B)^{N_2})
\end{aligned} \tag{1}$$

where $f(s) = E[s^{N_R}]$ defined for $0 \le s \le 1$, is the probability generating function of N_R, the total size of a standard Reed–Frost, chain-binomial epidemic. A closed expression for $f(s)$ is not known. However, for a given value of s, $f(s)$ may be calculated numerically on a computer and consequently P_G can be found.

Note that P_G, as given by Equation (1), underestimates the true probability that group 1 infects group 2, since there may be some back infection into group 1 from its other neighbouring groups. Although, unless P_B is large the discrepancy will be small. To obtain an upper bound for P_G we assume that all the foxes in group 1 become infected, i.e. that $N_R = N_1$, and, thus, Equation (1) becomes

$$P'_G = 1-(1 - P_B)^{N_1 N_2} \tag{2}$$

Equation (2) is independent of P_W since we have, in effect, set $P_W = 1$; however, provided P_W is reasonably close to one, P'_G should be a good approximation to P_G. This approximation will be frequently used in this chapter, and it is worthwhile ensuring that you are familiar with it.

We now assume that $N_1 = N_2 = N$. Table I shows the values of P_G and $P_{G'}$ for various combinations of values of P_W, P_B and N. The importance of fox group size is shown by this table as, for fixed (P_W, P_B), the group infection probability P_G can be seen to increase rapidly with group size N. Indeed, if the within-group infection probability P_W is close to 1, Equation (2) shows that $P_G \simeq N^2 P_B$, provided P_B is small.

The expected number of groups infected by a given infective group, $E[G]$ say, is clearly $4P_G$. However, if the epizootic has been progressing for some time, some of the groups infected by our given infective group will already have been

TABLE I

Cross Infection Probabilities P_G for Various Combinations of Group Size N, Within-group Infection Probability P_W and Between-group Infection Probability P_B, as Given by Equation (1)[a]

			$P_B = 0.05$		
			P_W		
N	0.2	0.4	0.6	0.8	1.0
2	0.115	0.133	0.150	0.168	0.185
3	0.198	0.258	0.313	0.354	0.370
4	0.297	0.421	0.513	0.554	0.560
5	0.411	0.599	0.697	0.721	0.723
6	0.530	0.756	0.832	0.842	0.842
7	0.643	0.869	0.915	0.919	0.919
8	0.742	0.936	0.961	0.962	0.962
9	0.820	0.971	0.984	0.984	0.984
10	0.876	0.987	0.994	0.994	0.994

			$P_B = 0.15$		
			P_W		
N	0.2	0.4	0.6	0.8	1.0
2	0.317	0.358	0.397	0.438	0.478
3	0.486	0.589	0.679	0.744	0.768
4	0.637	0.783	0.850	0.920	0.926
5	0.756	0.903	0.967	0.982	0.983
6	0.841	0.959	0.993	0.997	0.997
7	0.897	0.982	0.998	1.000	1.000
8	0.933	0.992	1.000	1.000	1.000
9	0.956	0.996	1.000	1.000	1.000
10	0.971	0.998	1.000	1.000	1.000

			$P_B = 0.25$		
			P_W		
N	0.2	0.4	0.6	0.8	1.0
2	0.486	0.536	0.585	0.634	0.684
3	0.676	0.770	0.850	0.904	0.925
4	0.808	0.905	0.964	0.987	0.990
5	0.858	0.963	0.992	0.999	0.999
6	0.935	0.985	0.998	1.000	1.000
7	0.962	0.993	0.999	1.000	1.000
8	0.978	0.997	1.000	1.000	1.000
9	0.987	0.999	1.000	1.000	1.000
10	0.992	0.999	1.000	1.000	1.000

[a] The columns with $P_W = 1$ yield the approximate group infection probability P_G' given by Equation (2).

infected. Indeed, for an advancing wave of infection about one-half of these infected groups will on average be already infected; thus, the expected number of groups freshly infected by our central infective group will be about $2P_G$.

To see this, consider a uniform wave of infection spreading North Westwards through our grid. By the time this wave meets our central group, the groups lying immediately to the south and west of this central group will already be infected and thus only the groups lying immediately to the north and east of the central group remain to be infected. In practice the situation is not quite as clear cut as this since owing to stochastic effects the wave of infection will only be approximately uniform. If the quantity $2P_G$ is less than or equal to 1, i.e. $P_G \leq \frac{1}{2}$, the epizootic will ultimately die out as the number of infected groups continually decreases, whilst if it is greater than 1, i.e. $P_G > \frac{1}{2}$, there will be a non-zero probability of a true epidemic. Thus the threshold value of $E[G]$ is about 2.

We shall describe some simulations of our model with $P_B = 0.1$ and $P_W = 0.8$. These values are fairly realistic for the hypothetical spread of rabies among fox populations whose inter- and intra-group contacts are similarly frequent to those pertaining within David Macdonald's study area near Oxford. As we increase N the value of $E[G]$ first becomes greater than the threshold value 2 when $N = 3$, and hence this is when we shall expect our epizootics to 'take off'.

D. RESULTS OF SIMULATIONS

We assumed that the group size N was constant throughout our 49×49 grid and for each of $N = 1, 2, \ldots, 9$, we simulated 10 epizootics starting from a single case in the central group. The epizootics were allowed to proceed until either they died out or the boundary of the grid was reached. Table II shows the number of simulated epizootics in each category. There is clearly a threshold group size between $N = 2$ and 3, which corresponds very well with the conjectured threshold of about 2 for $E[G]$.

It should be pointed out that this model is very similar to a model originally proposed by Bailey (1967, see also Bailey, 1975), in which he allowed spread to the eight nearest neighbours but the groups were all of size 1. His simulations showed a threshold value of about 0.3 for P_B, which gives a threshold value of 2.4 for $E[G]$. The nature of his threshold was not so distinct as ours, as he was varying a continuous parameter P_B whilst we have varied a discrete parameter N.

Returning to our simulations, Table III gives more details of those epidemics in which the group size was above the threshold.

As we increase the group size N the time for the epidemic to reach the boundary decreases until, when $N = 9$, the minimum of 24 time units to reach the boundary is nearly always achieved. However, for higher group sizes this faster rate of spread results in slightly less widespread epizootics when the boundary is reached.

TABLE II

Results of Simulations for Group Size $N = 1, 2, \ldots, 9$ with Parameter Values $P_W = 0.8$ and $P_B = 0.1$[a]

Group size (N)	Number dying out	Number reaching boundary
1	10	0
2	10	0
3	0	10
4	0	10
5	0	10
6	0	10
7	0	10
8	0	10
9	0	10

[a] Ten simulations were performed for each group size. Note the sharp threshold behaviour between $N = 2$ and $N = 3$.

These simulations clearly demonstrate the important effects of fox group size on the spread of rabies, under conditions for which the model is realistic, and so we shall now consider the consequences of control policies in which the group size is reduced.

E. CONTROL

We consider control policies that reduce the susceptible fox population in a region surrounding the initial case. We assume that N, the uncontrolled fox

TABLE III

Aspects of Simulated Epizootics that Reached the Boundary of the 49 × 49 Square Lattice[a]

Group size	Time to reach boundary	Total no. of groups infected	Proportion of foxes infected	No. of infective groups when boundary is reached	No. of rabid foxes when boundary is reached
3	43.6	894	0.35	99.5	133.1
4	34.1	1275	0.51	169.6	306.0
5	30.5	1336	0.53	189.5	429.6
6	28.1	1304	0.52	195.2	543.4
7	26.4	1273	0.51	193.8	654.8
8	25.3	1227	0.49	189.9	749.5
9	24.3	1119	0.48	181.1	840.7

[a] The figures given are the means of 10 simulated epizootics.

group size, is 5, $P_W = 0.8$ and $P_B = 0.1$ and that epizootics are initiated by a single rabid fox in the central group. The fox group size is well above threshold and consequently, to try to prevent an epizootic, the model 'control' reduces the fox population in an 'annulus' surrounding the initial case as shown in Fig. 1. No control is applied to the 12 groups immediately surrounding the initial case because in practice rabies is unlikely to be detected immediately and consequently an epizootic will have started to build up before we commence control (see Bacon, 1981). The shape of the control zone is that area which an epizootic would cover in time $d + 2$, where d is the control depth, if it was to spread radially at the maximum speed.

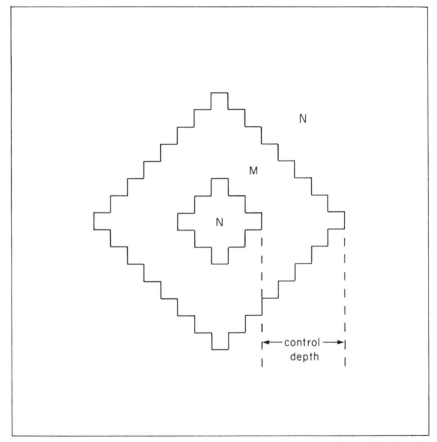

Fig. 1. Diagram showing zone (centre enlarged). Fox group size was reduced within the region labelled M. M and N are, respectively, the controlled and un-controlled fox group sizes (49 × 49 grid).

Note that the group size *M* within the control zone *must* be reduced to less than three, since otherwise the epizootic will be above threshold within the control zone! Table IV shows the number of simulations out of five in which the control was successful for various combinations of *M* and *d*. A control is considered successful if the disease does not reach the boundary of the grid.

Admittedly, the results in Table IV are based on only five simulations per control strategy and consequently little confidence can be placed in the results. Clearly, we can increase our confidence by doing more simulations, but this may not be a very fruitful use of computer time, since the fox population parameters (N, P_W, P_B) can vary considerably from one region to another. Thus, it is more profitable to develop a control simulation model with increased flexibility and this section has only been included as an intermediate illustrative step before proceeding to such a model.

III. General Control Model

A. INTRODUCTION

In Chapter 4, this volume, we have seen that the fox's social structure and territory size vary considerably from one habitat to another, even within the British Isles. The fox is an animal that adapts well to its environment; indeed, it is precisely its flexibility that has made it such a successful vector for rabies. Consequently, any control programme should take account of this adaptability of the fox and be able to accommodate the considerable flexibility of fox population parameters from one habitat to the next.

Our model gives all results concerning control depths in terms of the number

TABLE IV

Number of Simulations in Which Control was Successful out of Five Simulations per Control Strategy[a]

Control depth	Number of foxes per group in control zone	
	2	1
3	0	5
4	0	5
5	2	5

[a] A control was deemed successful if the boundary of the 49 × 49 square lattice was not reached by the simulated epizootic.

of groups that have to be controlled, and hence the variation in fcx territory size will not concern us, provided we convert correctly from group control depth (in units of territory size) to actual control depth (in kilometres) before applying control in the field. The wide range of possible values for fox group size and infection probabilities does cause concern, since for our control model of the previous section to cover all the possibilities we would require an inordinate amount of computer time. However, by making a few realistic approximations we arrive at the following highly flexible model.

B. BASICS OF MODEL

We consider control policies that reduce the susceptible fox population within a region surrounding the initial case, but we now develop a model that allows one set of simulations to estimate the efficacy of control strategies for any combination of control group size M and between-group infection probability P_B.

Consider two adjacent groups within the control zone, group 1 and group 2, say. When the within-group infection probability P_W is close to 1,

$$\begin{aligned} P(\text{group 1 infects group 2}) &= 1 - (1 - P_B)^{M^2} \\ &= P_G \text{ say,} \end{aligned} \tag{3}$$

to a very close approximation. For the control situations we are likely to encounter in Britain, P_W will usually be close to one, since foxes within the same group often share a sleeping den.

Now if the group size within the control zone is constant, then any rabid group will infect each of its four neighbouring groups independently of each other and with probability P_G, given by Equation (3). Thus, for spread within the control zone, the problem is reduced to one in which all the groups are of size 1. However, in the field, the group size within the control zone will not be constant but rather a random variable whose mean we may assume to be M. It can be shown that this variability results in a decreased group infection probability P_G and a positive correlation between a rabid group infecting any two given neighbours. Ball (1981) conjectured that this results in a decreased spread of rabies and performed some simulations that supported this hypothesis. Thus, a control that is successful with a constant group size M should also succeed when the group size is variable with mean M. Note further that the approximation used in Equation (3) will overestimate the true group infection probability, since it has assumed that all the foxes in group 1 become infected. This will also increase the probability of the successful spread of rabies with the consequence that our control model will again underestimate the probability of a successful control.

In most habitats the uncontrolled group size N is likely to be well above threshold. In such circumstances we make the following simple observations:

1. Rabies is likely to spread to most of the groups in the first line of control.

2. If rabies reaches the last line of control, then it will almost always spread outside the control zone and reach the boundary of the grid.

With this in mind we simulated epizootics amongst groups of size 1 on a 29 × 29 grid (reduced from 49 × 49 to save computer time), with the initial infective groups as shown in Fig. 2, until either they died out or they reached the boundary (see Fig. 2). Figure 2 also shows such an epizootic, and it can be seen that the minimum successful control zone has depth one greater than the maximum spread of rabies. In view of observation (2), we now deem a control policy

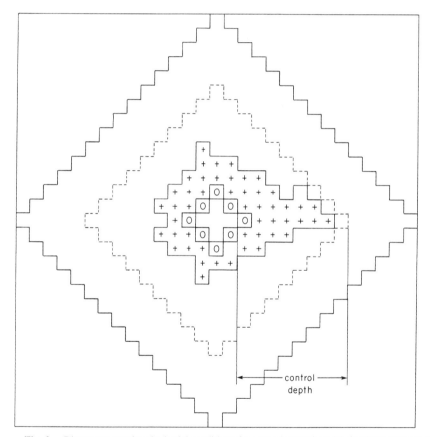

Fig. 2. Diagram portraying the initial conditions for general control model simulated epizootics (29 × 29 grid). Such a simulated epizootic is also shown, and the corresponding minimum control depth for the successful eradication of rabies is indicated. Initially infective group (○), subsequently infected group (+), boundary of control zone of minimum depth that will successfully eradicate rabies (- - -). Outside boundary is the boundary at which simulations were halted.

successful if it prevents rabies from spreading to the last line of the control zone. If the epidemic had reached the boundary then any control of depth 14 or less would have failed. Note that we are still assuming that the control zone has identical shape to that used in the previous section. To examine the dependence of the minimum successful control depth on P_G we use a technique of Hammersley and Handscomb (1964; Chapter 11) to produce linked simulations, in which one set of pseudo-random variables generates an epizootic for each value of P_G in the interval $[0,1]$.

C. DETAILS OF LINKED SIMULATIONS

For each simulation we generate a set $U = (U_{(i,j)}^{(k)} : 1 \leq i \leq 29, 1 \leq j \leq 29, 1 \leq k \leq 4)$ of independent random variables, each uniformly distributed on the interval $(0,1)$. $U_{(i,j)}^{(k)}$ is the minimum value of P_G required for the group at (i,j) to infect its kth neighbour (see Fig. 3), i.e. (i,j) infects k if and only if $U_{(i,j)}^{(k)} \leq P_G$; thus, for a given value of P_G, the probability (i,j) infects k is P_G, and all infections are independent, as required. Thus, one set of pseudo-random variables U generates an epizootic for any value of P_G in the interval $[0,1]$ and as we increase P_G the size of the epizootic is necessarily non-decreasing. Moreover, as we increase P_G, the size of the epizootic can only increase when $P_G \in U$ and consequently we need only generate epizootics for such vaues of P_G. More details of the linked simulations are given in Ball (1981), where it is shown that we can further reduce the set of values of P_G for which we need to generate epizootics. Note that our simulated epizootics for different values of P_G will be highly dependent, since they are derived from the *same* set of pseudo-random

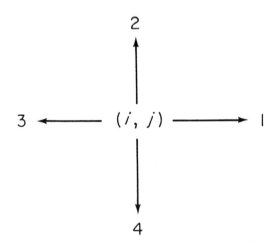

Fig. 3. Diagram illustrating the neighbours of the group at (i,j).

variables, but this does not cause concern since it is precisely this type of dependence that we are most interested in.

The success of a control policy of the type described in Section II is determined by the maximum spread of an epizootic, d^* say, defined by

$$d^* = \max_{(i,j)\in P} (|i - 15| + |j - 15|) \tag{4}$$

where P is the set of groups infected by the epizootic. d^* is simply the time taken for all the groups in P to become infected if the epizootic was to spread at its maximum possible rate. For each set of pseudo-random variables U, we obtain a "step function" depicting the dependence of d^* on P_G. The results of several simulations are combined to estimate probabilities relevant to the control of rabies.

D. RESULTS OF SIMULATIONS

We will use the results of 1000 simulations of the above model to answer the following questions:

1. For given control depth d and mean group size M within the control zone, what is the probability that the control will be successful?

2. For given control depth d, what is the maximum mean group size within the control zone so that the control has at least some predetermined probability α of succeeding?

For the ith simulated epizootic let $X_i(d)$, $d = 2,3, \ldots , 13$, be the minimum group infection probability P_G required for the epidemic to reach depth $d^* = d + 1$. For $P_G \in (0,1)$ define functions $U_i(P_G,d)$ by

$$U_i(P_G,d) = \begin{cases} 1 & \text{if } X_i(d) \leq P_G, \\ 0 & \text{otherwise} \end{cases} \tag{5}$$

Hence $U_i(P_G,d)$ is one if control of depth d is unsuccessful for the ith simulated epizootic and zero otherwise. Thus, if we have a total of n-simulated epizootics an unbiased estimate of the probability that control of depth d is successful is

$$\hat{p} = 1 - \frac{1}{n} \sum_{n=1}^{n} U_i(P_G,d) \tag{6}$$

where P_G is the group infection probability, which is related to the between-group infection probability P_B by equation (3). $\hat{p}$ is simply the proportion of simulation runs for which control of level M at depth d was successful.

Now let $P_d(\alpha)$ be the maximum value of P_G for which control of depth d has probability at least α of succeeding, and let $M_d(\alpha, P_B)$ be the mean group size corresponding to $P_d(\alpha)$ when the between-group infection probability is P_B. From Equation (3), we find that

$$M_d(\alpha, P_B) = [\ln(1 - P_d(\alpha))/\ln(1 - P_B)]^{1/2} \qquad (7)$$

and hence an estimate of $M_d(\alpha, P_B)$ immediately follows from an estimate of $P_d(\alpha)$.

For fixed control depth d let $X_{(1)}(d), X_{(2)}(d), \ldots, X_{(n)}(d)$ be the sample $X_1(d), X_2(d), \ldots, X_n(d)$ arranged in increasing order. An estimator of $P_d(\alpha)$ is then given by

$$\hat{P}_d(\alpha) = X_{([n(1-\alpha)])}(d) \qquad (8)$$

where for any positive number x, $[x]$ is the least integer greater than or equal to x. $\hat{P}_d(\alpha)$ is the maximum value of the group infection probability P_G for which the proportion of simulated epidemics in which control of depth d is unsuccessful is not greater than $1 - \alpha$.

Figure 4 shows for different values of P_G within the control zone, the minimum control depth required to have a specified probability $\alpha = 0.2, 0.4, 0.6$ and 0.8 of preventing rabies from spreading outside the control zone. Table V gives for different control depths d, the maximum value of P_G within the control zone $\hat{P}_d(\alpha)$, the corresponding group size, $M_d(\alpha, P_B)$ when $P_B = 0.1$ and the total number of foxes killed if the uncontrolled group size was five, for the control to have probability $\alpha = 0.9$ of succeeding. For the above set of parameter values control at the minimum depth is optimal in that it kills the least number of foxes to obtain the specified probabilities of success. It is worth noting that such a control policy will also cause less disturbance to the foxes' social system as a whole. As we decrease the between-group infection probability P_B towards zero, there will eventually come a point such that, *even in the absence of control,* the probability that an epizootic reaches the boundary of our grid will equal the specified probability of success, α. When P_B is slightly greater than this threshold-value control at maximum depth is optimal. Thus, the form of the optimal control policy depends critically upon the virulence of the epizootic.

This phenomenon concerning the form of the optimal control policy is interesting, but when the uncontrolled epizootic is only just above threshold, epidemics that break through the control will not necessarily reach the edge of the grid and consequently control at larger depths are greatly favoured. This was not taken into account when considering optimal policies and thus the conclusion obtained above must be treated very cautiously. However, we have already noted that the parameters appropriate for an epizootic in Britain are likely to be well above threshold and consequently under the conditions of our model, an intense localised control policy is probably preferable.

By making further approximations, it is possible to use the results of our linked simulations to obtain answers to the questions posed at the start of this section when the parameters are such that the epizootic is only just above threshold. Details of the methods involved can be found in Ball (1981), but further simulations are required to check the validity of the approximations entailed.

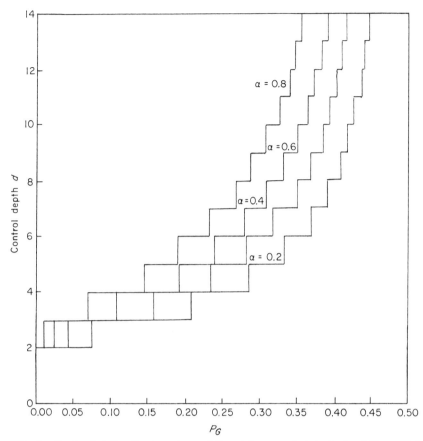

Fig. 4. Graphs depicting the dependence of the minimum control depth, to yield specified probability α of success, on the group infection probability P_G *within* the control zone; α = probability that the control is successful.

An example of the use of this figure is as follows.

Suppose that the uncontrolled group size N is 5, the between-group infection probability P_B is 0.1, and we wish to apply a control that reduces the fox group size to $M = 2$. How deep should our control zone be? From Equation (3), $P_G = 1 - (1 - 0.1)^{22} = 0.344$. We then draw a vertical line through $P_G = 0.344$ on the above graph, this cuts the $\alpha = 0.6$ curve at $d = 9$. Thus, a control depth of at least 9 will be required for the control to have a 60% chance of being successful.

IV. Modelling an Effect of Control: Altered Contacts

The evaluation of control strategies carried out in the previous sections have ignored any effect that a control policy might have on the surviving susceptible fox population. We have already noted in Section I that in the type of habitat for which our control model is appropriate, the fox population, in the absence of

TABLE V

Different Control Strategies Yielding a 90% Chance of Eradicating Rabies[a,b]

Control depth (d)	$\hat{P}_d(\alpha)$	Mean group size within the control zone, $M_d(\alpha, P_B)$	Total no. of foxes killed
2	0.005	0.220	95.6
3	0.053	0.720	154.1
4	0.111	1.059	220.7
5	0.162	1.296	296.3
6	0.192	1.424	386.2
7	0.240	1.612	474.3
8	0.264	1.704	580.1
9	0.282	1.774	696.8
10	0.303	1.851	818.7
11	0.315	1.894	956.6
12	0.325	1.931	1104.8
13	0.338	1.977	1257.6

[a] $\hat{P}_d(\alpha)$ is the maximum value of the group infection probability *within* the control zone for a control of depth d to have probability α of succeeding. Note that for the above parameter values, smaller depths of control require less foxes to be killed to achieve the same success rate.

[b] Probability that control is successful, $\alpha = 0.9$; between-group infection probability, $P_B = 0.1$; uncontrolled fox group size, $N = 5$

rabies, possesses a highly structured social system and clearly any control policy that kills foxes must distort this social system, probably in a manner which enhances the spread of rabies. Two possible disturbances immediately spring to mind, (1) that the killing of foxes will increase the interaction between the surviving foxes and (2) that if the control policy is sufficiently severe, complete groups of foxes will be wiped out resulting in fresh territory space becoming available, which will either be filled by itinerant foxes or absorbed into the territories of surrounding groups, the former being similar to (1) in that the newly resident itinerant foxes will probably have increased interaction with their neighbours. We will only study the effect of (1) on the success of a control policy.

Consider a control policy which reduces fox group size from N to M and write

$$M = (1 - \mathbf{i})N, \tag{9}$$

where $\mathbf{i}$ is the intensity of control. Let $P_B(p, \mathbf{i})$ be the probability that a given fox in one group infects a given fox in a neighbouring group when control is applied at intensity $\mathbf{i}$ and the between-group infection probability before control was p. Thus, we assume that the effect of control is a function of control intensity and not of the absolute number of foxes killed. The group infection probability within the control zone will now be approximately given by

$$P_G(p, \mathbf{i}) = 1-[1 -P_B(p, \mathbf{i})]^{(1 - \mathbf{i})^2 N^2} \tag{10}$$

We can thus incorporate the effect of control on the group infection probability into our previous control model by replacing the basic equation of that model, Equation (3), by Equation (10). However, to put this into operation, we first have to estimate the function $P_B(p, \mathbf{i})$, a non-trivial problem, for the solution of which we do not at present have the necessary data. We will, however, make some assumptions about $P_B(p, \mathbf{i})$ and examine their consequences, both in terms of the function $P_B(p, \mathbf{i})$ itself and also its effect on the control of a rabies outbreak.

We make the following assumptions:

1. $P_B(p,\mathbf{i})$ is a continuous function of p and $\mathbf{i}$.
2. Control of zero intensity has no effect on the between-group infection probability, i.e. $P_B(p,0) = p$ for all p such that $0 \leq p \leq 1$.
3. The between-group infection probability strictly increases with control intensity, i.e. for fixed p lying between 0 and 1, $P_B(p,\mathbf{i})$ strictly increases with $\mathbf{i}$.
4. Reducing the fox population in two stages has the same effect on the between-group infection probability as an equivalent single reduction, i.e. for all p and $\mathbf{i}$ lying between 0 and 1 the function P_B satisfies

$$P_B(p,\mathbf{i}) = P_B(P_B(p,\beta), 1-(1 - \mathbf{i})/(1 - \beta)) \tag{11}$$

for all β lying between 0 and $\mathbf{i}$.

From those four quite reasonable assumptions we can obtain the following results:

Result 1.   Control at maximum intensity results in the between-group infection probability being increased to its maximum value of 1, i.e. $P_B(p,1) = 1$ for all p lying between 0 and 1.

Result 2.   The function $P_B(p,\mathbf{i})$ is completely determined by its behaviour when $p = 0$, i.e. by $P_B(0,\mathbf{i})$, $0 \leq \mathbf{i} \leq 1$.

We shall not give formal proofs of these two results but note that the second follows almost immediately from the first, since given any p between 0 and 1 there exists, by the first result, a control intensity u such that $P_B(0,u) = p$, and hence from Equation (11)

$$P_B(P,\mathbf{i}) = P_B(0,1-(1 - \mathbf{i}) (1 -u)),   0 \leq \mathbf{i} \leq 1 \tag{12}$$

Under the assumptions we have made, decreasing the fox population by control measures affects the group infection probability in two ways. Firstly, the group sizes are reduced and thus there are fewer possible contacts between the two groups. In the absence of any effect of control, this will clearly decrease the group infection probability, but in the more realistic situation, which we are now considering, there will be an increased probability of contact between pairs of foxes that have survived the control policy. Whichever of these two effects is dominant will determine whether the control is worthwhile. Suppose that before control, the between-group infection probability is p and the group size is N. If an initial decrease in the susceptible fox population reduces the group infection probability P_G, the control will be marginally effective, otherwise it will be marginally countereffective. Expressed mathematically, we have that control will be marginally effective (countereffective) according to whether $\partial P'_G / \partial \mathbf{i}$, evaluated at $\mathbf{i} = 0$, is less (greater) than zero. From Equation (10), we have that control is marginally effective (countereffective) if

$$\left. \frac{\partial P_B}{\partial \mathbf{i}} \right| \mathbf{i}{=}0 < (>) - 2(1-p) \ln(1-p), \tag{13}$$

where ln is the natural logarithm.

From Equation (13), we observe that whether control is effective or not does not depend on the group size N. This is partially a consequence of our assumption that the effect of control depends only on the relative fox population reduction, i.e. on the control intensity and not on the absolute fox population reduction. The above observation permits us to set N equal to one in the following analysis, without losing any generality.

To proceed further we need to impose a particular form on $P_B(0,\mathbf{i})$, and it is convenient to use

$$P_B(0,\mathbf{i}) = 1 - (1 - \mathbf{i})^x, \qquad 0 \le \mathbf{i} \le 1, \tag{14}$$

where x is a positive constant. Application of Equation (12) to Equation (14) yields

$$P_B(p,\mathbf{i}) = 1 - (1 - p)(1 - \mathbf{i})^x, \qquad 0 \le p, \mathbf{i} \le 1. \tag{15}$$

Figure 5 shows typical graphs of $P_B(0,\mathbf{i})$ for the three cases, $x < 1$, $x = 1$ and $x > 1$. Note that if $x > 1$, then the low intensity control does most damage, whilst if $x < 1$, then it is the high intensity control that does most damage. From Equations (13) and (15), we have that control is marginally effective (countereffective) according to whether

$$p > (<) 1 - e^{-x/2}. \tag{16}$$

Now by assumption (3) $P_B(p,\mathbf{i})$ strictly increases with $\mathbf{i}$ and hence if $p \ge 1 - e^{-x/2}$, the group infection probability P_G will decrease with increasing intensity $\mathbf{i}$, whilst if $p < 1 - e^{-x/2}$, P_G will first increase and then decrease [since by result 1, $P_B(p,1) = 1 > 1 - e^{-x/2}$] with increasing $\mathbf{i}$. In both cases if we kill all the foxes, there can naturally be no spread of infection, i.e. $P_G(p,1) = 0$. The

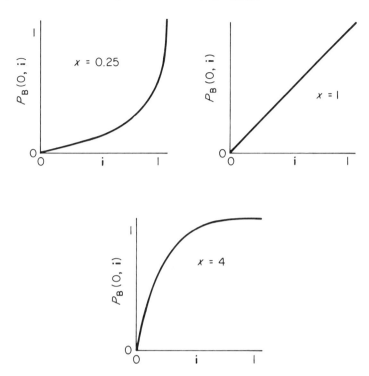

Fig. 5. Graphs showing the form of the dependence of the between-group infection probability on the intensity of control for the three cases $x < 1$, $x = 1$ and $x > 1$. $\mathbf{i}$ = control intensity; $P_B (0, \mathbf{i})$ = between-group infection probability after control of intensity $\mathbf{i}$; $P_B(0, \mathbf{i}) = 1-(1 - \mathbf{i})^x$, where x is a positive real constant.

two situations are illustrated in Fig. 6; it is the second case that we are most interested in, as there is a threshold intensity of control, $\mathbf{i}^*$, that has to be attained before control becomes effective.

The value of $\mathbf{i}^*$ is given by the only solution of $P_G(p,\mathbf{i}) = P_G(p,0)$ lying between 0 and 1, and from Equations (10) and (15), this is given by

$$\mathbf{i}^* = P_1^{-1} (1 - (1 - p)^{1/x}) \tag{17}$$

where $P_1^{-1}(\ )$ is the inverse of the function $P_1(\ )$ defined by

$$P_1(\mathbf{i}) = 1 - (1 - \mathbf{i})^{1/((1 - \mathbf{i})^{-2} - 1)} \tag{18}$$

A graph of $\mathbf{i}^*$ against p when $x = 1$, i.e. of $P_1^{-1}(p)$, is given in Fig. 7, from which we see that $P_1^{-1}(p)$ is closely approximated by the straight line

$$P_1^{-1}(p) = 1 - p/(1 - e^{-1/2}) \qquad 0 \le p \le 1 - e^{-1/2}, \tag{19}$$

and thus a good approximation to $\mathbf{i}^*$ is

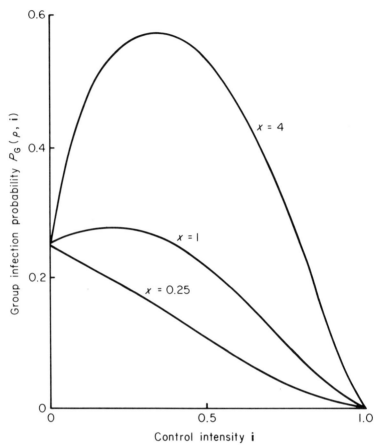

Fig. 6. Graphs showing the dependence of the group infection probability $P_G(p, \mathbf{i})$ on the control intensity $\mathbf{i}$, when prior to control the between-group infection probability was $p = 0.25$. x is a parameter describing how the between-group infection probability P_B varies with control intensity (see Fig. 5). Note that when $x = 0.25$, control is always effective, whilst for the other two cases control is only effective if its intensity is above a threshold level.

$$\mathbf{i}^* = [\,(1 - p)^{1/x} - e^{-1/2}\,/\,(1 - e^{-1/2})\,] \qquad 0 \leq p \leq 1 - e^{-x/2}. \quad (20)$$

We also see from Fig. 6 that when $x = 1$ the value of $\mathbf{i}^*$ can be quite large; indeed, when $p = 0.1$ (the value chosen in our simulations of Section II), we have to kill over 70% of the foxes to yield a reduction in the group infection probability P_G and, moreover, if $x > 1$ the situation is even worse. Admittedly, these results are highly dependent on the form we have chosen for $P_B(p, \mathbf{i})$, but it is qualitative, rather than quantitative, conclusions that we are most interested in, and our model has demonstrated the possible existence of a threshold level of control, below which all control is countereffective. It is interesting to note that I

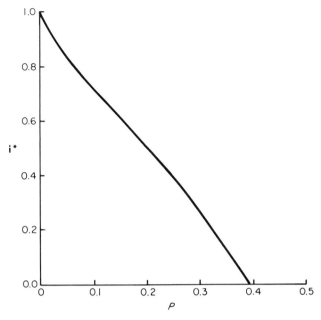

Fig. 7. Graph showing the dependence of the critical control intensity i* on the between-group infection probability *prior* to control p, when the 'shape' parameter x = 1. Control is only effective if it is of intensity at least i*.

obtained precisely the same conclusion from a one-dimensional model which incorporated the absorption of empty fox territories into neighbouring territories (Ball, 1981). It therefore seems likely that a threshold level of control will exist in real life rabies control and, moreover, we have seen that there is a distinct possibility that any intensity of control killing attainable in the field will be countereffective. Indeed, Bacon and Macdonald (1980) note an analysis by Ross, which showed that intensive killing of foxes ahead of the rabies front in France has at times accelerated the propagation of disease. In view of this, and of our control model, it seems preferable to bring about the required reduction in the susceptible fox population by oral vaccination of foxes against rabies, provided a sufficient reduction in the number of susceptibles can be achieved, since then there would be considerably less disturbance of the foxes' social system.

V. Conclusions

We have produced a model that clearly demonstrates the important role played by group size in the spread of rabies amongst foxes. The model also proved useful as the basis of an extremely flexible control model. However, this flexibility was only achieved by making a few quite reasonable approximations. All these approximations increased the spread of rabies and hence, provided our model is appropriate, any control policy will have a greater probability of succeeding in the field than that predicted by our model, although the difference will probably be quite small. However, some of the assumptions of our model were quite strict and we now briefly discuss some of its major shortcomings.

A. DISCUSSION

We have assumed that a rabid fox moves similarly to a normal fox, which resulted in our using a nearest-neighbour infection model. However, given any reasonable movement pattern for a rabid fox the role played by group size in the spread of rabies will be qualitatively similar, in that epizootics will only have a non-zero chance of 'taking off' if the group size is above some threshold, whose value will depend on the form of our model. In contrast, changing the movement pattern of a rabid fox could have dire consequences on the success of a control policy. For example, if a rabid fox moves erratically around covering vast distances we shall clearly require greater depths of control than those predicted by our model. Nevertheless, the slow rate of advance of the front of rabies through Europe, about 30–60 km/year (Anderson *et al.*, 1981), suggests that the spread of infection is generally of a nearest neighbour type. However, in the autumn juvenile foxes can cover considerable distances whilst dispersing. The main threat of such foxes to rabies control is the possibility that they might be incubating, or indeed transmitting, rabies. During these dispersal periods the spread of rabies is unlikely to be completely 'nearest-neighbour' and thus control zones of greater depth than usual will be required.

In our model we have made no distinction between 'paralytic' and 'furious' rabies cases, and until better knowledge of the movements of both types of rabid foxes is available, it seems sensible not to model the two types specifically. However, we note in passing that the two types of rabies are likely to contribute differently to the 'between-group' and 'within-group' infection probabilities, P_B and P_W, respectively. The furious rabid cases will probably be responsible for much of the between group transmission, whilst paralytic rabies for much of the within group transmission.

Our model has assumed that the parameters (N, P_n) and territory size are homogeneous over the 29×29 grid, whereas, in his studies of the Red Fox, Macdonald (1977) found that both group and territory size can vary considerably over quite a small region. The variation of fox population parameters can be classified into two types, namely heterogeneity and variability. Heterogeneity refers to the structured way in which these parameters vary over a given region, whilst variability refers to random fluctuations about this structure; thus heterogeneity is a global phenomenon and variability a local one. Variability by itself can easily be incorporated into our general control model but heterogeneity is another matter. Further, the latter is more important since a control policy can fail owing to rabies persisting in a small subpopulation of foxes. Heterogeneity in territory size is connected with lattice structure, since such a rigid grid structure cannot realistically accommodate different territory sizes. A non-lattice model would be preferable, but there has been little research into such models. It seems likely that qualitative results for lattice models, such as the existence of thresholds, will carry over to less regularly spaced populations (Mollison, 1977). However, this will not generally be the case for quantitative results, such as the probability of success of control policies. Indeed, it should be noted that qualitative results will be different for different types of lattice, e.g. the threshold group size might be different for triangular, square and hexagonal lattices.

Before we can use our control model in any real life rabies surveillance problem, we shall require estimates of the parameters (N, P_B) and also of the territory size for the region in which control is to be applied. Ball (1981) described methods of estimating P_B from radio-tracking data on foxes, whilst group size and territory size can be estimated by direct observation of foxes. However, unless they are already known for the region concerned, it will take a considerable time to obtain the above estimates, which will be rather embarrassing as it is clearly preferable to commence control as soon as a rabid fox is reported. In Chapter 11, this volume, I will suggest an alternative method of estimating these parameters, using data gathered from maps, which in spite of requiring considerably more research to make operable, should quickly yield the required estimates.

The major difficulty we have encountered in constructing our model is that of proceeding in the face of inadequate knowledge concerning the behaviour of rabid foxes. Good data on rabid foxes is the single quantity most urgently required by mathematical modellers, and until such data becomes available, the quantitative conclusions of our model should be viewed cautiously. Thus, apart from the qualitative conclusions, the main purpose of our present model is perhaps to provide a framework within which future models can be built once the relevant data become available.

Appendix. Symbols Used in Text, in Order of Appearance

P_W —*Within*-group infection probability—probability that a rabid fox infects a given susceptible fox *within the same* group.

P_B —*Between*-group infection probability—probability that a rabid fox infects a given susceptible fox belonging to a *neighbouring* group.

P_G —*Group* infection probability—probability that an infected group of foxes infects a given neighbouring group of foxes.

N —*Uncontrolled* fox group size.

M —Fox group size *within* the control zone.

Appendix (*Continued*)

d —Depth at which control is applied.

α —Required probability that rabies is eradicted by the control policy.

$P_d(\alpha)$ —Maximum value of P_G *within* the control zone for a control of depth d to have a probability at least α of succeeding.

$M_d(\alpha, P_B)$—Mean group size corresponding to a group infection probability of $P_d(\alpha)$ when the between-group infection probability is P_B.

i —Control intensity—proportion of foxes within the control zone that are killed by a control policy.

$P_B(p, i)$ —*Between*-group infection probability following control of intensity i when *prior* to control the between-group infection probability was p.

$P_G(p, i)$ —*Group* infection probability following control of intensity i when *prior* to control the between-group infection probability was p.

i^* —Threshold intensity of control, which has to be attained before control becomes effective.

Acknowledgement

This research was carried out whilst I was a research student in the Department of Biomathematics, University of Oxford. It is a pleasure to thank my supervisor, Professor P. Armitage, for his helpful advice and encouragement and the Medical Research Council for financial support.

References

Anderson, R. M., Jackson, H. C., May, R. M., and Smith, A. M. (1981). Population dynamics of fox rabies in Europe. *Nature (London)* **289**, 765–771.

Bacon, P. (1981). The consequences of unreported fox rabies. *J. Environ. Manage.* **13**, 195–200.

Bacon, P., and Macdonald, D. W. (1980). To control rabies: Vaccinate foxes. *New Sci.* **87**, 640–645.

Bailey, N. T. J., (1967). The simulation of stochastic epidemics in two dimensions. *Proc. Fifth Berkeley Symp. Math. Statis. and Prob.* **4**, 237–256. University of California, Berkeley and Los Angeles.

Bailey, N. T. J. (1975). "The Mathematical Theory of Infectious Diseases." Griffin, London.

Ball, F. G. (1981). Some statistical problems in the epidemiology of fox rabies. Ph.D. Thesis, University of Oxford.

Hammersley, J. M., and Handscomb, D. C. (1964). "Monte Carlo Methods." Methuen, London.

Macdonald, D. W. (1977). The behavioural ecology of the red fox, *Vulpes, Vulpes:* A study of social organisation resource exploitation. Ph.D. Thesis, University of Oxford.

Mollison, D. (1977). Spatial contact models for ecological and epidemic spread. *J. R. Stat. Soc. Ser. B.* **39**, 283–326.

Sensitivity Analysis of Simple Endemic Models

9

Denis Mollison

Department of Actuarial Mathematics and Statistics,
Heriot-Watt University,
Riccarton, Edinburgh, Scotland

I. Introduction

Simple mathematical models have had considerable success in explaining basic epidemiological features, such as threshold phenomena and cyclical outbreaks. This chapter presents a sensitivity analysis of some simple models for endemic diseases such as rabies, and shows that there are unresolved problems in making *quantitative* use of them, especially in the crucial area of evaluating control strategies.

This is not to say that it is wrong to look at simple models. On the contrary, what I try to do here is to go a step further in simplification and argue as far as possible in terms of the basic components which any model for endemic rabies must include. Such coarse data as exist for diseases like rabies can be used to confirm that we have included the essential components in our epidemic model, and to calibrate each such component correctly. It is much more difficult to get adequate data to determine the quantitative details of each component, yet these details are important if our model is to have predictive value.

I shall illustrate these problems mainly with reference to a basic differential equation model for endemic rabies introduced by Anderson *et al.* (1981; see also Anderson, 1981, 1982), and presented in this volume by Dr. Smith (Chapter 6); and particularly to the possibility of making quantitative use of this model, as

POPULATION DYNAMICS OF RABIES IN WILDLIFE

suggested by those authors. This rabies model differs from standard epidemic models (see e.g. Bailey, 1975) chiefly in including a density-dependent population growth term. This is a welcome improvement, as such a term is clearly important for a proper discussion of diseases like fox rabies in which the disease itself regulates the population density.

Anderson *et al.* cite as support for their model its predictions relating to (1) threshold densities, (2) contact rates between infectious and susceptible foxes, (3) average levels of prevalence of infection, (4) the 3- to 5-year cycle sometimes observed in fox populations infected with rabies, and (5) an association between unstable (i.e. cyclical) endemic conditions and areas of high carrying capacity. Encouraged by this agreement, they base a quantitative discussion of possible control strategies on their model.

The crucial model component for consideration of control, whether by vaccination or culling, turns out to be the *infection term*. These authors follow conventional lines in using a multiplicative term, βXY, for the rate of infection between susceptible and infectious populations of respective densities X and Y. Unfortunately, as I shall show here, the use of a multiplicative infection term in the case of varying population density makes strong implicit assumptions, which critically influence the conclusions on control strategies. However, once the importance of the exact form of the infection term is recognised, we can look for relevant observational evidence which will allow us a more reliably based discussion of control strategies.

The other two main components of a basic rabies model are the terms representing *population growth* and the *generation gap* of the disease (see Section II). We find that the level of prevalence and period of oscillations of the disease are fairly robustly determined, but that conclusions on the stability of oscillations are very sensitive to the detailed assumptions concerning these components.

The considerations presented here should also be relevant to a wide range of applications of simple epidemic models, the main theme being that the quantitative assumptions implicit in such models need careful consideration, especially if we wish to draw quantitative conclusions. The problem of controlling tuberculosis in badgers (see e.g. Henderson, 1982) is similar to that of rabies in foxes. The estimation of required vaccination rates in non-fatal diseases, such as measles and whooping cough, is cited as another example.

I shall also refer more briefly to other simple epidemic models, and to some factors which all these models omit, particularly spatial, stochastic and seasonal effects.

II. Components of Basic Epidemic Models

I here identify three basic components essential for modelling the endemic state of a disease such as rabies: (1) the population dynamics in the absence of disease, (2) the infectious contacts made by a diseased individual, and (3) the *generation gap* of the disease, that is the time interval between an individual's becoming infected and passing on the disease.

First are the population dynamics in the absence of disease. Diseases that are not usually fatal, such as human colds or measles, have little effect on population numbers; the latter can therefore be modelled separately. Often, it is reasonable to assume a constant equilibrium population, with deaths (from other causes) at a constant rate and births introducing fresh susceptibles occurring at the same constant rate.

In contrast, fatal diseases such as rabies will reduce a population below its usual level, and this may both increase the birth rate and decrease the death rate from other causes. We may reasonably assume that the *per capita net population growth rate* in the absence of disease, ϱ, is a decreasing function of the population density N, varying from a value r at low density to negative values at high densities. The population density K for which the net growth rate is zero defines the *carrying capacity* of the environment. For example, for their deterministic non-spatial model, Anderson *et al.* suggested $\varrho = r(1 - N/K)$, which yields the familiar logistic growth curve for a population below carrying capacity (in the absence of disease).

Second are the infectious contacts made by an infectious individual. Not surprisingly, the total number of potentially infectious contacts made by an infectious individual, sometimes called the *basic reproductive rate, C,* of the epidemic, is a crucial parameter. Indeed, for non-spatial models, in which homogeneous mixing of infectives and susceptibles is assumed so that in the initial stage of an epidemic almost all infectious contacts are with susceptibles and therefore successful, the basic threshold result states simply that the disease has a chance of spreading widely if and only if C is greater than 1. In models with more realistic (local) mixing, the probability of contacting another infective cannot be neglected, even in the earliest stages of an epidemic; C is still a crucial parameter, but its threshold value may be significantly greater than 1.

Unfortunately, the basic reproductive rate does not usually feature explicitly in epidemic models, but enters indirectly through the overall rate of infectious contacts, which is of course an important variable in analysis of such models. The relation between the two is quite straightforward, at least in the case of models with homogeneous mixing, and is as follows.

We take $\tau_2 = 1/\alpha$ to be the mean infectious period, so that an individual makes contacts at average rate αC while infectious; and assume that contacts are made indiscriminately among the population so that their probability of success is equal to the proportion of susceptibles in the population, X/N. Multiplying by the density of infectious individuals Y, we have that the overall rate of infectious contacts (per unit area) is $\beta X Y$, where $\beta = \alpha C/N$ is a constant which in general must depend on the population density and its relation to the carrying capacity, that is on N and K. Taking β to be a constant, as is often done (e.g. Bailey, 1975;

Anderson *et al.*, 1981), is equivalent to assuming that the reproductive rate $C = \beta N/\alpha$, i.e. that C is proportional to N and independent of K. [Indeed Bacon (see Chapter 7 of this volume) has explicitly used this relationship to produce a 'dimensionless' model, scaled relative to K.]

Third and last, is the *generation gap T*, defined as the time interval between an individual's becoming infected and passing on the disease. The generation gap's mean value τ is important in determining the speed with which an epidemic develops, and in endemic conditions is closely related to the level of prevalence, that is the mean proportion of the population suffering from the disease. Less obviously perhaps, the *variability* of the generation gap turns out to be important for such features as the dependence of an epidemic's velocity on population density, and for determining whether endemic conditions are stable or oscillatory.

It is important in principle to distinguish between the mean generation gap and the mean survival time after infection. However, the difference between the two in practical terms is usually small, at least for rabies where the infectious period is short compared with the latent period; and in several of the simplest models, including all those described in the next section (Equations 1–3), the generation gap and survival time are actually assumed to have the same distribution.

III. Some Basic Models and Their Assumptions

As described in the previous section, the models I shall discuss are each made from three basic components: *population growth, infection,* and the *generation gap* of the disease. In this section I shall first define some simple deterministic models, and then bring out some of the assumptions implicit in the particular form of components chosen for each of them.

In the model by Anderson *et al.* (1981) the densities of susceptible (X), incubating (I) and infectious (Y) individuals is as follows:

$$
\begin{aligned}
dX/dt &= \varrho X - \beta XY \\
dI/dt &= \beta XY - \sigma I - [(b+\gamma N)I] \\
dY/dt &= \sigma I - \alpha Y - [(b+\gamma N)Y]
\end{aligned}
\tag{1}
$$

where $N = X+I+Y$ is the total population density, and α, β, γ, σ and b are constants; ϱ denotes the *per capita* net population growth rate, which Anderson *et al.* take equal to $r(1-N/K)$, where K denotes the carrying capacity of the fox habitat. An interpretation of the constants β, α, σ and r, and of the corresponding constants in the following models [Equations (2) and (3)] is given later; for estimates, appropriate to fox rabies, of the values of all these constants, see Section IV. The terms in square brackets (involving the constants γ and b) relate to mortality from natural causes of incubating and infectious individuals; their effect is negligible in most respects, and discussion of the model will be much clearer if we omit them.

A somewhat simpler family of models is described by the equations

$$dX/dt = \varrho X - \beta'XV$$
$$dV/dt = \beta'XV - \alpha'V \qquad (2)$$

This equation covers several well-known models, in each case keeping β' and α' as constants. First, we can regard it as an epidemic model in which we fail to distinguish between incubating and infectious individuals; thus V replaces $I+Y$. If $\varrho = c/X$ we obtain a standard model for diseases such as measles (Bartlett, 1960) in which we assume the 'immigration' of susceptibles at constant rate c. For rabies it would be more appropriate to follow Anderson *et al.* in taking $\varrho = r(1-N/K)$. If we take the slightly different formula $\varrho = r(1-X/K)$, we have a special case of Verhulst's model, with V representing predators and X prey; while the simpler formula $\varrho = r$ similarly yields a special case of Lotka and Volterra's classic predator–prey model (see e.g. May, 1974, or Chapter 7, this volume).

So far, I have referred only to differential equation models. A possible alternative is to use a discrete-time model, such as the following, in which we have discrete generations of infectious individuals, at time intervals of fixed length τ:

$$X_{t+\tau} = X_t + (\rho X_t - \beta'X_tY_t)\tau$$
$$Y_{t+\tau} = \beta'X_tY_t\tau \qquad (3)$$

For *infection*, each of these models includes a conventional multiplicative term, βXY. As described in the previous section, this essentially amounts to taking the reproductive rate $C = \beta N/\alpha$; while the *effective reproduction rate*, the mean number of successful contacts, is $R = C. (X/N) = \beta X/\alpha$. Similarly, for Equation (2) we obtain $C = \beta'N/\alpha'$; for Equation (3), $C = \beta'\tau N$. Thus if we take β (or β') to be a constant, we are assuming that the reproductive rate C of the epidemic is proportional to N, and independent of K. These are strong assumptions, which go well beyond the observational evidence. The dependence of C on N and K is crucial for the evaluation of control strategies, as will be discussed in Section IV.

Each of the three models also includes a net *population growth* term ϱX, representing the excess of births over deaths from natural mortality. As already mentioned, Anderson *et al.* take $\varrho = r(1-N/K)$. The qualitative assumption here, that ϱ decreases from a value r in low-density populations to zero at the carrying capacity, is very reasonable and a welcome improvement on standard models. The quantitative assumption, that this decrease is linear with increasing population density N, has no particular justification, and we must be sceptical of any conclusions which depend on it.

Last is the distribution of the disease's *generation gap*. Here the three models make different detailed assumptions, in each case chosen to give the simplest mathematical equations. In each case the transfer rates out of certain states are assumed proportional to the numbers in those states. In the differential equation models, this amounts to assuming that the sojourn times in each state are exponentially distributed; while in discrete-time models they are assumed to be of fixed length or geometrically distributed.

Thus for Equation (2), the generation gap has exponential distribution with mean $\tau = 1/\alpha'$. For Equation (1), the terms σI and αY essentially assume exponential distributions for the incubation and infectious periods, respectively, with means $\tau_1 = 1/\sigma$ and $\tau_2 = 1/\alpha$; then the generation gap T has mean $\tau = \tau_1 + \tau_2$, and probability density function

$$[\alpha\sigma/(\alpha-\sigma)](e^{-\sigma t} - e^{-\alpha t}) \tag{4}$$

The discrete-time model [Equation (3)] assumes a fixed incubation period of length τ and an instantaneous infection period, so that the generation gap is of fixed length τ. This is clearly an extreme case; a more realistic discrete-time model for rabies will be mentioned in the discussion of Section V.

To sum up, the *infection term* involves a parameter β, which has traditionally been assumed to be a constant. The consequences of this assumption in the context of fox rabies will be examined in Section IV. The models discussed also include basic parameters r (the net *population growth rate* in low-density populations) and τ (the mean *generation gap*), which can both be estimated fairly reliably from observations. The detailed forms of the population growth and generation gap terms are less easy to estimate from data, and all the models considered here make simple assumptions based on mathematical convenience. As we shall see in Section V, some features of the models depend principally on r and τ and are thus insensitive to the modelling details, while others are not.

IV. Control Strategies and the Reproductive Rate

The first two points of observational evidence cited by Anderson *et al.* (1981) relate to threshold densities, and contact rates between infectious and susceptible foxes.

Firstly, they note evidence that there exists a threshold value K_T for the carrying capacity K, below which rabies cannot become endemic (their estimate is $K_T \approx 1$ per km²). This supports the common assumption that the contact rate between foxes increases with K, but not necessarily the further assumptions implicit in the βXY infection term, i.e. that the reproductive rate $C = N/K_T$.

Secondly, the authors cite observations suggesting that the contact rate between normal foxes at around the threshold population density, βK_T, is approximately equal to the death rate α of infectious foxes, as predicted by their model. However, it is axiomatic that at the threshold population density (if such exists) each infected fox gives rise on average to one secondary case. Thus if foxes are rabid for an average period of 5 days, they must in these conditions contact on average one susceptible every 5 days. The prediction that $\beta K_T = \alpha$ is thus not dependent on their particular model.

Two notes of caution should be sounded here. Firstly, we really need data on the rates of contacts by rabid rather than normal foxes. Secondly, if we take a model which more accurately reflects the local structure of the population, e.g. a stochastic lattice model, we will find that the deterministic model's assumption that $R \approx C$ when $N \approx K$, i.e. that initially almost all infectious contacts are with susceptibles, is incorrect; in fact R may be significantly lower than C because the few infectious cases tend to be clumped together. Thus $\beta K_T = \alpha$ is not strictly correct, the threshold value of C being rather greater than unity for a more accurate model (see Mollison, 1981, or Chapter 12, this volume). In this context, it should be noted that the definition of Anderson et al. of the basic reproductive rate is also unsatisfactory in that it ignores the difference between contacts within and outwith a fox's family.

However, ignoring these complications, we may sum up by saying that the evidence of the existence of a threshold population density, together with '$\beta K_T \approx \alpha$', support the general form of the infection term, but not necessarily its quantitative detail, especially its implicit assumption that β does not depend on N or K. But if we do assume the quantitative form, this evidence serves to calibrate our model.

This is a convenient point at which to summarise the calibration of all three models [Equations (1–3)] for the case of fox rabies. For Equation (1), Anderson et al. estimate $r \approx \frac{1}{2}$ year^{-1}. They take $\tau_1 = 28$ days and $\tau_2 = 5$ days for the mean incubation and infectious periods, respectively, leading to $\sigma = 1/\tau_1 = 13$ year^{-1}, $\alpha = 1/\tau_2 = 73$ year^{-1}, and $\tau = \tau_1 + \tau_2 = \frac{1}{11}$ years. The threshold population density K_T is estimated ≈ 1 per km^2, as mentioned previously, so that using $\beta K_T \approx \alpha$ we have that $\beta \approx \alpha = 73$. For Equations (2) and (3), the corresponding estimates are given by $\alpha' = 1/\tau = 11$ year^{-1}, and $\beta' K_T \approx \alpha'$, so that $\beta' \approx \alpha' = 11$.

We now turn to the discussion of control strategies. Simply put, the aim of any control strategy must be to reduce the effective reproductive rate R to less than unity. As we have seen, the use of a βXY infection term by Anderson et al. implicitly assumes that $R = X/K_T$ and, thus, immediately implies the core of their conclusions, namely that a control policy will succeed if and only if it reduces the density of susceptibles below the threshold carrying capacity K_T.

Consider first a vaccination programme among an undisturbed population, where the density N is equal to the carrying capacity K, and K is greater than K_T. If we vaccinate a proportion p, the density of susceptibles will be $(1-p)K$, so that according to Anderson et al. (1981) the vaccination programme will succeed if and only if $p > 1 - K_T/K$. (Note that the more complex spatial simulation model of Berger (1976) also assumes a βXY infection term, and therefore not surprisingly leads to numerical conclusions in good agreement with this.) Experiments cited by Anderson *et al.* suggest that the maximum achievable value of p for foxes is about $\frac{2}{3}$, leading to the conclusion that vaccination alone can only be effective if K is less than about $3K_T$. However this conclusion depends on the assumption that contact rates are proportional to density ($C = N/K_T$). This does not seem a realistic assumption for territorial animals such as foxes, since the number of *neighbours* of a fox family will increase only slightly if at all as the population density increases. If, for instance, we take C proportional to $\sqrt{N}$ [i.e. $C = \sqrt{(N/K_T)}$], we find that vaccination will be successful if $p > 1 - \sqrt{(K_T/K)}$; so that for the same vaccination success rate ($p = \frac{2}{3}$), we would predict that the disease can be prevented in populations of density up to $9K_T$ rather than $3K_T$.

The effects of culling (or of a mixed programme of vaccination and culling) are more difficult to assess. Anderson *et al.* (1981) consider two types of culling policy, of which the 'constant effort' strategy seems the most relevant, the alternative of quota culling being more appropriate to red herring (May, 1981). In any case, their main conclusion is that control by culling will succeed if and only if the population density is held down below K_T. This assumes that contact numbers in a population held down to density K_T will be the same as in an undisturbed population in territory of carrying capacity K_T. There are obvious ecological reasons why this might not be so. For instance, when $N = K_T << K$, competition between foxes for available food will be much reduced, tending to reduce contacts; while on the other hand, families will be broken up by the culling, and this social disturbance is likely to cause more contacts. The poor record of practical attempts at control by culling, to which Anderson *et al.* refer, suggests that the latter may be the stronger effect. Of course, rabies is itself a culling policy of sorts, so that observations of equilibrium densities in endemic areas will be of use, especially in areas where the carrying capacity can be estimated. However, the effect on the contact rate will depend on the method of culling: whether it kills one fox at a time or whole families, and whether it selects relatively more itinerant or settled foxes. Quantitative conclusions clearly require more evidence.

V. Endemic Equilibrium and Oscillations about It

Anderson *et al.* (1981) cite three pieces of evidence relating to the population growth rate and generation gap: namely, the observed level of prevalence, the period of oscillations, and their stability. The first of these concerns the *level of prevalence,* that is the proportion of incubating plus infected cases when the disease is in endemic equilibrium. This can be more simply explained without reference to any particular model as follows: in equilibrium, the net population growth rate ϱX (in their model $\varrho = r(1-N/K)$), and the transition rates from susceptible to incubating, incubating to infectious, and infectious to dead, must all be equal. It is easily deduced that the ratio $X:I:Y$ (susceptibles : incubating : infectious) must be approximately $\varrho^{-1}:\sigma^{-1}:\alpha^{-1}$ (approximately because natural mortality among infected cases is here neglected). If we let τ denote the mean generation gap (as previously), we then have that the level of prevalence is approximately $\varrho\tau$. Thus we need only the qualitative assumption, that ϱ varies from a value r when $N \ll K$ down to 0 when $N = K$, to predict that levels of prevalence in endemic areas will vary up to a maximum of $r\tau$. In fact, the cited observation that levels of prevalence in endemic areas lie in the range 3–7%, together with the relatively exact estimate for τ, $\approx \frac{1}{11}$ (years), suggests values of r up to about $\frac{3}{4}$ (per head per year), slightly higher than the authors' estimate of $r \approx \frac{1}{2}$. However, the evidence available does not appear adequate to determine the detailed form of ϱ.

The period of oscillations also turns out to depend principally on the two parameters r and τ (rather than primarily on r alone as suggested by Anderson *et al.*). For instance, for all the models defined previously [Equations (1) to (3)], we find that oscillations close to the equilibrium point have period approximately $T_0 = 2\pi\sqrt{(\tau/\varrho)}$, $\approx 2\pi\sqrt{(\tau/r)}$ for endemic areas of stable rabies where we may assume $\varrho \approx r$ and for oscillations further from equilibrium the period rises in each model. Taking the authors' figures ($r = \frac{1}{2}$, $\tau = \frac{1}{11}$), we find that periods of around 3 years upwards are predicted in each case.

All these models share the authors' assumption that the disease's effective reproduction rate R is proportional to the density of susceptibles, $R = X/K_T$. It is easy to analyse oscillations near equilibrium without making this assumption, and it is found that their period is approximately $T_0 g^{-\frac{1}{2}}$, where $T_0 = 2\pi\sqrt{(\tau/\varrho)}$ as previously, and $g = (X/R)(dR/dX)$, evaluated at the equilibrium value X_0. For instance, if R is proportional to $X^{1/n}$ instead of to X, the period is increased by a factor of $\sqrt{n}$. Thus observed periods of 3–5 years suggest that R does indeed increase with population density, but are also equally consistent with a considerably slower than linear dependence of R on X.

The form of the population growth term ϱX has much less influence on the period. Whether we assume $\varrho = r(1-N/K)$, or take any of the three alternative forms for ϱ mentioned following Equation (2), makes very little difference to the period, at least for small oscillations.

Lastly, Anderson *et al.* cite evidence of a tendency for unstable, i.e. cyclical, dynamic behaviour to be associated with areas of high carrying capacity, $K \gg K_T$. This supports the use of a density-dependent growth term, as in their model or Verhulst's equations, rather than the constant birth rate of the Lotka–Volterra model or the constant growth term of the epidemic with immigration. Qualitatively, their use of a more realistic growth term thus appears to be an improvement on previous deterministic epidemic models, though it should be noted that cyclical behaviour can arise through the seasonal and stochastic factors which they neglect (Bartlett, 1960; Stirzaker, 1975). However, the quantitative details of their model are very sensitive to their precise assumptions concerning both the population growth rate and the distribution of the generation gap. For instance, while their model is unstable for K greater than $K_c \approx 9K_T$, the discrete-time model [Equation (3)] is unstable when $K > K_c = 2K_T$. It is not clear that the discrete-time model, with its fixed generation gap, is a worse approximation than their model, which assigns a probability of about $\frac{1}{4}$ to the generation gap's being shorter than the minimum observed value (12 days). Clearly we need to model the distribution of the generation gap better if we are interested in the conditions for stable population dynamics. A more realistic generation gap distribution, intermediate between the fixed gap of the discrete-time model and Equation (4), will presumably lead to intermediate values for K_c. (For instance, a discrete-time model with geometrically distributed incubation period, and constant infection period of 1 week so that the minimum generation gap is 2 weeks—yields $K_c \approx 5.6K_T$.)

Unfortunately, the value of K_c is also sensitive to the form of the per capita growth rate ϱ, which is difficult to estimate from observations. For instance, K_c will be significantly lower if ϱ, instead of declining linearly as the population density N increases, is near constant for low values of N, decreasing rapidly to zero as N nears K. In the extreme case, where $\varrho = r$ for $N < K$, and $\varrho = 0$ for $N > K$, we find that $K_c = K_T$, i.e. that endemic conditions are always unstable. The formula $\varrho = r(1 - (N/K)^z$, is suggested by R. M. May (personal communication), with values of z perhaps between 2 and 3. Figure 1 shows the dependence of K_c/K_T on z for Equation (1). Remembering that seasonal and stochastic factors may also tend to increase instability, K_c does seem likely to be less than Ander-

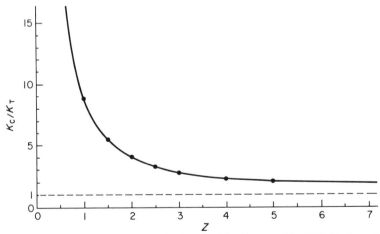

Fig. 1. The dependence of K_c/K_T on z for Equation (1), when $\rho = r[1 - (N/K)^z]$ (values of r, α, β and σ as given in Section III).

son *et al.*'s value of approximately $9K_T$, but it is clear that no quantitative conclusions can be drawn at present.

VI. Conclusions

The cardinal virtue of a simple model is that it should be possible to see clearly which assumptions lead to which conclusions. Judged by this criterion, even the simplest models for endemic disease are too complex when considered as a whole.

What I have tried to do here is to show how such models can be dissected into their basic components, and that much of the discussion of their behaviour can be conducted in terms of these components. This dissection clarifies the implicit assumptions which are present in even the simplest models, and makes it easier to assess the dependence of any conclusions on those assumptions.

The most crucial questions concern the likely success of various possible control strategies. This turns out to depend almost entirely on the infection term alone and in particular on its assumptions as to how the basic reproductive rate C will change under the strategy considered. It becomes clear that if we are to make reliable predictions for the control of fox rabies, we need more information on the dependence of C on the population density N and the carrying capacity K. It should not be too difficult to investigate these factors, except that, ideally, studies of rabid foxes are required.

Further difficulties may however arise when we consider the effects of heterogeneous mixing. This is perhaps best illustrated by the example of non-fatal diseases, such as measles and whooping cough, where the population density is not affected by the disease, so that the dependence of C on N and K is of less importance. For such cases, a simple argument due to Dietz (1975) suggests that, when the disease is in endemic equilibrium, C can be estimated as $\approx 1+L/A$, where L is the mean lifetime and A the mean age of contracting the disease. It is easy to construct a model in which the population consists of groups relatively isolated from each other, where the apparent reproductive rate as estimated from Dietz's formula is essentially determined by the contacts between groups rather than between individuals. The true reproductive rate can be much lower, since it only takes $C \approx 3$ to ensure that the introduction of the disease to a 'virgin' group will infect practically all ($> 95\%$) of it (see also Chapter 8; this volume).

Returning to rabies models, we have seen that both the mean level of prevalence and the period of any oscillations about it are determined fairly robustly by the net population growth rate at low densities, r, and the mean generation gap, τ; being $\approx r\tau$ and $2\pi\sqrt{(\tau/r)}$; respectively. The stability of oscillations is a much less robust phenomenon, being particularly sensitive to the way the net population growth rate depends on population density, an aspect on which it is difficult to find adequate data.

Even the more robust features considered here may also be sensitive to the effects of heterogeneous mixing associated with the spatial factor omitted from our present discussions (see Chapter 12, this volume).

References

Anderson, R. M. (1981). Infectious disease agents and cyclic fluctuations in host abundance. *In* "The Mathematical Theory of the Dynamics of Biological Populations II" (R. W. Hiorns and D. Cooke, eds.), pp. 47–80. Academic Press, London.

Anderson, R. M. (1982). Fox rabies. *In* "Population Dynamics of Infectious Diseases: Theory and Applications" (R. M. Anderson, ed.), pp. 242–261. Chapman & Hall, London.

Anderson, R. M., Jackson, H. C., May, R. M., and Smith, A. (1981). Population dynamics of fox rabies in Europe. *Nature* **289**, 765–771.

Bailey, N. T. J. (1975). "The Mathematical Theory of Infectious Diseases," 2nd ed. Macmillan, New York.

Bartlett, M. S. (1960). "Stochastic Population Models." Methuen. London.

Berger, J. (1976). Model of rabies control. *In* "Mathematical Models in Medicine" (J. Berger, W. Buhler, R. Repges, and P. Tautu, eds.). *Lect. Notes Biomath.*, No. 11, pp. 75–88. Springer-Verlag, Berlin and New York.

Dietz, K. (1975). Transmission and control of arbovirus diseases. *In* "Epidemiology" (D. Ludwig and K. L. Cooke, eds.), pp. 104–121. SIAM, Philadelphia, Pennsylvania.

Henderson, W. M. (1982). The control of disease in wildlife when a threat to man and farm livestock. *In* "Animal Disease in Relation to Animal Conservation" (M. A. Edwards and V. McDonnell, eds.), pp. 287–297. Academic Press, London.

May, R. M. (1974). "Stability and Complexity in Model Ecosystems," 2nd ed. Princeton Univ. Press, Princeton, New Jersey.

May, R. M. (1981). Mathematical models in whaling and fisheries management. *In* "Some Mathematical Questions in Biology" (G. F. Oster, ed.), Vol. 2, Am. Math. Soc., Providence, Rhode Island.

Mollison, D. (1981). The importance of demographic stochasticity in population dynamics. *In* "The Mathematical Theory of the Dynamics of Biological Populations II" (R. W. Hiorns and D. L. Cooke, eds.), pp. 99–107. Academic Press, London.

Stirzaker, D. R. (1975). A perturbation method for the stochastic recurrent epidemic. *J. Inst. Math. Appl.* **15**, 135–160.

Pattern Analysis of the Case Occurrences of Fox Rabies in Europe

10

B. McA. Sayers
A. Jane Ross
P. Saengcharoenrat
Department of Electrical Engineering,
Imperial College,
London, England

B. G. Mansourian
World Health Organization,
Geneva, Switzerland

I. Approach

This chapter addresses the problem of analysis and interpretation of the spatio-temporal and longitudinal patterns of case occurrences of fox rabies in several of the recent European outbreaks. The aim is to achieve an operational description of the way the epizootic spreads, interpreted in the light of known factors, such as season or geofeatures of various kinds. A *pattern* is, in effect, any recognizably organized feature in a record—single or multidimensional. The strategy of

235

pattern analysis is to establish the existence and character of any pattern in the record and then to link the pattern or its features to other factors that might be important in understanding or describing the record or, in the present example, in identifying factors that influence the spread of rabies and that may also be relevant to control measures.

One specific assumption is involved in the spatio-temporal analysis: the individual monthly (say) record of the case locations of the disease can be treated as a statistical sample in the classical sense. Each sample is regarded as one example of case occurrences drawn from a conceptual underlying source that is seen as generating cases randomly, subject to a specific case occurrence density distribution. Such a generating source or process is conceptually capable of producing an infinite set of examples of monthly case occurrences. If the properties of the process could be imagined to remain constant, the successive monthly examples of case occurrences observed in practice would constitute different samples from the underlying process—varying randomly in detail but exhibiting the same underlying density distribution pattern. (Naturally, in the real data, seasons change as the months progress and the epizootic translates across geographic regions with changing density of susceptibles and varying ecology. So the real data cannot be treated as time stationary.) Accordingly, it is the task of analysis to estimate the conceptual underlying case occurrence density distribution and to identify its apparent changes with the passage of time: as the seasons alter, as the outbreak moves across different geographic regions and as the case intensity evolves.

Both spatial and temporal dimensions enter into the data records, so two different lines of analysis can be considered; both involve a general *disaggregation* procedure. The data can be separated into individual and sequential time segments for spatial analysis or by region, for longitudinal analysis. Another kind of disaggregation of the data can be achieved by separating translational effects from case evolution effects. All of these methods will be discussed here.

II. Data Pre-processing

Given suitable records of the case occurrences in terms of case location and date (the question of data validity is not considered here), it is necessary to carry out some preliminary pooling of the data (in the time domain) and smoothing (in the spatial domain) in order to acquire spatio-temporal records in an appropriate form for analysis. For the data studied here, the possible geographic locations of cases were organised into a cartesian grid of elementary spatial (geographical) cells, each approximately 4×4 km. Case occurrences were compiled monthly into these cells, and most of the detailed illustrations used below are based on a 32×32 grid.

The spatial distribution of case occurrences often exhibits a substantial month-

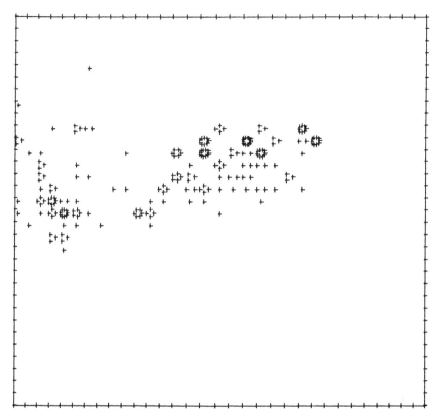

Fig. 1. A quarterly record of successive case occurrences of confirmed fox rabies in a study area 133 × 133 km.

by-month variability (Fig. 1), and there are two factors that apply. First, the expected statistical variability due to sampling effects will cause a partly random dispersal of case occurrences around whatever focus of cases (concentration of infectivity) is operative throughout the area of study. Second, the normal processes of the infection of susceptibles will result both in the evolution of the outbreak (case occurrence numbers will wax or wane) and in its geographical translation. The statistical sampling variability, which could otherwise mask any systematic characteristics of the epizootic to a greater or lesser extent, can be reduced by the usual process of data pooling: in this situation, by pooling successive monthly case counts in individual spatial cells. But if the longitudinal pooling is excessive, systematic variations of the epizootic due to evolutionary or translational effects would be masked. In consequence, empirical trials are needed to optimise the choices; at present, there is no evidence that challenges a quarterly pooling as a good choice.

Turning to the need for spatial smoothing, two factors again are relevant.

Some cases will certainly have been missed, whether the data were collected by actively searching for rabid animals or by recording spontaneous reports; smoothing will reduce this contribution to randomness although it will not alter the systematic bias in mean case numbers. Further, some variability will be introduced by statistical sampling effects and again, spatial smoothing should reduce the influence of this factor. Of the various methods of spatial smoothing that have been tested, the use of a smoothing profile with broadly Gaussian form in two dimensions is probably as satisfactory as any, but, provided that the smoothing does not extend too far, the detailed profile is not important.

These procedures have been used in studying records from West Germany, Denmark, Italy and France. (Various examples are discussed later), starting with the estimation of spatial case occurrence density in the form of the pooled, smoothed spatial data, usually displayed as a contoured pattern.

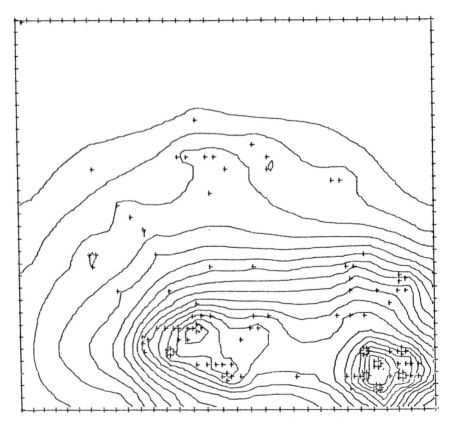

Fig. 2. Contours of estimated case occurrence density in 5% steps referred to the maximum estimated case density as 100%. The raw data has been pooled over 3 months and smoothed by a spatial filter (Sayers *et al.*, 1977).

III. Spatial Patterns of Case Occurrence Density

Figure 2 shows an example of estimated case occurrence density for a specific 3-month period, produced from the pooled and spatially-smoothed raw data. Two features are evident: a small number of local maxima of case occurrences, and the more broadly spread lower level contour boundaries that encompass and smooth out local irregularities of case occurrence density. The former can be interpreted as indicating foci of infectivity; low contour levels of case occurrence can be treated as 'global' estimates of the current scope of the outbreak. Thus, both focal and global views of the epizootic can be obtained through this approach and separately studied as a function of time. The focal approach proceeds by locating the important local maxima of estimated case occurrence density in each quarterly record and forming up the successive focal locations into the most evidently continuous pathways (trajectories) depicting how each inferred focus of infectivity translates with the passage of time. The global approach selects a specific contour level, chosen to encompass the bulk of estimated occurrences, say down to 50% or so of the maximum case density estimated. The description is based on a study of the spatial alterations in this contour level (the forward segment represents the advancing wavefront of the outbreak) as time passes. In both cases it is interesting to examine the changes in the light of possible seasonal and geographic correlates: terrain, natural or man-made obstacles, and geological or other environmental factors.

A. A 'Focal' Description

It has been observed that the locations of local maxima of estimated case occurrence density often tend to be positioned, in successive quarterly periods, as if they lie on systematic pathways. Figure 3 illustrates such a series of successive estimated case density contours. This particular data records the progress of the epizootic through a study area (133 × 133 km) in Baden Württenberg (Federal Republic of Germany) between 1963 and 1971 (Sayers *et al.*, 1977) spreading roughly from northwest to southeast, with 3000 cases or so confirmed during that period. The foci appear to translate systematically but with quite variable rate and direction. Accordingly, it is useful to link the indicated locations graphically to delineate systematic pathways and to treat these pathways as trajectories of infectivity in the manner shown in Fig. 4A. Several main trajectories can be identified as the epizootic moves down from the (top left) northwest corner of the region, together with some short duration pathways. Two of the trajectories appear to terminate on the north bank of the River Danube (I,II; Fig. 4B), whereas two others (III,IV) evidently cross the river and continue to progress southwards. North of the river (Fig. 4A), a circulating trajectory traverses the Suabian Jura during quarterly periods 19 (third quarter 1967) to 32 (last quarter 1970), indicating a secondary outbreak in that region.

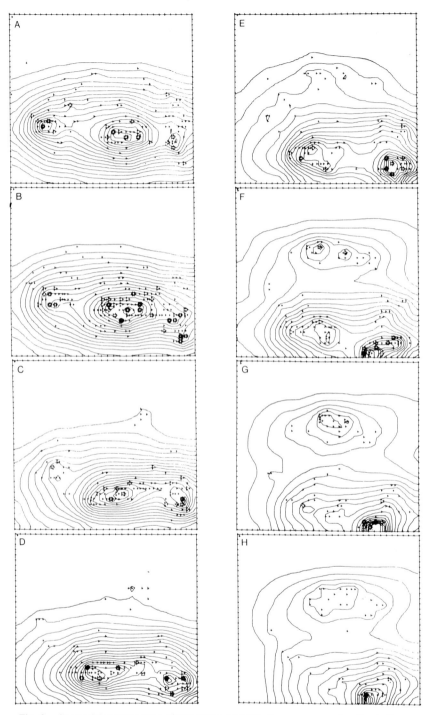

Fig. 3. Sequential contour maps of successive quarterly case occurrence densities in the same study area, normalized to the maximum individually in each quarter. From Sayers *et al.*, 1977.

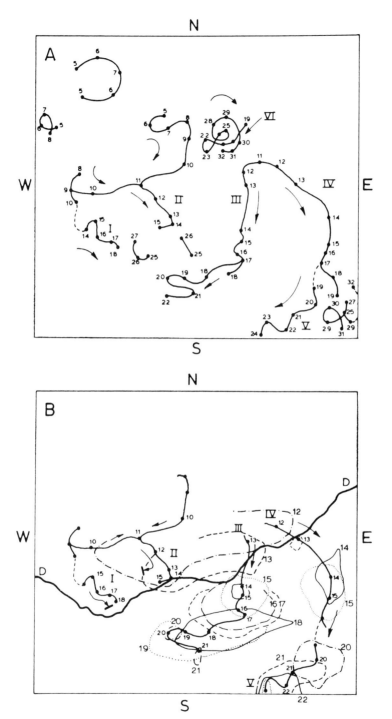

Fig. 4. (A) Trajectories of the apparent movements of separate foci. (B) Trajectories with superimposed 80% contours showing the changes as the trajectories cross the River Danube. From Sayers *et al.*, 1977.

The two major trajectories that are shown to cross the Danube can be clarified by close inspection of the contours of estimated case occurrence density in the relevant quarterly periods. In Fig. 4B, the 80% contour (a convenient level) during quarterly period 12 is very widely distributed; in fact it corresponds to the north bank of the Danube (Fig. 5). During period 13, however, the same contour level on trajectory IV is extremely circumscribed, indicating a much smaller spatial spread of the dominant infectivity. In later periods, the focus translates and enlarges. These observations are consistent with a broad advancing wavefront that approaches the river from the north, a small focus of infectivity appearing shortly afterwards, near a bridge, on the south bank of the river. The outbreak subsequently translates southwards and spreads.

A similar picture can be associated with the other trajectory (III), which crosses during quarter 14. Taken together with the observations about trajectories I and II, these illustrate how rivers (and other geofeatures) can act as a natural barrier to forward propagation, which cannot always be traversed, but in some instances lead to lateral transmission.

B. A 'Global' or Wavefront Description

In order to specify wavefronts and their velocities in an advancing epizootic, it is useful to consider a different aspect of the estimated case occurrence density in successive quarterly periods. We consider sequential contours corresponding to a

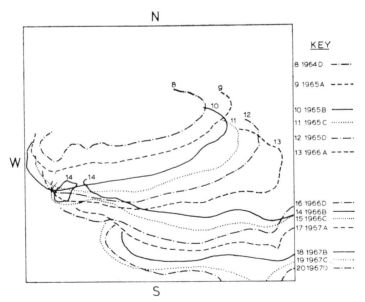

Fig. 5.   Same area as Fig. 4. The advancing front of the epizootic as represented by the 55% (of maximum) contour levels for a number of successive quarterly periods. From Sayers *et al.*, 1977.

fixed level of estimated case occurrence measured with respect to, say, the quarterly maximum intensity. For this purpose it is appropriate to consider contour levels at say 50% of the maximum, or thereabouts; this has the effect of overcoming local irregularities of estimated case distribution and leads to an overall view of the way the epizootic has spread.

Figure 5 shows the 55% of maximum contour level for each of 13 successive quarterly periods. The directional change of the progressive movement between periods 13 and 14 is actually attributable to the river crossing, as evidenced more clearly in the focal trajectories. Nevertheless, this figure does make it clear that general directional changes and velocities could be specified, on the large scale, from this type of presentation.

In the case of the French data, much more consistent propagation takes place—systematic movement is towards the south and southwest, once the epizootic is established in the northwestern segment of the country, as expected for a primary outbreak. Given the 50% constant-level estimated contours shown in Fig. 6, it is possible to seek correlated factors that might account for the form of

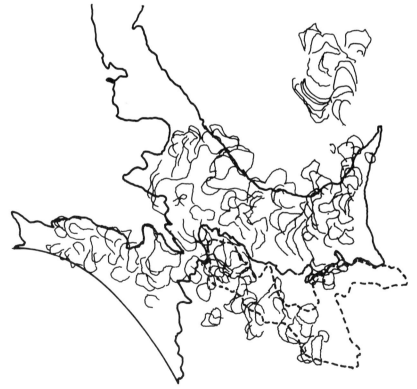

Fig. 6. Contour lines (for 50% of maximum) for successive quarters in France overlaid on the indicated region of surface limestone.

the propagation. In fact, it is interesting to relate these contours to overall topographical features in the regions concerned.

The area of high case occurrence density shown in Fig. 6 actually corresponds quite closely with the existence of a broad ridge of limestone with elevations up to 600 (m). The area concerned is characteristically diverse in landcover and vegetation, in distinction to the low occurrence density areas, having more uniform landcover. Alluvial regions (Rhine or Rhone Valleys) often exhibit low case densities of fox rabies. However, limestone substrata have been consistently linked with high and persistent levels of rabies infection and for the most part, higher altitude and greater diversity of vegetation are associated with high case densities. Thus, the geological substrata, elevation and diversity of land use are likely factors affecting the general extent of the spread and direction of propagation (see Ball, Chapter 11, this volume, for further comment).

However, recurrent or persistent infection constitutes a different situation. As seen for the German data in Fig. 4A and B, the later periods exhibit a circulating trajectory that tracks back over its earlier path (again in a region of limestone substrata) and naturally, the constant level contours then show little systematic temporal development: a focal description is more appropriate.

IV. Longitudinal Analysis: Variations with Time

Two of the possibilities for pattern analysis concern the time variations of case occurrence numbers: a study of case evolution patterns in space after removal of the translational component, using trajectory information, and a study of the longitudinal case occurrence pattern in circumscribed regions disregarding the spatial characteristics of the epizootic.

A. Case Occurrence Evolution Patterns

Given the estimated case occurrence density pattern for sequential quarterly periods, the inferred foci of infectivity on each trajectory can be located; then it becomes possible to analyse sequential patterns of the spatial spread as a function of season or terrain, freed from the effects of translation—by collecting case occurrences around the appropriate focus and by displaying them relative to the position of their appropriate focus. Accordingly, this corresponds to the pattern of evolution of the disease case occurrences.

Figure 7 shows the typical case evolution patterns for 4 years in respect to the four quarters of each year. Only the 50% contours are shown and, since these contours are normalized, the effect of fluctuations in magnitude are suppressed; only spatial pattern changes from quarter to quarter are indicated. Naturally, it is not essential to use normalised data, in which case the effects of several factors

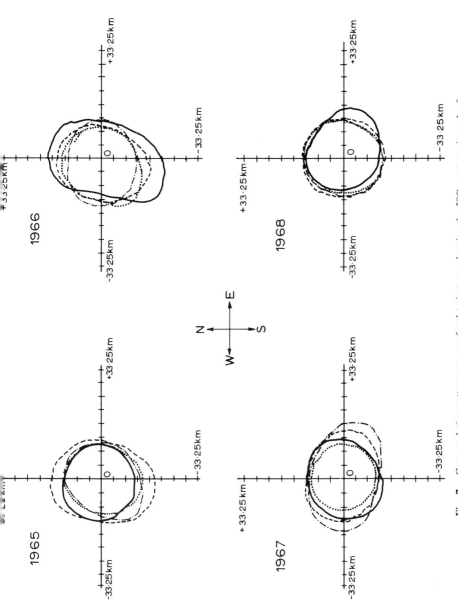

Fig. 7. Case evolution patterns on one focal trajectory, showing the 50% contours in each of four successive quarters for 4 years, after removal of the translational component.

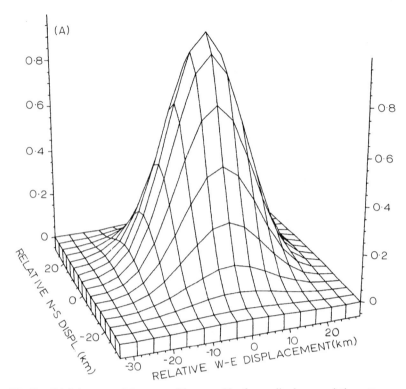

Fig. 8. (A) Coherent spatial average of the ensemble of normalized case evolution patterns, each centered on the focal location for the relevant quarter. (B) Coherent spatial standard derivation of the normalized case evolution ensemble.

may interact, but in the present records, the major discernable factor is the occasional change of orientation, with some evidence of alterations in the range of spread. When normalised data are used, it becomes possible to estimate the coherent average profile of the spread of case occurrences, so as to confirm the way cases spread out around the hypothesised foci.

A typical result appears in Fig. 8A and B. The isometric plots show the average profile (and SD) of the normalised case distributions, freed from any translational component. The actual form of the profile is unsurprising, and the greatest ensemble variability is observed to occur at the steepest part of the average profile, where the ensemble coefficient of variation is about 0.25, a relatively small figure for data of this type.

B. Longitudinal Patterns of Regional Data

It is assumed that, by appropriate spatial segmentation, regions of spatially stable data can be determined. A typical record of monthly cases in a region is

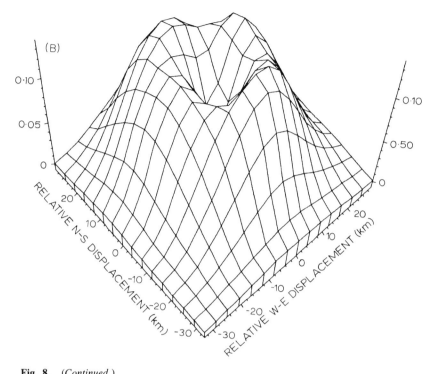

Fig. 8.   (*Continued.*)

shown in Fig. 9. The major observable pattern feature is a variable magnitude recurrent transient that runs throughout the record. The recurrent fluctuations are characteristic of these records. The strategy of analysis is to determine the average pattern and typical variability of the recurrent fluctuations; if any consistent pattern emerges, the detailed profile and the features of its recurrence will be of interest.

The data have been treated on a monthly basis in the examples shown here and a coherent average formed from all of 24 sub-regional records. In this context 'coherent' means that the maxima were aligned with respect to their times of occurrence, so that an ensemble of some 200 short record segments can be formed, each centered on an individual clear maximum in the record and lasting about $2\frac{1}{2}$ years or so as chosen. Since the record segments are aligned, it is feasible to form the average pattern of the segments by calculating mean case numbers and their standard deviation for each month before, at and after the maximum. The coherent average pattern (Fig. 10A) is roughly symmetrical, over about 8–10 months, rising from an average regional level of 10 cases per month up to about 25 with a standard error peaking at some 1.5 cases. It is therefore recognized that the different segmental records exhibit a very closely similar

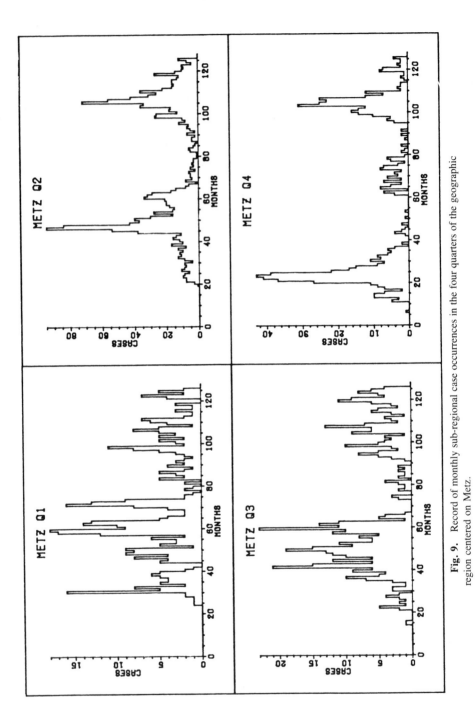

Fig. 9. Record of monthly sub-regional case occurrences in the four quarters of the geographic region centered on Metz.

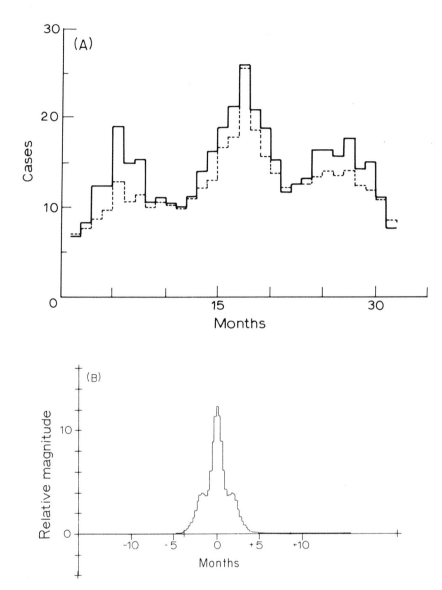

Fig. 10. (A) The coherent average profile (– – –) and standard deviation (——) of the longitudinal records in 24 sub-regions, each record in the ensemble being centered on a local case occurrence maximum. (B) The microepidemic profile extracted from the coherent average after removing the estimated contribution of the background.

pattern. Accordingly, two steps are appropriate: (1) to design a method for the objective detection of the occurrence locations of the standard pattern thus identified and for determining their magnitudes and (2) to establish how much these patterns contribute to the overall records.

Because of the nature of the recurrent patterns, it is convenient to envisage them as miniature outbreaks; the term *microepidemic* will be used here, without any implication beyond that of a brief recurrent outbreak. So we now consider how to determine the location and magnitude of the individual microepidemics, assuming that the complete record is indeed made up of the summation of various microepidemics, as isolated in Fig. 10B.

1. Detecting Microepidemics

Detecting the presence of a microepidemic requires a process that will, preferentially, turn the record into a series of variable magnitude *spikes* occurring at the locations of the microepidemics and having magnitudes proportional to the size of the individual microepidemics. Within limits, this can be achieved. The method is referred to as *inverse filtering*. The basis of the scheme is to pass the record through a numerical 'filter', designed in such a way that the individual microepidemics are each turned into the required sharp spike-like form. Inevitably, this accentuates the random fluctuations in the record, so some compromises are needed in the design of the numerical filter.

The principle of the inverse filter is as follows: it is imagined that the observed pattern of the microepidemic is the result of physical and biological processes acting consistently on a narrow occurrence impulse $e(t)$. This impulse is of course conceptual, but, given the right circumstances (minimal high-frequency noise in the records), it is possible to transform a record in which a microepidemic occurs into such an impulse $e(t)$ centered at the occurrence. Given a choice of the impulsive pattern, the transfer function that turns this into the microepidemic average profile can be computed and so can its inverse, which would operate on the average profile to generate the chosen impulsive pattern. This impulsive pattern $e(t)$ is treated, accordingly, as a 'target' function. When the complete monthly data sequence of the actual case occurrences is applied to the inverse filter, the output should comprise a series of these target patterns located at the sites of any indicated microepidemics and weighted according to their magnitudes.

More precisely, the average microepidemic profile, $s(t)$, is thus envisaged as the output of a linear system whose input is a narrow pulse $e(t)$, which approximates a unit impulse function. The system frequency response that turns the conceptual $e(t)$ into the actual $s(t)$ is determined as

$$H(\omega) = S(\omega)/E(\omega)$$

where $S(\omega)$ and $E(\omega)$ are the Fourier transforms of $s(t)$ and $e(t)$, respectively. The second step is to form the inverse filter $H^{-1}(\omega)$ and to apply to it any epidemic

$p(t)$ to generate an output $i(t)$, in which the constituting microepidemics would be enhanced, appearing as sharp pulses. With this kind of signal, forming and utilising the inverse filter can be a frequency-domain operation.

This procedure has been implemented by using the discrete fast Fourier transformation algorithm on 128-point (monthly) records. The target function $e(t)$ was taken to be a Gaussian curve of the form $e(t) = \exp(-t^2/2\sigma^2)$, where σ is the standard deviation. Empirically, it was found that σ could be taken to be between 0.5 and 1.0 weeks and, further, that the particular choice of σ within this interval does not affect the results significantly.

The resulting inverse filter was applied to all of the 24 sub-regions. During this process and also during reconstruction, Fourier-band limited interpolation has been used to extend the length of the inverse filter output by 4 times from 128 to 512, by adding zeroes as extra spectral terms, prior to the inverse Fourier transformation leading to the output signal from the inverse filter. This method simplifies the visual identification of maxima indicating the presence and location of microepidemics. Typical results are shown in Fig. 11, in which it is clear that a series of approximate target functions is indeed generated. Evidently, there should be little difficulty in determining both location and magnitude of the individual microepidemics that are indicated. So the approach does seem to lead to consistent results, which thus justify further consideration.

2. Reconstructing the Longitudinal Records

The appropriate next step is to attempt the reconstruction of individual complete records by using the microepidemic profile together with magnitude and

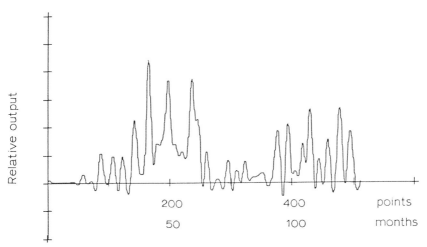

Fig. 11. An example of the output from an inverse filter (Metz Q3) designed to locate, and identify the magnitude of, microepidemic occurrences; the maxima of the output fix both the estimated locations and magnitudes.

location information obtained from the inverse filter; we assign to each location a standard (interpolated) microepidemic profile of the indicated magnitude, and summate.

Figure 12A and B allows a comparison of reconstructed and original records. It can be seen that the reconstruction has captured both form and details of the observations. Accordingly, the microepidemic model can be regarded as a valid

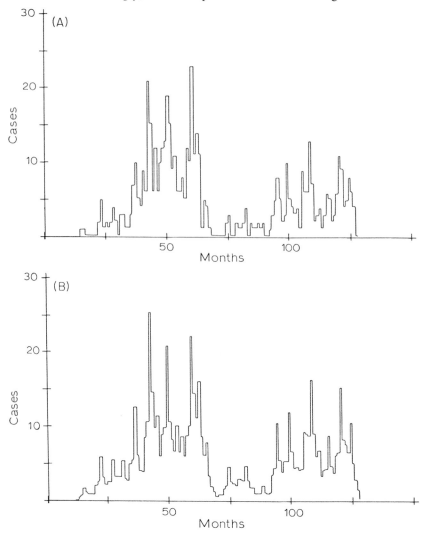

Fig. 12. Raw data (A) and reconstructed (B) records for comparison. The latter were reconstructed by summating microepidemic profiles having location and magnitude as indicated by the inverse filter output.

basis for describing these records. It is particularly interesting that a quite standard pattern of the microepidemics emerges from the analysis and that it is only necessary to assign the correct location and magnitude to the occurrences to achieve a good representation of the real data. On this evidence, the form of each individual transient outbreak is thus independent of its magnitude; if this feature of the longitudinal patterns is found to occur generally, it would carry significant implications for the detailed biological dynamics of rabies propagation.

However, we limit discussion here to certain elementary features of the patterns of microepidemic occurrences such as their sequential magnitudes and inter-event intervals. In brief, the mean interval between microepidemic events in this data is 4.9 months, and the first serial-correlation coefficient of interval is 0.56, a fairly substantial value. The first-order interval histogram has a slightly skewed unimodal form and a mode of 4.0 months. It has not been possible to confirm any relation between the duration of an inter-event interval and the magnitude of the immediately following microepidemic. The microepidemic magnitudes themselves are, however, not significantly correlated except by virtue of their seasonal and similar factors.

V. Comment

The temporal and spatio-temporal analysis carried out here has been effective in drawing attention to several hypotheses that are consistent with the known facts and that fit data other than those used in their generation. A focal basis for propagation is suggested by analysis of the sequences of the contour plots representing quarterly spatial case occurrence data. It is feasible to separate case occurrences on the basis of their nearest apparent focus of infection, and the average spatial profile of case clustering around the focus is approximately symmetrical. In longitudinal detail, this spatial distribution around the nearest focus shows limited systematic changes with season and terrain apart from magnitude variations; however, other workers may be interested to examine the details of case evolution more closely.

Longitudinal analysis of the regionally-segmented data suggests a microepidemic hypothesis—that longitudinal propagation takes place through a sequence of microepidemics exhibiting a more-or-less standard shape of transient rise and fall of the case-occurrence rates. Relationships between successive microepidemics can be investigated because it is possible to detect and quantify the occurrences objectively, using the microepidemic model and a procedure such as inverse filtering to locate occurrences.

As the microepidemic profile model is evidently capable of representing the records closely, the significance of this fact needs exploration. It should be remarked that the microepidemic model is more than simply a convenient means for describing the record. All fluctuating records naturally exhibit recurrent maxima and minima, but there is no reason to presume that the pattern of rise towards, and decrease from the maximum should be anything other than highly variable. However, the real rabies data behave quite differently: the pattern of the recurrent maximum is relatively stable and independent of size. Indeed, when the individual patterns are normalized prior to coherent averaging, the standard deviation down the ensemble of individual patterns is small (typically 0.25 in this data). This suggests that the stable recurrent pattern is a property of the data, not merely a convenient way of looking at the particular kind of fluctuation. On this basis, it would appear that the possible biological significance of the micro-epidemic pattern can reasonably be sought. Certainly, it would not be difficult to propose mechanisms to account for the property, if and as this became appropriate.

Acknowledgements

Some of the work mentioned above has been supported by the MRC and the ARC. The assistance of Mr. K. Paulat and Mr. P. Baxter is gratefully acknowledged. Dr. K. Bögel (WHO, Geneva) and Dr. L. Andral (C.N.E.R., Melzeville) have made their data available for this study, and their assistance is gratefully acknowledged.

References

Sayers, B. McA., Mansourian, B. G., Phan Tan, T., and Bögel, K. (1977). A pattern analysis study of a wild-life rabies epizootic. *Med. Inf.* **2,** 11–34.
Sayers, B. McA., Saengcharoenrat, P., and Mansourian, B. G. (1983). Longitudinal patterns in detected occurrences of fox rabies: A microepizootic hypothesis. To be published.

Front-wave Velocity and Fox Habitat Heterogeneity

11

Frank G. Ball[1]

Department of Biomathematics,
University of Oxford,
Oxford, England

I. Introduction

It is well known that geographical features, such as rivers, motorways and towns, considerably affect the course of a rabies epizootic. For example, in

---

[1]Present address: Department of Mathematics, University of Nottingham, University Park, Nottingham, NG7 2RD England.

POPULATION DYNAMICS OF RABIES IN WILDLIFE

Chapter 10 of this volume, Sayers gave an analysis of the current German rabies epizootic, which showed that foci of infection were held up for a period by the river Danube, becoming more diffuse, until eventually rabies crossed the river, forming highly concentrated foci of infection on the opposite bank. A similar analysis of the present French rabies epizootic showed that the foci of infection followed a belt of limestone running southwest across France. Both of these analyses, although using quantitative methods to describe the spread of rabies, have related this spread to geographical features in a qualitative manner. In this chapter I shall describe a preliminary quantitative analysis in which I attempt to relate the velocity of the fox rabies front through France to geographical features by using a multiple regression model. I should emphasize the word preliminary, since our aim is to discover whether such a quantitative analysis is feasible, rather than to produce a definitive solution to the problem. Indeed, such a solution is unlikely to exist.

There have been two accounts of quantitative analysis of rabies epizootics in the literature, both of which have attempted to relate reported incidence of rabies to geographical features. Jackson (1979) used a contingency table analysis in an attempt to relate the reported incidence of rabies in Europe to various habitat classes, as found fron an indicator species analysis, see Section IV. A study on such a wide scale as this is clearly plagued with many difficulties, not least the considerable variation in reporting patterns from one country to another; nevertheless, she managed to show a significant dependence between reported incidence and habitat type, with reported incidence being higher than expected in patchy habitats and lower than expected in homogeneous habitats, such as arable regions and grasslands. Lineback (1980) used a regression model in an attempt to relate the reported incidence of rabies in the States of Kentucky, North Carolina, Tennessee, Virginia and West Virginia to land-use-related explanatory variables. He found that the reported incidence of fox rabies was significantly partially correlated with the area of cropland and the logarithm of the distance from limestone, the reported incidence increasing with the former and decreasing with the latter, thereby endorsing the results of Ross's study described earlier. However, the results of the above two analyses should be viewed cautiously since they both ignored any spatial autocorrelation that might be present amongst the data, see Appendix 2.

We chose to examine front-wave velocities for the three following reasons.

1. They are highly relevant to forecasting future spread, and thus the control of rabies epizootics.

2. A knowledge of how front-wave velocity varies with fox parameters, such as territory size and group size, would increase our understanding of the dynamics of fox rabies spread, thus assisting us with identification of relevant models.

3. The reporting of such cases is more likely to be consistent. The first front

wave is novel and a greater proportion of the cases are likely to be reported; thus, there might be fewer local reporting biases than in subsequent cases.

II. Description of the Rabies Data

We shall analyse data on the reported incidence of rabies in France during the period from March 1968 to June 1978.[2] Rabies was reported amongst 19 different species of animal, but since the Red Fox was the predominant vector, accounting for about 80% of all cases, we shall restrict our analysis to fox rabies. For each rabies case we are given, amongst other things, the town at which it was reported (usually the nearest town to where the carcass was found), together with the reporting date. Thus, the spatial and temporal resolution of the data is low, since for the former the reporting town might be some distance from the location of the carcass, whilst for the latter some time will have elapsed between the death of an animal and the discovery of its body.

For the purpose of our study, we divided the region of France in which rabies was reported into grid squares of length 20 km (see Fig. 1). The choice of 20-km squares was dictated to a lesser extent by the spatial resolution of the rabies data and to a greater extent by the time involved in recording map attributes for the subsequent analyses. Figure 2 shows the number of fox rabies cases reported in each of the grid squares. Note that fewer cases are reported around the periphery of the study region than in the centre. In the eastern area of the study region this is because only part of the grid squares lie in France (only French rabies cases are reported in these squares), whilst in the western area the grid squares had not experienced the full force of the epizootic by June 1978. In the next section we shall estimate front-wave velocities from the times of the first reported case in each grid square; thus, the above partial reporting will not adversely affect our velocity estimates in the western area but may result in overestimates in the east.

III. Estimating Front-wave Velocities

In the previous chapter, Sayers described an extremely sophisticated method of estimating the front wave of a rabies epizootic at any given time, from which estimates of front wave velocity could easily be obtained. However, his method is very complex, and it is worthwhile to see whether simpler empirical methods will suffice. One such method is that of Bögel et al. (1976), who noted that rabies spread from north to south through their German study region and thus by

---

[2]Data were kindly supplied by Dr. Andral of Centre d'Etude sur la Rage, Maezeville, France.

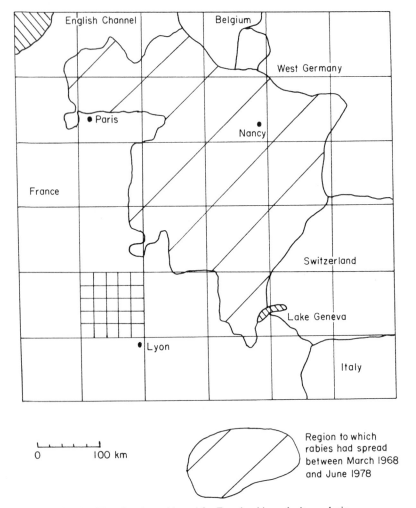

Fig. 1. Map showing grid used for French rabies velocity analysis.

dividing the region into north–south strips, they were able to estimate the front wave at any given time by joining the most southerly cases in neighbouring strips by a straight line. Unfortunately, this method is not appropriate for our French data, as the rabies front did not propogate in a uniform direction. Both of these methods estimate front-wave velocities by first estimating the front wave at successive points in time. We shall now describe a procedure to estimate them directly.

Using the grid described in Section II (see Fig. 1), we record for each grid square the time that rabies was first reported in that square, measured in months

```
                              3
        1              3   2  12   2
   26  7  4  1      2   8   8  20  16   9
 1 29 30 35 59 59  20   7  19  26  42  77  26  25  10   8
 1  5 49 60 68 69  34   8  23  29  36  66  46  71  29  35   7
 2 24 16 32 75 56  18  13  18  30  41  42  67  69  50  43  30  17   3   8   2  13
   25 10  7 64 23  15   4   9  22  32  37  61  68  94  57  18  23  77  36  28   8   4
 1                      5  19  54  50  36  58 116 123  37  21  32  55   6  10
                   3    4  16  83  67  33  64  88 106  82  73  23  56   5
              2  1  1  19  45 128 135  40 117  64  54  39  80  89  69   6
              1  2 14  53  73  83  60  34 163  90 111  84  94 137  65   4
              2  2 48 107  92  63  69  43  56 133 143  86  68  74  43   1
              1 17 42  53  55  67  32  81  47  63 126  72  37  86  37
         1     40  6 41  34  37  34  41  59  60  41  53  33  18  47  47  11
              19 15 45  52  35  53  50  54  56  54  56  61  30  42  36  15
               4 14  7  25  23  52  66  38  44  53  61  42  49  18
                  1    18  29  77  28  37 117 117  88  66  32   2
                  2     2  20  45  17  28  12  75  50  26  10
                       1  16  19   2   2  65  50  32  30
                                      2  59  38  14
                                     13  22  33  20
                                     42  31  25   8
                                     20  12  29
                                      1   2
                                          6
```

Fig. 2.   Reported incidences of fox rabies in France between January 1968 and May 1978.

after December 1968, i.e. January 1969 = 1, January 1970 = 13 etc. If we fit a surface to these points, then we are able to estimate front-wave velocities as follows: Let $t = f(x,y)$ be the equation of our surface, with respect to a pair of coordinate axes. For each point (x,y) we draw the contour of this surface that passes through (x,y) and calculate the directional derivative of the function $f(x,y)$ along the normal to this contour at (x,y) in the direction of increasing t, i.e. we calculate how fast the function $f(x,y)$ is changing in direction of its steepest ascent from (x,y). The reciprocal of this derivative yields an estimate of front-wave velocity through (x,y).

Specifically, if we let

$$b = \frac{\partial f}{\partial x}(x,y) \qquad \text{and} \qquad c = \frac{\partial f}{\partial y}(x,y)$$

then the front-wave velocity through (x,y) has magnitude $V = \sqrt{(b^2 + c^2)}$ and direction $\theta = \tan^{-1}(c/b)$.

In practice, we will not know the shape of the 'first incidence' surface so we approximate it locally by a quadratic, which we estimate from the data as follows: For a given grid square we record the time that rabies was first reported in that square and the eight surrounding squares, as follows:

$$
\begin{array}{ccc}
77 & 74 & 71 \\
81 & 77 & 72 \\
81 & 76 & 75
\end{array}
$$

and fit the quadratic

$$t = a + bx + cy + dx^2 + exy + fy^2$$

by ordinary least squares, taking our given square as the origin. In fact, because of the orthogonality of the above design, it is only necessary to fit a plane. An estimate of front-wave velocity is then given by the previous formulae; for our example we have $V = 61.9$ km/year with a bearing of 244°.

Figure 3 shows the front-wave velocities, estimated by this method, for each of the grid squares having rabies reported in it and the eight surrounding squares. If rabies was not reported in each of the eight surrounding squares, then no velocity estimate was calculated for that square. The velocities shown in Fig. 3 seem, apart from a few outliers, quite reasonable since their magnitudes are clustered in space, as one would expect, and their directions yield a front moving in a direction varying between south and west, as suggested by an earlier descriptive analysis of Toma and Andral (1977). The large magnitude of some of the estimated velocities is not too surprising since they are estimates of the instantaneous front-wave velocities, and the observed front-wave velocities over a period of time will be smaller owing to the front not propagating in a straight line. Moreover, one should remember that they are based on reported, rather than actual cases, and consequently might be appreciably affected by local reporting patterns.

IV. Map Attributes and a First Analysis

A. MAP ATTRIBUTES

The aim of this study is to relate the front-wave velocities estimated in the previous section to fox habitat heterogeneity. To this end we require some way, preferably quantitative, of describing the various types of fox habitats present in France. Clearly, the preferable course of action would be to firstly draw up a list of important habitat variables and then go out into the field and measure them at sample points taken from each grid square. This has not so far been carried out, though the results of our subsequent analyses will suggest that such a study is

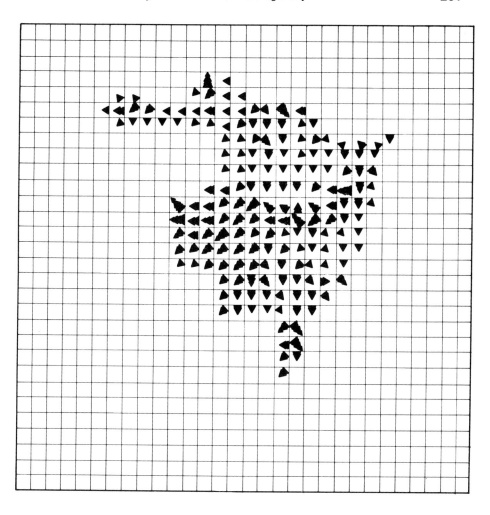

Fig. 3. Estimated front-wave velocities for French fox rabies.

< 25 km/year

25-50 km/year

50-100 km/year

7100 km/year

imperative if we are going to obtain a proper understanding of the ecological mechanisms underlying the spread of rabies, and thus a real chance of eradicating it once it has become endemic. In the mean time another solution is required, and recent studies at the Institute of Terrestrial Ecology Merlewood Research Station have shown that attributes read off maps can be used to provide a useful method of land classification. We thus chose to use map attributes to attempt to explain the large variation in fox rabies front-wave velocities.

We recorded for each grid square in which rabies was reported the presence or absence of a variety of different map attributes. A list of the attributes recorded is given in Appendix 1. Note that many of the attributes are mutually exclusive in that the presence of one necessarily implies the absence of another. Indicator species analysis (ISA) was then applied to these recorded attributes and each grid square was allocated to one of 16 classes. The ISA method classifies the grid squares into groups, such that grid squares within the same group portray similar map attributes. The classification is hierarchical; at each stage the analysis splits each group into two new groups, according to the location of grid squares along the first axes of a weighted reciprocal averaging (see Hill *et al.*, 1975 and Hill, 1973). Although the ISA divided the grid squares into 16 groups, which we shall call land classes, we decided for our analysis to split the grid squares into only eight groups, since otherwise some land classes would contain very few representative grid squares. Figure 4 summarises the major land features used by the ISA in dividing the grid squares, whilst Fig. 5 shows the spatial distribution of the initial 16 land classes.

B. A ONE-WAY ANALYSIS OF VARIANCE

As a preliminary statistical analysis we performed a one-way analysis of variance to determine whether mean front-wave velocity varies significantly from one land class to another. We fitted the following model by the standard method.

$$Y_{i,j} = \mu + T_{(i,j)} + \epsilon_{i,j} \tag{1}$$

where $Y_{i,j}$ is the estimated velocity of front wave through grid square (i,j); μ is the constant and $T_{(i,j)}$ is the effect of land class of grid square (i,j) on velocity. We then performed a second analysis in which the $Y_{i,j}$ were the natural logarithms of the estimated velocities. The F statistics for testing whether the land class effects $T_{(i,j)}$ are all zero or not were respectively, 2,429* and 4.104**, both with 7 and 170 degrees of freedom.[3] Histograms of the estimated residuals for both these models are given in Fig. 6, whilst estimated first-order spatial autocorrelations of these residuals were $\rho_X = 0.31$, $\rho_Y = 0.30$ and $\rho_X = 0.40$, $\rho_Y = 0.49$, respectively [ρ_X is the estimated correlation between the residual at grid square (i,j) and that at grid square $(i,j+1)$, assuming that the correlation structure is spatially stationary]. Thus, although taking logarithms yielded more 'normal' residuals, it also increased their spatial autocorrelation; consequently, we have to decide

---

[3]Throughout this chapter, * means a statistic is significant at the 5% level and ** at the 1% level. When appropriate, the absence of stars means that the statistic is not significant at the 5% level.

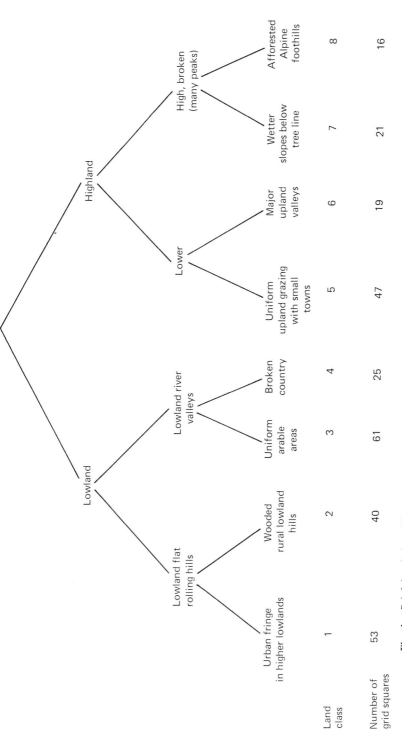

Land class	1	2	3	4	5	6	7	8
Number of grid squares	53	40	61	25	47	19	21	16

Highland

Lowland

Lowland flat rolling hills

Lowland river valleys

Lower

High, broken (many peaks)

Urban fringe in higher lowlands

Wooded rural lowland hills

Uniform arable areas

Broken country

Uniform upland grazing with small towns

Major upland valleys

Wetter slopes below tree line

Afforested Alpine foothills

Fig. 4. Brief description of French land classes used in the analyses together with the number of grid squares in each class.

```
                                        6
            5                    1   9   9   9
        4   5   5   5        6   9   9  12   1   9
    6   5   5   7   7   8    5   6   5   6   4   3   3   1   1   9
    5   6   5   5   5   5    5   5   3   6   3   1   3   1   1   1   1
    5   5   7   6   6   6    7   5   6   6   6   4   1   1   5   2   1   1   1   9   2   8
        7   7   5   6   5    5   5   5   6   3   3   1   1  12   1   1   2   9   2   1           7
    7                            6   6   6   2   1   4   1   1   1   2   1   1   8   8   8
                             3   6   6   3   3  12   1   1   1   2   9  10  10   8
                5   5   5    6   3   3   4   3   4  15   1   1  10  10  16   7
                6   6   6    3   3   4   3   3   4   9   1   9  10  13  11  11
                5   2   6    3   2   3   3   3   9   9   9  10  10  16  11  11
                5   6   2    4   3   4   3   3   9   2   9  10  13  10   7
        5       6   1   9    3   3   9   2   3   3   2   2   9   9  12   7  11
                2   9   1    1   2   9   9   2   4   1   9   9   2   9  11  15
                3  11  10   10  12   6  12   7   5   9  14  14  13  13
                   10       10  10   9   7   7   5  12  14  13  13  15
               10           10   9  12   7   7  12  14  13  13  15
                            10  12   8   6   7  14  14  13  15
                                         7  14  13  15
                                        12  15  15  15
                                        15  13  15  15
                                        11  14  15
                                        14  15
                                        14
```

Fig. 5. Diagram showing the distribution of French land classes. In the analyses, land classes 1 and 2 became land class 1, 3 and 4 land class 2, . . . , 15 and 16 land class 8.

whether it is preferable to have residuals which are patently non-normal or an increased spatial autocorrelation. However, even if we choose the former, there is still considerable spatial autocorrelation, which should be taken into account in our analysis. The phenomenon of spatial autocorrelation is clearly very important, and in Appendix 2 we give an account of its effect upon least squares regression, together with a description of Papadakis' method, which we shall use to adjust for spatial autocorrelation.

In the mean time, it is worth ensuring that we are familiar with the concept of spatial autocorrelation. The model we envisage is one in which the front-wave velocity of rabies is decomposed into two additive components, a deterministic component relating mean front-wave velocity to the values of map attributes and a stochastic component describing the random fluctuations about that mean. It is the second of these two components that contains any spatial autocorrelation. If the residual random errors are correlated, the assumptions of ordinary least squares are violated and alternative techniques should be considered. With spatial autocorrelation the residuals are correlated according to some spatial pattern,

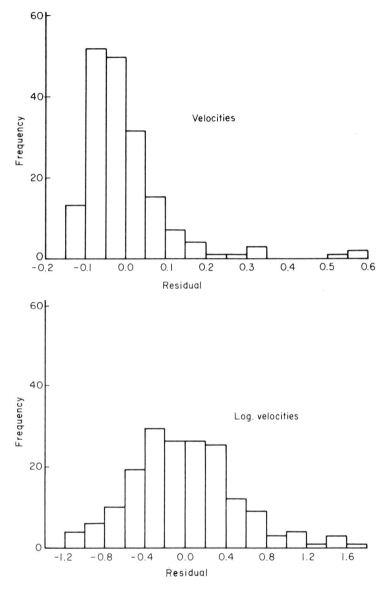

Fig. 6. Histograms of estimated residuals for one-way ANOVA model for effect of land class on front-wave velocity.

the form of which can be exploited to provide the before-mentioned alternative techniques.

It is important to realise that providing the model is correct, the spatial autocorrelation as described previously is not influenced by the distribution of land classes within our lattice grid, but rather it is induced by our method of estimating front-wave velocities and perhaps also by the mechanism governing the spatial spread of rabies. However, if we had assumed that the residual in a grid square was influenced by the observed velocities in neighbouring squares, rather than the residuals in those squares, then the distribution of land classes within the lattice could induce correlation between the regression residuals. In such circumstances, a clustered pattern of land classes would yield a higher degree of spatial autocorrelation than a more random pattern, since the residual at a given grid square will be influenced by the cluster type in which it is contained and consequently with a clustered pattern one would expect regions of high, and regions of low, residuals. Of course, there would still be spatial autocorrelation induced by the velocity estimation scheme.

We adjusted for spatial autocorrelation using the Papadakis method as outlined in Appendix 2, avoiding edge effects by restricting our analysis to interior grid squares. We iterated the analysis until successive estimates were equal to five decimal places. The results are outlined in Tables I–IV, the final column of Tables I and III giving the number of grid squares used in the analysis for each land class, whilst the estimate of the effect of land class i is the estimate of the

TABLE I

Estimates of Parameters in Analysis of Variance Model with Actual Velocities[a]

	Initial ANOVA	Papadakis (1 iteration)	Papadakis (19 iterations)	n_i
Land class				
1	0.128	0.148	0.149	28
2	0.186	0.177	0.167	33
3	0.144	0.161	0.161	14
4	0.184	0.178	0.178	3
5	0.203	0.188	0.179	25
6	0.117	0.119	0.125	5
7	0.125	0.138	0.131	6
8	0.146	0.161	0.160	1
Covariate regression coefficients				
γ_1		0.111	0.116	
γ_2		0.421	0.416	

[a] n_i = number of grid squares of 'land class' i.

TABLE II

Analysis of Variance Table for Model with Actual Velocities

Before adjustment Source	DF[a]	SS[a]	MS[a]	F[a]
Land classes	7	0.116	0.017	2.070
Residual	107	0.858	0.008	

After 1 iteration Source	DF	SS	MS	F
Land classes	7	0.040	0.006	1.024
γ_1, γ_2	2	0.388	0.194	34.819[b]
Residual	105	0.585	0.006	

After 19 iterations Source	DF	SS	MS	F
Land classes	7	0.027	0.004	0.731
γ_1, γ_2	2	0.429	0.214	41.304[b]
Residual	105	0.545	0.005	

[a] DF, degrees of freedom; SS, sums of squares; MS, mean square; F, F statistic.

[b] Significant at the 1% level.

mean front-wave velocity through a grid square of land class i. We see from Tables II and IV that for both models the effect of the Papadakis adjustment is to reduce the significance of the difference between land class effects, clearly a consequence of the high positive spatial autocorrelation present in the first analysis, as indicated by the considerable significance of the parameters γ_1 and γ_2 in subsequent covariance adjusted analyses.

We see from Tables I and III that for both models (actual and logarithm velocities) the Papadakis adjustment is having very similar effects on the estimates of mean land class effects in that usually, for a particular land class, they are either both increased or both decreased. Note also that, since only interior grid squares are being used, some land classes have very few representative grid squares and hence the estimates of their effects will have relatively high mean square errors. This, together with the non-significant results obtained with the previous analyses, suggests that an alternative approach might be preferable, and accordingly we shall use a multiple regression model in an attempt to relate front-wave velocities directly to the map attributes. However, we should not be too disappointed with the lack of success of the analysis of variance model, since it is not inconceivable that the map attributes most influencing the ISA will be quite different from those most influencing the front-wave velocity of rabies.

TABLE III

**Estimates of Parameters in Analysis of Variance Model
with Logarithms of Velocities**[a]

	Initial ANOVA	Papadakis (1 iteration)	Papadakis (26 iterations)	n_i
Land class				
1	−2.120	−2.074	−2.089	28
2	−1.756	−1.896	−1.958	33
3	−2.035	−1.932	−1.890	14
4	−1.698	−1.877	−1.911	3
5	−1.799	−1.907	−1.941	25
6	−2.244	−2.300	−2.278	5
7	−2.083	−2.042	−2.049	6
8	−1.924	−1.914	−1.936	1
Covariate regression coefficients				
γ_1		0.176	0.184	
γ_2		0.378	0.351	

[a] n_i = number of grid squares of 'land class' i.

V. Multiple Regression Models

A. THE BASIC MODEL

We now describe the analysis of a multiple regression model in which we attempted to relate front-wave velocities to map attributes. It was clearly not feasible to use all 103 map attributes given in Appendix 1; indeed, to do this would be inappropriate since many of the attributes are mutually exclusive and, moreover, several attributes may refer to the same environmental feature, e.g. attributes 18–34 in Appendix 1 all refer to altitude. We thus decided to combine some attributes and ignore others; the resulting set of explanatory variables used on our analysis is shown in Table V.

We shall describe the analysis using the logarithm of front-wave velocities as they produced 'more normal' residuals in our earlier analysis, but similar results, which we shall summarise later, were obtained when the velocities themselves were used.

We first fitted the model

$$\log V_{i,j} = \alpha_1 + \sum_{k=2}^{18} \alpha_k x_{i,j}^{(k)} + \varepsilon_{i,j} \qquad (2)$$

TABLE IV

Analysis of Variance Table for Model with Logarithms of Velocities

Before adjustment Source	DF[a]	SS[a]	MS[a]	F[a]
Land classes	7	3.384	0.483	2.299*
Residual	107	22.503	0.210	
After 1 iteration Source	DF	SS	MS	F
Land classes	7	1.171	0.167	1.289
γ_1, γ_2	2	12.254	6.127	47.188**
Residual	105	13.633	0.130	
After 26 iterations Source	DF	SS	MS	F
Land classes	7	0.291	0.132	1.086
γ_1, γ_2	2	13.160	6.580	54.284**
Residual	105	12.727	0.121	

[a] DF, degrees of freedom; SS, sums of squares; MS, mean of squares; F, F statistic.
* Significant at the 5% level.
** Significant at the 1% level.

where $V_{i,j}$ is the front-wave velocity through grid square (i,j), $x_{i,j}^{(k)}$ is the value of the kth explanatory variable in grid square (i,j), α_k is the regression coefficient of the kth explanatory variable and $\epsilon_{i,j}$ is the residual in grid square (i,j). The resulting estimates of $\alpha_1, \alpha_2, \ldots, \alpha_{18}$ are shown in Table VI together with their standard errors and t statistics for individually testing whether a given attribute has a significant effect on front-wave velocity, i.e. whether $\alpha_k = 0$. A step-down backward regression algorithm, which at each step eliminated the least significant explanatory variable, was then used until the remaining explanatory variables were all significant at the 5% level; the results are given in Table VII.

B. SEASONAL EFFECTS

Figure 7A gives a plot of the signs of the estimated residuals for the full model of Equation (2), whilst the estimated spatial correlogram of these residuals is given in Table VIII. There was clearly considerable spatial autocorrelation amongst the residuals, for which we will have to correct. However, before doing

TABLE V

List of Explanatory Variables Used in Multiple Regression Analysis

1	Constant
2	Mean air temperature
3	Average rainfall
4	Altitude
5	Major river or canal present[a]
6	Major road or motorway present[a]
7	Main railway present[a]
8	City–town score[b]
9	Alluvial[ac]
10	Cretacious–Jurassic[ac]
11	Triassic[ac]
12	The rest[ac]
13	Arable land[d]
14	Meadows and permanent grass[d]
15	Fruit trees or vines[a]
16	Woods and forests[d]
17	Urban non-agricultural land[a]
18	Soil, rough grazing[d]

[a] Presence–absence variable score 1 if present, 0 if absent.
[b] City = 4, major town = 3, minor town = 2, small town = 1; summed over grid.
[c] Geological attributes.
[d] Score 1 if covers between 0 and 10% of grid square; score 2 if covers between 10 and 50% of grid square; score 3 if covers greater than 50% of grid square.

so, we first incorporate a seasonal effect into our model to see whether the omission of such a factor will explain the previous spatial autocorrelation. To this end we fit the following model:

$$\text{Log } V_{i,j} = \alpha_1 + \sum_{k=2}^{18} \alpha_k x_{i,j}(k) + a \sin(t_{i,j}\pi/6) + b \cos(t_{i,j}\pi/6)$$
$$+ c \sin(t_{i,j}\pi/3) + d \cos(t_{i,j}\pi/3) + \varepsilon_{i,j}$$

where $t_{i,j}$ is the number of the month that fox rabies was first reported in grid square (i,j), (January = 1, Februrary = 2, etc.). The terms in $(t_{i,j} \pi)/6$ correspond to a yearly cycle and those in $(t_{i,j} \pi)/3$ to a 6-month cycle. The resulting analysis is shown in Table IX, where it is seen that the seasonal effects are not significant; hence, we now proceed with a Papadakis adjustment for spatial autocorrelation.

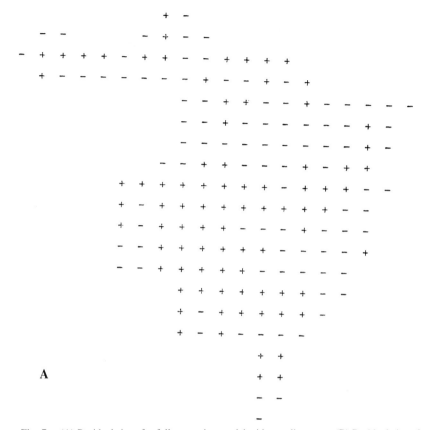

Fig. 7. (A) Residual signs for full regression model with no adjustment. (B) Residual signs for full regression model with single Papadakis iteration (continued).

Even though the seasonal effects proved not significant in the previous analysis, it was thought that they might become significant once the spatial autocorrelation was adjusted for; consequently, we performed a Papadakis iteration, with all 18 explanatory variables plus yearly and 6-month cycles in the regression model. Convergence of the Papadakis iterative scheme was considerably slower than in the analysis of variance model; indeed, it was never achieved for any of the regression models. Figure 8 shows the variation of the residual sum of squares with the number of iterations for the previous model, with and without seasonal effects. Note that although convergence appears to have been achieved rather rapidly for the model with seasonal effects, this is not convergence in the strict mathematical sense, since a closer examination of the graph shows that the residual sum of squares, slowly but steadily, increased with successive iterations after the seventh iteration. However, for most practical purposes convergence

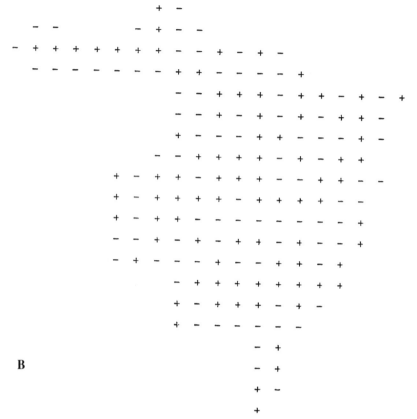

B

Fig. 7.   (*Continued.*)

can be said to have been achieved. In view of the slow rate of any convergence, we decided to terminate the iterations as soon as the residual sum of squares began to increase. We thus stopped the iteration of the full model with seasonal effects after seven iterations and tested the significance of the 6-month and yearly cycles by removing them in turn from the regression model, but still using the same residuals in the covariance adjustment. The resulting F statistics were 0.34 on (2153) degrees of freedom for 6-month cycles and 1.11 on (2155) degrees of freedom for yearly cycles. We again concluded that there is no significant seasonal effect. This is not too surprising since the front wave of rabies will usually take at least 6 months to cross a grid square of length 20 km, and, thus, any seasonal effects will tend to be smoothed out.

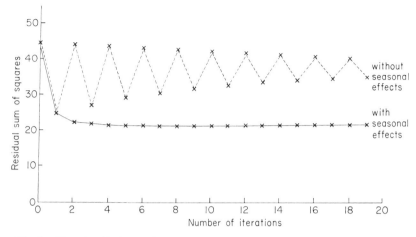

Fig. 8. Plot of residual sum of squares against number of Papadakis iterations for full model with and without seasonal effects.

C. PAPADAKIS' ADJUSTMENT

We now returned to the initial regression model with all 18 explanatory variables, but no seasonal effects, and performed a Papadakis iteration, which was stopped after a single covariance adjustment. Backwards regression was then performed until all retained explanatory variables became significant, the same residuals in the covariance adjustment being used throughout, and the covariate coefficients γ_1 and γ_2 being constrained to remain in the model. This final constraint was, in fact, redundant since γ_1 and γ_2 remained in the model in any case, again emphasising the considerable spatial autocorrelation present amongst the residuals. The results of the previous backward regression are given in Table X. Note that the Papadakis adjustment has simply resulted in two further explanatory variables being removed from the final model, following backward regression (compare Tables VII and X).

We now briefly examine the success of the Papadakis method in compensating for the spatial autocorrelation present in the data. Table VIIIb gives, for the model with all 18 explanatory variables, the estimated correlations amongst the residual following a single covariance adjustment; whereas Fig. 7B shows the signs of these estimated residuals. The residuals referred to here are those in the analysis of covariance model. This table and figure should be compared with Table VIIIA and Fig. 7A. Clearly, the Papadakis adjustment has not removed all the spatial autocorrelation amongst the residuals, though it should be borne in

TABLE VI

**Estimates of Coefficients of Explanatory Variables
in Full Regression Model with No Covariance Adjustment**

Variable	Coefficient	Standard error	t_{159}
Constant	−2.353	0.539	4.368**
Temperature	−0.252	0.213	1.180
Rainfall	−0.002	0.003	0.725
Altitude	0.001	0.000	2.654**
River or canal	−0.026	0.096	0.273
Motorway	−0.016	0.097	0.164
Railway	−0.188	0.092	2.059*
City score	−0.031	0.032	0.967
Alluvial	−0.030	0.124	0.242
Cretacious–Jurassic	0.042	0.131	0.322
Triassic	0.005	0.131	0.037
The rest, geology	−0.434	0.152	2.848**
Arable land	0.020	0.072	0.277
Meadows	−0.072	0.056	1.278
Fruit trees or vines	−0.162	0.092	1.755
Woods and forests	0.005	0.078	0.066
Urban non-agricultural land	−0.179	0.096	1.856
Soil, rough grazing	0.004	0.055	0.079

Estimate of residual variance = 0.279 with 159 degrees of freedom

* Significant at the 5% level.
** Significant at the 1% level.

mind that the estimated residuals of a regression model are necessarily correlated. However, the covariance adjustment has considerably reduced the spatial autocorrelation, and thus more emphasis should be placed on that model when interpreting the results.

D. COLLINEARITY

We have spent a considerable time incorporating the spatial autocorrelation into our analysis, but as yet we have ignored the considerable collinearity present amongst some of the explanatory variables. For example, railways tend to follow valleys and thus are unlikely to be present in regions of high altitude. This collinearity will not unduly affect the predictive aspect of the full regression model, nor will it necessarily invalidate the estimated regression coefficients of that model, though they will probably be correlated and have increased variances. However, it can cause considerable difficulties when interpreting the results of a backward regression, since if a group of explanatory variables is

TABLE VII

Estimates of Coefficients of Explanatory Variables
Following Backward Regression of Model with No Covariance Adjustment

Variable	Coefficient	Standard error	t_{171}
Constant	−2.045	0.112	15.454**
Altitude	0.001	0.000	4.064**
Railways	−2.087	0.081	2.589*
The rest, geology	−0.476	0.137	3.487**
Fruit trees or vines	−0.193	0.087	2.229*
Urban non-agricultural land	−0.185	0.093	1.986*

Estimate of residual variance = 0.271 with 171 degrees of freedom

* Significant at the 5% level.
** Significant at the 1% level.

highly autocorrelated then it is likely that only one of them will be retained in the
final set of significant variables, and it will be somewhat arbitrary which one is
retained. Moreover, if instead another variable in that intercorrelated group was
constrained to remain in the regression, the final model might be appreciably
different.

TABLE VIII

Estimated Spatial Correlogram for Residuals of Full Regression Model with No Adjustment
and with Single Papadakis Iteration[a]

	A. No adjustment					
	x lag					
	0	1	2	3	4	5
y lag						
−5	0.218	0.065	0.021	0.099	0.073	0.014
−4	0.117	−0.027	−0.004	0.081	0.028	0.120
−3	0.259	0.072	0.107	0.051	0.115	0.052
−2	0.381	0.067	0.081	0.031	0.051	0.014
−1	0.485	0.080	−0.124	−0.204	−0.076	−0.088
0	1.000	0.380	0.014	−0.141	−0.054	−0.106
1	0.485	0.226	0.063	−0.121	−0.190	−0.142
2	0.381	0.202	0.117	−0.150	−0.167	−0.150
3	0.259	0.128	0.073	−0.078	−0.099	−0.157
4	0.117	0.001	−0.034	−0.165	−0.078	−0.175
5	0.218	0.070	0.100	−0.133	−0.091	−0.128

(continued)

TABLE VIII (*Continued*)

B. Single Papadakis iteration

			x lag			
	0	1	2	3	4	5
y lag						
−5	0.253	0.088	0.140	0.032	0.053	0.015
−4	−0.002	−0.120	−0.051	0.028	−0.250	0.222
−3	−0.009	0.005	0.157	−0.053	0.056	−0.166
−2	0.194	−0.090	0.094	0.073	0.036	0.078
−1	−0.139	0.154	−0.115	−0.114	0.009	−0.068
0	1.000	−0.112	−0.033	−0.034	0.152	0.010
1	−0.139	−0.126	0.007	0.060	−0.173	0.053
2	0.194	−0.071	0.149	−0.140	0.066	−0.129
3	−0.009	0.002	−0.001	0.114	0.072	−0.134
4	−0.002	−0.184	−0.023	−0.109	0.085	−0.095
5	0.253	−0.078	0.077	0.034	0.071	0.028

[a] The table shows the estimated correlation between a residual in one grid square and the residual in a grid square that is displaced by the *x* and *y* lags from it.

Some authors have suggested overcoming this problem by performing a principal components, or some similar analysis, on the explanatory variables *prior* to multiple regression. I hesitate to recommend such an approach since, unless the resulting components have some environmental meaning, considerable difficulties will be encountered in interpreting the resulting regression model. A more instructive approach would be to examine the correlation matrix of the explanatory variables, discover which variables are highly correlated and perform several

TABLE IX

Testing for Seasonal Effects in Full Regression Model without Covariance Adjustment

Model	Sum of squares	df
A Variables 1–18 plus yearly and 6-month cycles	43.913	155
B Variables 1–18 plus yearly cycle	44.023	157
C Variables 1–18	44.425	159

Hypothesis test	F	df
Test for 6-month cycles (B versus A)	0.19	2,155
Test for yearly cycles (C versus B)	0.72	2,157

TABLE X

Estimates of Coefficients of Explanatory Variables
Following Backward Regression of Full Model with Single Papadakis Iteration

Variable	Coefficient	Standard error	t_{171}
Constant	−2.189	0.096	22.838**
Altitude	0.001	0.000	5.282**
The rest, geology	−0.309	0.105	2.965**
Urban non-agricultural land	−0.235	0.072	3.276**
Covariance adjustments			
γ_1	0.292	0.035	8.337**
γ_2	0.265	0.041	6.659**

Estimate of residual variance = 0.161 with 171 degrees of freedom

**Significant at the 1% level.

backwards regressions, in which different members of sets of highly correlated explanatory variables are dropped from the analysis at the appropriate stages; the results of these backwards regressions should then be interpreted together rather than individually. If we wish to use our model for *predictive* purposes, rather than as a means of discovering the environmental factors underlying the spread of rabies then it would be incorrect to use principal components, since (1) they do not automatically provide good predictors and (2) no economy of description is achieved, since in obtaining the principal components we are using *all* the original variables.

However, in spite of these objections, it was decided to perform such an analysis, which was to be seen as an additional tool in interpreting the data. Rather than using principal components, we used the axis scores of the reciprocal averaging underlying the indicator species analysis described in Section IV,A, which are nearly uncorrelated. The scores on the first five such axes were related to the logarithm of the front-wave velocity by a multiple regression model. No correction for spatial autocorrelation was made, and the results are shown in Table XI.

From Table XI, we see that only the first and third axis scores were significant at the 5% level. The first axis score gave a general indication of the altitude of a grid square, with a high score indicating a high altitude, whilst the second axis described the general relief, with a high score indicating rugged topography and a low score more rolling country. The third axis unfortunately seemed to yield no simple interpretation. It is important to note that the significance of the first axis score agrees nicely with the importance of altitude in our previous analyses.

TABLE XI

**Estimates of Coefficients of Explanatory Variables for Multiple
Regression of the Logarithm of Front-wave Velocity on Reciprocal
Averaging Axis Scores, with No Correction for Spatial Autocorrelation**

Variable	Coefficient	Standard error	t_{172}
Constant	−2.252	0.421	5.351**
Axis 1	0.010	0.003	4.186**
Axis 2	−0.003	0.003	1.189
Axis 3	−0.008	0.002	4.257**
Axis 4	0.007	0.004	1.543
Axis 5	0.001	0.004	0.186

Estimate of residual variance = 0.276 with 172 degrees of freedom[a]

[a] Degrees of freedom in this table differ from those in some other tables as a grid square was inadvertently omitted from earlier analyses.
** Significant at the 1% level.

E. INTERPRETATION

We now give a possible interpretation of our analyses, but before doing so, it should be emphasized that the proportion of variation explained by our models is not high, being about 20% for the full regression model with logarithms of front-wave velocities. This is hardly surprising since (1) it is extremely unlikely that the logarithm of front-wave velocity will be *linearly* related to the set of map attributes we have chosen and (2) there are likely to be several factors influencing the spread of rabies not included in our model, e.g. fox control policies. The low proportion of variation explained does not invalidate the results of our analyses but warns us to be cautious with our conclusions. It also tells us to place greater emphasis on the qualitative results of the analysis than on the quantitative results; thus we would not expect our model to yield accurate predictions of front-wave velocities, but we should be able to determine whether front-wave velocities increase or decrease with the values of various explanatory variables. As mentioned previously, we should interpret the analyses as a whole, rather than individually.

A summary of the final set of explanatory variables for the two backward regression models previously described and for the equivalent models with actual front-wave velocities, which, incidentally, resulted in slightly less spatial autocorrelation, is given in Table XII. An encouraging feature of these results is that they are quite similar for the four models and hence in spite of the exploratory nature of the Papadakis adjustments, we can still have reasonable confidence in

TABLE XII

Summary of Backward Regression Results for Various Models[a]

	Without Papadakis' adjustment	With Papadakis' adjustment
Log velocities	Altitude$^+$ Railways$^-$ The rest, geology$^-$ Fruit trees or vines$^-$ Urban non-agricultural land$^-$	Altitude$^+$ The rest, geology$^-$ Urban non-agricultural land$^-$
Actual velocities	Altitude$^+$ Railways$^-$ The rest, geology$^-$	Altitude$^+$ Railways$^-$ The rest, geology$^-$

[a] A + (−) indicates that the estimated multiple regression coefficient of the corresponding explanatory variable was positive (negative).

the results. We shall interpret these results in terms of habitat richness and a nearest-neighbour contact model for the spread of rabies. In poor habitats, such as Cumbrian moorland, fox territories tend to be large, and consequently nearest-neighbour spread will result in high front-wave velocities, whilst in rich habitats, such as the rural suburbia of Boars Hill, Oxford, territories tend to be small and nearest-neighbour spread will result in low front-wave velocities. The factors affecting fox territory sizes are not fully understood, although the availability of food clearly plays a major role (Macdonald, 1980; see also Chapter 4, this volume). From Table XII, we see that altitude was a significant variable in all the models and that it always had a positive partial correlation with front-wave velocity. This supports the previous interpretation since an increase in altitude, with all other factors remaining constant, will probably result in larger fox territories. A similar explanation can perhaps be given to the lower velocities in grid squares containing fruit trees or vines. The effects of rivers–canals and railways on front-wave velocities could be because they are natural barriers to fox movement and, hence, to the spread of rabies. Though this is reasonable for rivers–canals, and indeed has been noted by Ross (1981) and Sayers et al. (1977, also Chapter 10, this volume), it is not so for railways, since railway banks are known to be a favourite haunt of foxes. However, this would suggest that territories adjoining railways would be small, and we could perhaps invoke our previous argument. The lower velocities in grid squares containing urban non-agricultural land is probably owing to the lack of town foxes in France. 'The rest' geology is an attribute characteristic of a broken topography and small fields, the type of habitat where one might expect small fox territories and thus low front-wave velocities. Finally, it is worth noting that the regression coefficients, given in Table VI, for the full model without covariance adjustment generally support the hypothesis that rabies spread is of the 'nearest-neighbour' type, as indeed does the analysis of the reciprocal averaging axis scores.

VI. Concluding Discussion

As stated in the introduction, the analysis presented here is only a preliminary one and hence could be improved in many ways, some of which I now outline.

A. VELOCITY ESTIMATES

Firstly, it would be instructive to compare the results of our velocity estimation method with those of a more sophisticated method, such as that of Sayers *et al.* (1977). Care should be taken though, as the schemes are estimating slightly different velocities. Our method estimates the velocity of the extreme front of fox rabies, whilst the method of Sayers *et al.* estimates the velocity of propagation of a contour containing a fixed proportion, α say, of smoothed cases. Thus, for α sufficiently large, the two methods should give similar results. It would also be interesting to examine the consistency of our velocity estimates under changes in the size, location and orientation of the underlying grid. Clearly, with too fine a grid the estimates of front-wave velocity will be unduly affected by reporting biases, whilst too coarse a grid will smooth out the heterogeneity in front-wave velocities, which we wish to study. We noted in Section III that our estimated front-wave velocities contained some possible outliers, which should be investigated further; indeed, some of these velocities should perhaps be removed from our subsequent analyses.

B. COLLINEARITY AND SPATIAL AUTOCORRELATION

Our regression analysis was hindered considerably by the spatial autocorrelation present in the data and, to a lesser extent, by the collinearity amongst the explanatory variables. As far as collinearity is concerned, it would be instructive to examine the correlation matrix of the explanatory variables and to perform several backward regressions as outlined in Section IV, D. Turning to the problem of spatial autocorrelation we saw that the Papadakis method was partially successful in that it removed a fair proportion of the spatial autocorrelation amongst the residual. However, difficulties occur when we attempt to give a meaning to the values of the covariance adjustment coefficients, γ_1 and γ_2. This, in itself, is a difficult problem since it is not known under what error structures the Papadakis method yields good estimates. However, a first-order spatial autoregressive model is clearly favoured, but all the obtained estimates of γ_1 and γ_2 violate the stationarity of such a model, although this might be owing to a variable missing from the regression.

C. MODEL IDENTIFICATION, FURTHER ANALYSIS AND PREDICTION

An important reason for performing empirical studies of rabies epizootics is that the results will often aid model identification, since the behaviour of front-wave velocity with fox population parameters, such as group size and territory size, is distinctly different for various fox rabies models. We have seen that the results of the front-wave velocity regression analysis are consistent with a nearest-neighbour epidemic model, though, of course, they do not prove that such a model is correct. It would be worthwhile to carry out similar regression analyses on other aspects of rabies epizootics, such as intensity and persistence. The results of these analyses will either increase our confidence in the nearest-neighbour epidemic model or make us reconsider the assumptions of that model.

It would be instructive to examine the predictive ability of the model presented here by using the estimated regression coefficients to forecast the velocities of spread of French fox rabies after May 1978 and comparing the results with the observed velocities. A similar exercise could be done with a model to predict the future intensity of rabies, and if both models proved successful in a forecasting capacity, then they could be used in conjunction by a rabies surveillance team to highlight regions in whch to concentrate control.

D. ESTIMATING PARAMETERS OF MECHANISTIC MODELS

In Chapter 8, this volume, we used a nearest-neighbour epidemic model to evaluate the efficacy of various control strategies. However, in order to use such a model in real life rabies surveillance, it would be necessary to obtain estimates of fox population parameters, such as group size, territory size and infection probabilities. At present, the only method of obtaining these estimates is from extensive field work involving the radio tracking of foxes. Clearly, in the event of a rabies outbreak in Britain, it would be advantageous, and most likely essential, to obtain these estimates rapidly, which will not be possible if there have been no radio-tracking studies of foxes in the region concerned. We have seen how front-wave velocities of a rabies epizootic can be related to map attributes, and it seems likely that the before-mentioned fox population parameters could also be related to map attributes. Thus, given the results of radio-tracking studies in a few carefully chosen habitat environments, we could estimate the above fox population parameters and then relate them, via a regression model, to map attributes. This final regression model could then be used to estimate those parameters, from map attributes, in regions for which there have been no radio-tracking studies. The success of Macdonald *et al.* (1981) in estimating fox densities from map atrributes suggests that this approach might be feasible.

E. HABITAT HETEROGENEITY
AND MECHANISTIC MODELS

In spite of its preliminary nature, our analysis has clearly demonstrated that habitat heterogeneity significantly affects the velocity of a rabies front, and thus the course of an epizootic. Previous mechanistic models of rabies have always assumed a spatially homogeneous environment. Our analysis does not necessarily invalidate the use of such models since (1) at present their main use is in predicting qualitative rather than quantitative behaviour and (2) our analysis shows heterogeneity between 20 × 20 km grid squares, whilst the mechanistic model might be on a much smaller scale. However, if in the future we wish to use mechanistic models to quantitatively describe the spread of rabies over an appreciably sized region, then the results of this chapter show that it would be imperative to incorporate any heterogeneity in fox population parameters into the model. Clearly such a model of a real life rabies epizootic will be peculiar to the region concerned, but in the meantime it would be instructive to simulate rabies amongst various artificial heterogeneous regions to increase our understanding of the role played by habitat heterogeneity in the spread of rabies.

Appendix 1. List of Map Attributes Used in French
Rabies Velocity Analysis

Attribute	Attribute number
Climate	
Mean air temperature	
10°–15°C	1
5°–10°C	2
0°–5°C	3
−5°–0°C	4
Average annual rainfall	
10°–50°mm	5
50°–100°mm	6
100°–200°mm	7
200°–400°mm	8
Latitude	
Most northerly band	9
Northern band	10
Southern band	11
Most southerly band	12
Distance from Atlantic coast	
Most westerly	13
Westerly	14
Central	15

Easterly	16
Most easterly	17
Altitude	
Land below sea level present	18
0–100 m	
<50%	19
>50%	20
100–200 m	
<50%	21
>50%	22
200–500 m	
<50%	23
>50%	24
500–1000 m	
<50%	25
>50%	26
1000–1500 m	
<50%	27
>50%	28
1500–2000 m	
<50%	29
>50%	30
2000–3000 m	
<50%	31
>50%	32
Maximum spot height	
>3000 m	33
Minimum spot height	
>4000 m	34
Mark the highest and lowest points in the square and join these by a straight line	
Slope line length	
<3 mm	35
3–6 mm	36
6–9 mm	37
>9 mm	38
Aspect line direction	
North	39
East	40
South	41
West	42
Hill behind slope	
none present	43
< 500 m	44
<2000 m	45
<3000 m	46
>3000 m	47
Rivers and lakes	
Major river	48

(*continued*)

Appendix 1. (*Continued*)

Minor river	49
River source present	50
River length	
<6 mm	51
>6 mm	52
Large (>20 km²) lake(s) present	53
Small (<20 km²) lakes present	54
Canals present	55
Roads and cities	
Motorway present	56
Motorway present in adjacent square	57
Trunk road	
<6 mm	58
>6 mm	59
Minor road	
<6 mm	60
>6 mm	61
Main railway present	62
Minor railway present	63
City present	64
City present in adjacent square	65
Town(s) size 1 present	66
>1 Town size 3	67
Town(s) size 2 present	68
Town(s) size 3 present	69
Major town in adjacent square	70
Coastline	
<6 mm	71
>6 mm	72
Geology	
Dotted (alluvial)	
centre	73
<2 surrounds	74
≥3 surrounds	75
Cross-hatched (Cretacious–Jurassic)	
centre	76
<2 surrounds	77
≥3 surrounds	78
Square-hatch (Triassic)	
centre	79
<2 surrounds	80
≥3 surrounds	81
The rest	
centre	82
<2 surrounds	83
≥3 surrounds	84

Agriculture
　Arable land
　　<10%   85
　　10–50%   86
　　>50%   87
　　　Meadows and permanent grass
　　<10%   88
　　10–50%   89
　　>50%   90
　Fruit trees or vines present   91
　Market gardens present   92
　Woods and forests
　　<10%   93
　　10–50%   94
　　>50%   95
　Upland grazing (white on map)
　　<10%   96
　　10–50%   97
　　>50%   98
　Urban non-agricultural land present   99
　Rural non-agricultural land present   100
Soils
　Rough grazing (yellow on map)
　　<10%   101
　　10–50%   102
　　>50%   103

Appendix 2. Spatial Autocorrelation and Papadakis' Method

A fundamental assumption of any ordinary least squares analysis, such as the one-way analysis of variance analysis of Section IV, B, is that the observational errors $\varepsilon_{i,j}$ are mutually independent. If in fact the residuals $\varepsilon_{i,j}$ are autocorrelated, then the ordinary least squares analysis is upset, since (1) the residual variance will be under (over) estimated according to whether the correlation is positive (negative) and hence we are more (less) likely to find an attribute significant than is implied by the nominal significance levels and (2) if, for example, a presence–absence variable is only present in a region of high residuals its effect might be considerably overestimated. In practice, the error structure is usually assumed to be stationary over the grid and thus if the experiment were repeated our presence–absence variable might then only be present in a region of low residuals.

Consequently, what we are really saying in (2) is that estimates of effects can have far greater variances than predicted by the theory assuming independent residuals. Whereas (1) will always be a problem, usually with positively-correlated residuals, (2) is most likely to be a nuisance when some presence–absence variables are only present in a few grid squares; however, in analyses of the type we are performing such variables are often clustered in space, e.g. see Fig. 5, which will confound with the error structure to enhance the likelihood of (2).

Cliff and Ord (1981) give the following as the most likely causes of spatial autocorrelation:

1. The regression function is not linear.
2. An explanatory variable is missing from the regression.
3. The regression model has a correlation structure, i.e. spatial autocorrelation is actually present and not induced in our model!

We would expect (3) to be the major of these three causes in our analysis of variance model, since our velocity estimation procedure would induce some spatial autocorrelation, and further it is highly plausible that the system governing the spread of rabies is such that a high velocity through one square leads to a high velocity through the next. However, we should not ignore (1) and (2); clearly, (1) plays some role as can be seen by the different results obtained with logarithm and actual velocities. Also, the lack of any seasonal element in our model suggests that (2) might be having an effect as well. Indeed, it is quite likely that there will be a seasonal effect since for example, one would expect higher front-wave velocities during the autumn dispersal of juvenile foxes; in a later model we shall admit this possibility.

Having concluded that spatial autocorrelation is present amongst our data, we must decide how we are going to incorporate it into our analysis. Two possibilities are, firstly, to decide on a particular form for the error structure and try to fit it to the data and, secondly, to use an empirical method, in which no particular error structure is assumed, though some will be more favoured than others. In the former, we could hypothesise a system for the spread of rabies and use this, together with our velocity estimation scheme, to evaluate the form of the error structure. Although this is very attractive in principle, in practice evaluating the error structure could be fairly intractable mathematically and consequently it is probably preferable to assume straight away a particular form for the error structure, such as a scheme in which the *direct* dependence is only nearest neighbour, i.e. a first-order scheme. However, having decided upon a form for the error structure, estimating the parameters involved and constructing hypothesis tests still present considerable difficulties. Moreover, this whole approach can be dangerous since the results might be highly sensitive to the assumed error structure. Consequently we chose to use an empirical method, but the interested reader is referred to the works of Bartlett (1976), Besag (1974), Cliff and Ord (1981) and Ripley (1981), and the references contained therein, for details of analysing regression models in the presence of an assumed form of spatially correlated residuals.

Padadakis (1937) proposed a method for estimating treatment effects in ran-domised agricultural field experiments in which the ordinary least squares esti-mates are adjusted by an analysis of covariance on the residuals of neighbouring plots (see also Bartlett, 1938). (A *randomised experiment* is one in which within blocks treatments are allocated randomly to experimental units). If the residuals are spatially autocorrelated then this method can give estimates of treatment effects with considerably lower mean square errors than those obtained by ordi-nary least squares (Atkinson, 1969; Bartlett, 1978). We shall use Papadakis' method to adjust for spatial autocorrelation amongst the residuals in our analyses of front-wave velocities of fox rabies. Such an analysis is in a sense exploratory since clearly the conditions of our velocity analysis differ from those of the before-mentioned field trials. We now briefly outline the method as it would be applied to the model

$$y_{i,j} = \alpha + \beta x_{i,j} + U_{i,j} \tag{3}$$

where $y_{i,j}$ is the velocity in grid square (i,j); $x_{i,j}$ is the value of an explanatory variable in grid square (i,j): $U_{i,j}$ is the residual in grid square (i,j).

In ordinary least squares the $U_{i,j}$ are assumed to be independent normal ran-dom variables each with zero mean and variance σ^2, $N(0,\sigma^2)$ say. However, in our model they possess some unknown spatial correlation structure. To apply Papadakis' method, we first obtain estimates $(\hat{\alpha}_0, \beta_0)$ of (α,β) by ordinary least squares and hence obtain an estimate of the residual in the (i,j)th grid square by

$$\hat{U}_{i,j} = y_{i,j} - \hat{\alpha}_0 - \beta_0 x_{i,j} \tag{4}$$

We now fit the model

$$y_{i,j} = \alpha + \beta x_{i,j} + \gamma_1(\hat{U}_{i-1,j} + \hat{U}_{i+1,j}) + \gamma_2(\hat{U}_{i,j-1} + \hat{U}_{i,j+1}) + \epsilon_{i,j}. \tag{5}$$

where the $\epsilon_{i,j}$ are independent $N(0,\sigma^2)$ random variables, by ordinary least squares; the resulting estimates, $(\hat{\alpha}_1, \beta_1)$ say, are called the covariance adjusted estimates of (α,β). The logic behind this method is that the inclusion of (γ_1, γ_2) will to some extent correct for any correlation between the residual in the grid square (i,j) and its neighbouring residuals.

The method can be iterated by calculating a new set of residuals from Equation (4) with $(\hat{\alpha}_0, \beta_0)$ replaced by $(\hat{\alpha}_1, \beta_1)$ and then fitting the model into Equation (5) with these new residuals, the process being repeated until, hopefully, con-vergence, is achieved. To increase the possibility of convergence, at each stage of the iteration we add a constant to each of the residuals to make them have zero mean. Note that it is a consequence of ordinary least squares that the first set of residuals as given by Equation (4) will necessarily have zero mean.

It is possible to construct approximate hypothesis tests on the parameters (α, β) in the usual way from the ANOVA table for the model in Equation (5). We can perhaps also use this table to test hypotheses such as $\gamma_1 = \gamma_2 = 0$, that is, that there is no spatial autocorrelation amongst the residuals. However, it must be stressed that these tests are only approximate since the assumptions for ordinary least squares are clearly not met in the model given by Equation (5). Indeed, a simulation study by Beeyendeza (1981) suggested that the before-mentioned test for spatial autocorrelation is optimistic, as opposed to conservative, whilst tests for the effect of explanatory variables are usually quite good, provided the design matrix and error structure are not confounded, as would be the case if our model contained a spatial trend element.

There will be difficulties with edge effects since it is not possible to calculate residuals of all four nearest neighbours for those grid squares on the boundary of the region in which front-wave velocities were estimated. Two ways of circumventing this problem are (1) to restrict the analysis to those grid squares having velocities estimated in all four neighbouring grid squares or (2) make a sensible estimate of residuals, when they are not available, for the nearest neighbours of those grid squares on the before-mentioned boundary. One such method for (2) is as follows: if, for example, $\hat{U}_{i,j-1}$ is present but $\hat{U}_{i,j+1}$ absent, then, we estimate $\hat{U}_{i,j+1}$ by $\hat{U}_{i,j-1}$. If $\hat{U}_{i,j-1}$ and $\hat{U}_{i,j+1}$ are both absent, then we estimate $\hat{U}_{i,j-1} + \hat{U}_{i,j+1}$ by $\hat{U}_{i-1,j} + \hat{U}_{i+1,j}$, where in this final sum if, for example, $\hat{U}_{i-1,j}$ is absent it is estimated by $\hat{U}_{i+1,j}$. Note that since there are no 'island' grid squares with front-wave velocity estimates, we can use this method to estimate all the residuals required by Equation (5).

Acknowledgements

This research was carried out whilst I was a research student in the Department of Biomathematics, University of Oxford. It is a pleasure to thank my supervisor, Professor P. Armitage, for his helpful advice and encouragement and the Medical Research Council for financial support. Dr. P. Bacon kindly assisted with collecting the map attribute data.

References

Atkinson, A. C. (1969). The use of residuals as a concomitant variable. *Biometrika* **56**, 33–41.
Bacon, P., and Macdonald, D. W. (1981). Habitat and the spread of rabies. *Nature (London)* **289**, 634–635.
Bartlett, M. S. (1938). The approximate recovery of information from field experiments with large blocks. *J. Agric. Sci.* **28**, 418–427.

Bartlett, M. S. (1976). "The Statistical Analysis of Spatial Pattern." Chapman & Hall, London.

Bartlett, M. S. (1978). Nearest neighbour models in the analysis of field experiments. *J. R. Stat. Soc. Ser. B* **40**, 147–174.

Beeyendeza, J. (1981). An investigation into the effects of spatial autocorrelation in least-squares estimation. M.Sc. Thesis, University of Sussex.

Besag, J. E. (1974). Spatial interaction and the analysis of lattice systems. *J. R. Stat. Soc., Ser. B* **36**, 192–236.

Bögel, K., Moegle, H., Knorpp, F., Arata, A., Dietz, K., and Diethelm, P. (1976). Characteristics of the spread of a wildlife rabies epidemic in Europe. *Bull. W. H. O.* **54**, 433–447.

Cliff, A. D., and Ord, J. K. (1981). "Spatial Processes, Models and Applications." Pion, London.

Hill, M. O. (1973). Reciprical averaging an eigenvector method of ordination. *J. Ecol.* **61**, 237–249.

Hill, M. O., Bunce, R. G. H., and Shaw, M. W. (1975). Indicator species analysis, a divisive polythetic method of classification, and its application to a survey of native pinewoods in Scotland. *J. Ecol.* **63**, 597–613.

Jackson, H. C. (1979). A contribution to the study of fox rabies in relation to habitat in Europe. M.Sc. Thesis, Imperial College, University of London.

Lineback, N. G. (1980). A model of rabies diffusion. *Southeast. Geogr.* **20**, 1–15.

Macdonald, D. W. (1980). "Rabies and Wildlife, a Biologist's Perspective." Oxford Univ. Press, London and New York.

Macdonald, D. W., Bunce, R. G. H., and Bacon, P. J. (1981). Fox populations, habitat characterisation, and rabies control. *J. Biogeogr.* **8**, 145–151.

Papadakis, J. S. (1937). Méthode statistique pour des expériences sur champ. *Bull. Inst. Amel. Plantes Salon* No. 23.

Ripley, B. D. (1981). "Spatial Statistics." Wiley, London.

Ross, J. (1981). Rabies spread and land classes in France. *In* "Habitat Classification, Fox Populations and Rabies Spread" (P. J. Bacon and D. W. Macdonald, eds.), Merlewood Res. Dev. Pap. No. 81. Institute of Terrestrial Ecology, Grange-over-Sands, Cumbria, England.

Sayers, B. McA., Mansourian, B. G., Phan Tan, T., and Bögel, K. (1977). A pattern analysis study of a wild-life rabies epizootic. *Med. Inf.* **2**, 11–34.

Toma, B, and Andral, A. (1977). Epidemiology of fox rabies. *Adv. Virus Res.* **21**, 1–36.

Spatial Epidemic Models: Theory and Simulations

12

Denis Mollison
Kari Kuulasmaa[1]
Department of Actuarial Mathematics and Statistics,
Heriot-Watt University,
Riccarton, Edinburgh, Scotland

I. Introduction

The aim of this chapter is to survey theoretical results on spatial models for epidemics, and to discuss how they can help us in understanding, and if possible controlling, diseases such as rabies. In the first half of this chapter we give a general survey of work on spatial models for epidemics. In the second half we discuss some simulations carried out by Kuulasmaa (1983), aimed at exploring general aspects of endemic fox rabies; these provide evidence of the importance of incorporating stochastic and spatial features. We conclude with some discus-

[1]Present address: National Public Health Institute, Mannerheimintie 166, SF-00280 Helsinki, Finland.

sion of the relations between simple general spatial models as considered here, and more detailed specialised models such as those described in other chapters by Bacon, Ball, and Voigt and Tinline.

We first introduce the three main aspects of epidemics with which we shall be concerned, namely *thresholds, velocities* and *endemicity*.

A population is said to be 'above threshold' for a particular disease if, once started, the disease has a chance of spreading widely through the population; and 'below threshold' if it will die out with only a small proportion of the population infected. The practical problems are to identify when a population is above threshold when threatened by a particular disease such as rabies, and to estimate whether various control strategies, such as vaccination or culling, could bring the population below threshold.

The second question, of velocities, relates to how fast the disease will spread if it does become established (in an above threshold population), and how this depends on factors such as the territorial range of individuals. Practical questions include the likelihood of success of a spatially selective control strategy, such as clearing a control zone of a certain width in front of the epidemic.

The third question, of endemic behaviour, is the most difficult theoretically because our models must allow for the introduction of new susceptibles, without which the disease would die out. Here again the most important practical questions relate to the possible elimination of the disease. However, because of the greater difficulties of modelling, we need first to improve our understanding of spatial endemic models. For instance, the pattern of endemic fox rabies in Europe shows much spatial heterogeneity ('wandering patches', see e.g. Sayers, Chapter 10, this volume), and it is an important question how much this is due, if at all, to heterogeneities in the population.

II. Theory of Spatial Models

A. BASIC SPATIAL MODELS

We begin by introducing a simple spatial epidemic model motivated by the study of fox rabies. Rabies, especially among the fox population of western Europe, is a disease which spreads through local interactions among territorial animals. It therefore seems important that our model should be *spatial* and *stochastic,* and should include the *carrying capacity* or some other kind of limit on the population density. Models which are non-spatial or deterministic, or which allow populations of unbounded density, are not fully adequate (Mollison, 1981); although they have been and will continue to be extremely useful as stepping stones towards better, more complex, models.

We envisage space as a two-dimensional array of sites (see Fig. 1); in the

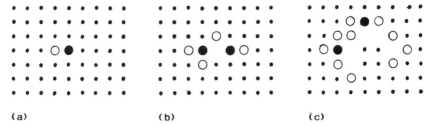

Fig. 1. The spatial epidemic model of Equation (1). (a) Part of the two-dimensional array of sites shown just after the start of an epidemic outbreak: this started with a single introduced infectious individual (●), who has now infected one neighbour (now incubating, marked ○). All other sites are still occupied by susceptibles (•). (b) The same sites, a little later: the site originally infected is now vacant (   ), and there are several incubating (○) and infectious (●) individuals. (c) Still later: note that two sites which had become vacant have now been recolonised by susceptibles.

context of fox rabies, these may be taken to represent square territories. Each site may either be empty (E), or occupied by an individual who may be susceptible (X), incubating (I), or infectious (Y). The development of the epidemic is then prescribed by stochastic change rates (formally 'instantaneous transition rates' or *ITRs*: when we say that a possible change has ITR equal to λ, we mean that in any short interval of time dt, the probability of its occurring is λdt), as follows:

	Change	Change rate	
Infection	$XY \rightarrow IY$	$\beta/4$	
Becoming infective	$I \rightarrow Y$	σ	(1)
Death	$Y \rightarrow E$	α	
Recolonisation	$EX \rightarrow XX$	$r/4$	

Here β is the overall rate at which an infective makes contacts; the change rates α and σ correspond exactly to those of the simple deterministic non-spatial model described in Chapter 9 [Equation (1)], this volume, and lead to a generation gap with probability distribution given by Equation (4) of Chapter 9 (a sum of two exponential distributions), with mean $\tau = 1/\alpha + 1/\sigma$. The 'recolonisation' term represents population regrowth, net of natural mortality (see later).

A simpler alternative model, corresponding to Equation (2) of Chapter 9, omits the incubating state:

	Change	Change rate	
Infection	$XY \rightarrow YY$	$\beta'/4$	
Death	$Y \rightarrow E$	α'	(2)
Recolonisation	$EX \rightarrow XX$	$r/4$	

Here the infectious period and the generation gap both have exponential distribution with mean $\tau = 1/\alpha'$.

In both models, the spatial element is involved in the other two types of change. Thus *XY* indicates a pair of neighbours, one of whom is susceptible and the other infectious; the first type of change represents infection of the former by the latter. Since each individual has four neighbours (see Fig. 1), each infectious individual will be making potentially infectious contacts at an overall rate β [for Model (1), β' for Model (2)], these contacts being divided equally among its four neighbours, and of course succeeding only if the neighbour chosen is susceptible. The parameter β thus corresponds to βN, in the simple non-spatial models described in Chapter 9 (Equations 1–3). Similarly, the parameter r, which represents the per capita net population growth rate at low densities, corresponds roughly to the parameter r of those models (but see comments in Section III,C). An important concept in spatial models is the *contact distribution* (Mollison, 1972, 1977), which describes the spatial distribution of the potentially infectious contacts made by an infectious individual. Here we have taken the contact distribution as concentrated on an individual's four nearest neighbours. This simple distribution is probably adequate at least for the initial exploration of endemic conditions, but if we are interested in the velocity of spread of an epidemic, as in Section II,C, we will need to allow for longer range contacts as well. In models for endemic conditions, we need a secondary contact distribution as well, to describe the process of recolonisation of empty sites: here this has also been assumed to be a nearest-neighbour distribution, and again in a more detailed analysis we should consider the effect of allowing for longer range movements by recolonising animals.

The type of model introduced here is about as simple as seems possible for a stochastic spatial model suitable for endemic disease. Ideally, one would like to achieve a broad understanding of such models, and then introduce further realistic details, such as seasonal and social variability. However, even such simple models are not well understood, and initially we shall go in the other direction, and consider the problems of thresholds and velocities in the context of even simpler models.

B. SPATIAL MODELS: THRESHOLDS

The 'threshold' for a disease has been defined previously as the dividing line between conditions in which the disease will die out with only a small proportion of the population infected, and conditions in which there is a chance of the disease spreading widely through the population. This should perhaps be called the 'pandemic threshold', to distinguish it from the 'endemic threshold', which may be defined as the initial conditions such that the disease will persist indefinitely. The endemic threshold, to which we shall return in Section II,D, will depend crucially on the rate of regrowth of the susceptible population, and will in general be higher than the pandemic threshold.

In considering the basic (pandemic) threshold it seems reasonable in the first instance to neglect the regrowth of susceptibles, since this is slow compared with the initial velocity of the disease. (A detailed analysis of this requires consideration of the rate of advance of the front, its depth, and the typical dispersal distances of each year's young foxes.) If we do neglect the regrowth of susceptibles, we can simplify our analysis of threshold conditions in one important respect. It is then possible at least in the slightly simplified models usually studied, to make a *list* of each individual's potential contacts (in a stochastic model, this will involve random choices) without having to consider time or whether that individual will in fact be infected. The set of those eventually infected by the disease then consists precisely of those for whom we can find a 'chain of infection', with each individual in the previous one's list, which begins with one of those initially infected. Thus, if we are only interested in who will and who will not be infected, as we are when considering thresholds, we need take no direct account of the time structure.

The classic threshold theorem is due to Kermack and MacKendrick (1927). It refers to a non-spatial deterministic epidemic model with homogeneous mixing, and says that a pandemic will occur if and only if the basic reproductive rate C, which is essentially the average size of each individual's list, is greater than unity. The further the population is initially above threshold, the further the remaining susceptibles at the conclusion of the pandemic will be below threshold (Kermack and Mackendrick, 1927; Kendall, 1965).

A similar stochastic model behaves similarly, except that there is a chance that the disease will fail to get established even though the population is above threshold. The probability of failure can be estimated by comparison with a simpler model which allows an unlimited pool of suceptibles, and is approximately C^{-Y_0}, where Y_0 is the number initially infected (Whittle, 1955; Kendall, 1965).

In models incorporating the introduction of fresh susceptibles, the disease may either settle into endemic equilibrium, or into a cyclic pattern, with each peak of infection behaving much like one of Kermack and McKendrick's pandemics (Bartlett, 1960; see also Chapters 6, 7 and 9 of this volume).

We next turn to models for spatially distributed populations. Most work on the velocity of epidemics has been restricted to one-dimensional models (see next section). However, it can be shown for quite a general class of models that pandemics in one dimension are impossible, provided only that infectious cases are subject to eventual removal (F. Kelly in discussion of Mollison, 1977, pp. 318–319). While this is a rather theoretical result (there does appear to be a 'pseudo-threshold' above which the disease can spread a great distance), it suggests that for a realistic consideration of thresholds we do need to study two-dimensional models.

We consider here only models without recolonisation of empty sites. Perhaps the simplest case is that where the infectious period is of fixed length, rather than exponentially distributed as in Models (1) and (2) of the previous section. This is because in this case the infections made by an individual are statistically independent, each having probability p say. The epidemic model is therefore formally equivalent to the well-known *bond percolation* model of physics, which has threshold value $p_0 = \frac{1}{2}$ (Broadbent and Hammersley, 1957; Kesten, 1980). The threshold value of the basic reproductive rate is then $C_0 = 4p_0 = 2$. If, on the other hand, the infectious period is extremely variable, we tend towards the following case: with probability p the infectious period is very long and the individual infects all four neighbours, while with probability $1-p$, the infectious period is very short and it infects none. This corresponds to *site percolation,* for which the critical value p_0 has been estimated to be 0.6; thus in this case C_0, which is again $4p_0$, is equal to 2.4. For intermediate infectious periods, we may suspect that C_0 will lie between these two values, i.e. between 2 and 2.4. By using a comparison technique for epidemic models which differ only in the distribution of their infectious periods, Kuulasmaa (1982) has shown that this is true for all such distributions. In particular, it is true for the exponential distribution, as in Models (1) and (2) (without recolonisation, i.e. with $r = 0$), and simulations show that for this case $C_0 \approx 2.12$.

These results refer to the case where each individual only interacts with its four nearest neighbours. Asymptotic results (e.g. Ball, 1983) suggest that C_0 will be closer to unity when the number of potential contacts is larger.

C. SPATIAL MODELS: VELOCITIES

The velocity of spread of a disease will clearly depend to a large extent on the *contact distribution,* which describes the spatial distribution of the potentially infectious contacts made by an individual. This dependence has only been studied in any depth for very simple one-dimensional models, namely *simple epidemics,* in which infected individuals remain permanently infective: this corresponds to Model (2) with $\alpha' = 0$ (r is then irrelevant, since sites never become vacant). This work is reviewed in Mollison (1977). There has also been some thorough work on two-dimensional models with the contacts restricted to an individual's nearest neighbours, mostly on percolation models; this field is reviewed by Smythe and Wierman (1978).

Most work even in the one-dimensional case has been on deterministic models, in the form of nonlinear convolution or diffusion equations. These can be shown (McKean, 1975; Mollison, 1977) to be closely related to 'linear' stochastic models, which make the simplifying but unrealistic assumption of an unlimited pool of susceptibles, and in which the density of infectives consequently can grow exponentially. It is thus perhaps not surprising that these deterministic models turn out to be a poor guide to the behaviour of more realistic stochastic models.

The earliest work on velocities appears in two classic papers which appeared independently in 1937, one by Fisher and the other by Kolmogoroff, Petrovsky and Piscounov. Their work concerned the advance of an advantageous gene but translates fairly straightforwardly to epidemic models. They used a diffusion approximation rather than a contact distribution, which yields a characteristic velocity of $\beta\sigma\sqrt{2}$; here β is the rate at which individuals make contacts, and σ the standard deviation of the contact distribution. For the exact model the characteristic velocity is rather higher, varying between about $1.5\beta\sigma$ and $1.85\beta\sigma$ for contact distributions with mainly local concentration; but for more widely spread distributions, the characteristic velocity may be infinite, so that the epidemic spreads at arbitrarily increasing speed (Mollison, 1972, 1977; the exact condition for finite velocity is that the contact distribution should have exponentially bounded tails). In cases where the velocity is finite, the behaviour of the corresponding linear stochastic model is unrealistically well-behaved (see Mollison, 1977, esp. pp. 323–324).

For the stochastic simple epidemic model itself, the velocity can be shown to be infinite only if the contact distribution has infinite standard deviation. Simulations confirm that the manner of advance is less regular than for the linear model; indeed, for intermediate contact distributions (with finite standard deviation but with tails not exponentially bounded), the epidemic appears to advance in a mixture of steady progress and 'great leaps forward' (Mollison, 1972). Where the linear model (and the deterministic simple epidemic) have finite velocity, however, the stochastic simple epidemic advances in a relatively steady manner, at a rather lower velocity than the linear process. The difference in velocity appears to be greatest when an individual's potential contacts are concentrated on a small number of neighbours, the ratio being over 3 to 1 in the extreme case where an infective can only contact a single individual to either side.

In two dimensions, for the linear stochastic model and its associated deterministic models, the velocity in each direction can be found simply from the one-dimensional analysis, and thus varies between about $1.5\beta\sigma'$ and $1.85\beta\sigma'$ for contact distributions with exponential tails, where σ' denotes the standard deviation of the contact distribution in the direction considered (that is, of the projection of the contact distribution in that direction).

A number of results have been obtained for simple stochastic epidemic models, particularly percolation models, showing that the infected area expands with a characteristic shape and velocity; if, as in lattice models, the contact distribution is direction dependent, the velocity will not be exactly the same in each direction (Richardson, 1973; Mollison, 1978; Schürger, 1980). Actual velocities have only been estimated from simulations. As in one dimension, they appear to be significantly lower than for linear or deterministic models. For instance, for nearest neighbour contact distributions, simulations suggest that the velocity is $0.83\beta\sigma'$ on a square lattice and $0.89\beta\sigma'$ on a hexagonal lattice; on an irregular lattice the velocity is found to be a little higher (P. J. Green, in discussion of Mollison, 1977, pp.317–318). [Incidentally, for nearest neighbour models with just one individual at each site, the velocity is proportional to the *crinkliness* of the boundary of the infected area (Mollison, 1974; see also Downham and Green, 1977).] As to contact distributions without exponentially bounded tails, the conditions for the simple epidemic in two dimensions to have finite velocity are unknown.

The work discussed so far concerns continuous-time models, in which an infective makes contacts at rate β from the moment at which it becomes infected. What little is known of simple epidemics with different time structure, as for instance with a fixed generation gap between the infection times of an infective and its victims (i.e. a discrete-time model), suggests that similar results will hold as regards velocities and the conditions to ensure a finite velocity. However, velocities will no longer be simply proportional to the infectiousness of individuals, as measured by β or some similar parameter; the velocity is likely to rise more slowly than proportionately, the exact relation depending on the contact distribution.

For epidemics with removal [Model (2) without recolonisation, i.e. $r = 0$], the velocity of the linear and deterministic models is approximately $\sqrt{(1 - \alpha/\beta)}$ times the velocity of the model without removal (D. G. Kendall, in discussion of Bartlett, 1957, pp. 64–67; Atkinson and Reuter, 1976). For the nonlinear stochastic model, however, unpublished simulations by one of the authors suggest that the reduction in velocity is rather greater. Some of these simulations, incidentally, show a pattern in which the front breaks down into a number of 'arcs of infection' (as conjectured by D. G. Kendall, in discussion of Bartlett, 1957, pp. 64–67), with no infectives on the stretches in between. However, this seems to occur principally in simulations where the epidemic is dying out.

D. SPATIAL MODELS: ENDEMICITY

In discussing thresholds in Section II,B, we restricted attention mainly to the initial spread of a disease in the case where removed individuals are not replaced. If the infection is to become *endemic*, it is of course essential that new susceptibles should be introduced.

One of the simplest spatial models exhibiting endemic behaviour is the 'contact process' introduced by Harris (1974) (there are two surveys by Griffeath, 1979, 1981; see also Durrett and Griffeath, 1982). This process may be regarded as a simplified version of Model (2) in which infectives, instead of being removed and leaving vacant sites, simply recover and become susceptible again. We thus have the following:

	Change	Change rate	
Infection	$XY \rightarrow YY$	$\beta'/4$	
Recovery	$Y \rightarrow X$	α'	(3)

[Note that this is nearly the same as is obtained by setting $r = \infty$ in Model (2).] For this process the parameter $\lambda = \beta'/4\alpha'$ has a threshold value λ_0, which (for a two-dimensional model) is known to lie between $\frac{1}{3}$ and 1 [Holley and Liggett, 1978; Harris, 1974; the lower bound here can be improved marginally, to 0.359 (Griffeath, 1975, p. 191)]. Above this threshold value, the process may tend to a stochastic equilibrium in which both infectives and susceptibles are present.

An apparently rather similar model, but exhibiting very different behaviour, is that introduced by Williams and Bjerknes (1972) for two competing cell populations. In this model 'susceptibles' can replace neighbouring infectives, so that the process is symmetrical between the two types:

$$
\begin{array}{lcc}
 & \text{Change} & \text{Change rate} \\
\text{Infection} & XY \rightarrow YY & \beta'/4 \\
\text{'Recovery'} & Y \rightarrow X & \alpha'
\end{array}
\tag{4}
$$

Even though this model includes the introduction of new susceptibles, it appears to have only trivial equilibria. If $\beta < \alpha$ the infection is certain to become extinct (Kelly, 1977b) (we are assuming that the initial set of infectives is finite). If $\beta > \alpha$ the infection may survive forever, but in that case the infected area expands as an approximate disk of linearly growing radius (i.e. at fixed velocity), so that all sites eventually become infected (Bramson and Griffeath, 1980, 1981).

Few theoretical results are available for even the simplest models for endemic disease, such as our Model (2). One technique which is worth mentioning is that of 'balance equations,' in which we consider the density of each type of individual and of each type of pair of neighbours: for instance, let $\pi(Y)$ denote the proportion of infected sites, and $\pi(XY)$ the density of neighbouring XY pairs. In endemic equilibrium, if such is possible, the creation and removal of infected cases must be in balance: thus, taking into account the change rates of Model (2), we have that

$$
\alpha'\pi(Y) = (\beta'/4)\pi(XY)
\tag{5}
$$

Such equations, together with the fact that all such proportions must lie between 0 and 1, can be used to find bounds on the parameter values for which endemic equilibrium is possible [note that $\pi(XY) = $ density $= 2 \times$ (proportion of XY pairs), so that $0 \leq \pi(XY) \leq 2$]. For instance, we can show that $\lambda_0 > \frac{1}{3}$ for Model (2) (Kuulasmaa, 1983; this approach was applied to Harris's contact process by Clifford and Sudbury, 1979).

In the next section we report the results of some simulations. One final technique which is worth mentioning derives from physics, and lies in a sense intermediate between theory and simulations. In this approach a specific model, usually a power law, is derived heuristically, and parameter values are then estimated from simulations. This yields surprisingly precise values for parameters such as λ_0 for various percolation type processes (Grassberger, 1983). While this approach is not strictly rigorous, it must at least be regarded as producing very interesting conjectures.

III. Simulations of a Spatial Model for Endemic Fox Rabies

A. METHODOLOGY

Simulations of the endemic models introduced previously [Models (1) and (2) of Section II,A] have been performed on a finite rectangular area (typically of 60 × 60 sites). To avoid edge effects, we assume that the pattern repeats outside the rectangle considered. (In precise mathematical terminology, we identify opposite pairs of edges of the rectangle, so that our area is topologically a torus.)

It is convenient to look on the process of infection from the susceptible's point of view. At any moment, each susceptible is independently subject to an infection at rate $\beta/4$ times the number of neighbouring infectives. In this way unsuccessful infections are omitted, and hence a considerable amount of computing time is saved. The filling of vacant sites by reproduction of neighbouring susceptibles works in a similar way. In Model (1), incubating sites are liable to becoming infected, with change rate σ, and infectives to becoming vacant at rate α; in Model (2) we only have infective sites, which are liable to become vacant at rate α'.

Since, given the present state of the process, the types of the sites change in independent Poisson processes, the time to the next change in the process has exponential distribution with mean 1/(sum of the change rates of the sites). Furthermore, the probability that the next change occurs at a given site is the ratio of the change rate for that site to the total change rate, independently of the waiting time. Hence we can first decide what is the next change and then, if we are interested in it, find out the time of this change. In practice, since the number of changes will be large in any period of interest, we usually get very accurate timing by taking the time between successive changes to equal the mean value, 1/(total change rate).

The simulation algorithm used is the following:

1. Give the necessary initial values. The main arrays needed are TYPE and RATE, where TYPE(I,J) indicates the current type of site (I,J), and RATE(I,J) indicates its change rate (ITR). Also, a variable TOTALRATE for the total change rate is needed. We store the time in variable TIME.

2. Let TOTALRATE = $\Sigma_{I,J}$ RATE(I,J).

3. Choose the site, (I,J) say, where the next change occurs; the probability of choosing this particular site is RATE(I,J)/TOTALRATE.

4. Replace TYPE(I,J) by its new value and update RATE for (I,J) and its neighbours.

5. Increase TIME, for exact timing by a random value from the exponential distribution of mean 1/TOTALRATE, or for approximate timing, simply by 1/TOTALRATE.

6. Output as required: for instance, proportions of different types of sites, or a plot of the state of the process to printer, VDU or film.

7. To continue the simulation, go to step 2; otherwise

8. The simulation is concluded.

B. SIMULATION RESULTS

Simulations of both models were carried out for a wide range of parameter values. These are presented here with an assumed timescale such that the generation gap of the disease matches rabies data, as were the non-spatial models of Chapter 9. Thus for Model (1) we take $\sigma = 13$, $\alpha = 73$ (year^{-1}); while for Model (2) we take $\alpha' = 11$. We shall plot the infectivity in terms of $\mu = \beta/\alpha$ [for Model (1), $= \beta'/\alpha'$ for Model (2)], since this ratio to a good approximation determines the basic reproductive rate of the infection, $C \approx \mu/(1 + \mu/4)$ (the approximation involved here is that we neglect the possibility of infecting two or more susceptibles in succession on the same neighbouring site).

Both models show broadly similar patterns. If the infection is started from an initial focus, it spreads at first with a fairly regular front, behind which occurs a 'silent' phase (compare Macdonald, 1980, Fig. 3.5, showing the advance of rabies in France). This regularity disappears in the subsequent endemic phase, and one can no longer observe any direction for the infection, except very locally.

The simulations indicate that there is a unique endemic equilibrium for certain parameter values. Figure 2 shows the estimated proportions of susceptibles and infected cases in this equilibrium. [Note that for Model (1) the proportion of incubating cases in equilibrium is always $\frac{73}{13} \approx 5.6$ times the proportion of infective cases.] The size of the simulation area has no observed effect on the mean proportions, but it does affect their fluctuation (see below).

Except possibly for very low values of r, there is a clear critical value C_0 of the basic reproductive rate, such that for $C < C_0$ extinction is certain. For larger values of r, the critical value C_0 is close to its theoretical lower bound of $\frac{4}{3}$ (see Section II,D); for values of r appropriate to fox rabies ($r < 1$), C_0 is considerably higher.

When r is large, and C near C_0, the proportion of empty sites is negligible. This supports the conjecture that for such values the process can be approximated by Harris's contact process. In particular, we would then have that $\inf_r C_0(r)$ is the same as the critical C_0 of Harris's process, for which the best known lower bound is $4 \times 0.359 = 1.44$.

Figures 3 and 4 show states of the two models in apparent equilibrium, in each case for two different choices of parameters. These patterns are again reminis-

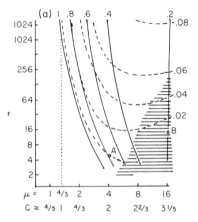

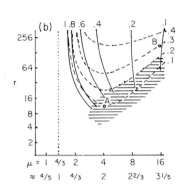

Fig. 2. Estimated proportions of susceptibles (——) and infected cases (– – –) in endemic equillibrium, for Models (1) and (2). In the shaded regions fluctuations of the proportions are significant on a 60 × 60 lattice. (a) Model (1), with $\alpha = 73$, $\sigma = 13$. The horizontal scale is given in terms both of $\mu = \beta/\alpha$ and of the (approximate) basic reproductive rate $C \approx \mu/(1 + \mu/4)$. Simulations with the parameter values marked A and B are shown in Figs 3 and 4. (b) Model (2), with $\alpha' = 11$. Similarly, with $\mu = \beta'/\alpha'$.

cent of those observed in real endemic conditions (compare for instance, Macdonald, 1980, Figs 3.5a and 5.18).

The relative proportions, in equilibrium, of each type of site deserve further comment; we shall denote them here simply by (e.g.) X rather than $\pi(X)$. The basic balance equations for equilibrium are then, for Model (1),

$$\beta XY q_{XY} = \sigma I = \alpha Y = rEX q_{EX} \qquad (6)$$

and for Model (2),

$$\beta' XY q_{XY} = \alpha' Y = rEX q_{EX} \qquad (7)$$

Here q_{XY} denotes the density of neighbouring XY pairs relative to the expected value assuming homogeneous mixing ($= 4XY$), and similarly for q_{EX}; setting the q's both $= 1$ we thus recover the balance equations for the non-spatial models of Chapter 9. The level of prevalence, $(I + Y)/X$, is then not $Er\tau$ as found for the non-spatial model, but q_{EX} times as much. Typically, we find a lower level of prevalence; for example, for the parameter values of Fig. 3a, $q_{EX} \approx 0.4$, and the level of prevalence averages 3%, compared with an expected value from the non-spatial analysis of nearly 8%.

From Eq. (6) we can also deduce that $X = 1/(\mu q_{XY})$. The tendency of Xs and Ys to avoid each other appears even more marked than that of Xs and Es. Again in Fig. 3a, we find that $q_{XY} \approx 0.3$, so that the proportion of susceptibles is approximately 80%, rather than 25% as expected assuming homogeneous mixing. The low values of q_{XY} can be attributed to a combination of factors. A new infective is likely to begin with fewer than average susceptible neighbours (for a start, the site which infected it is unlikely to be susceptible again yet); and if it infects one it is similarily unlikely to get a replacement, so that an individual who has been infectious for some time is even less likely to have susceptible neighbours (this latter factor has already been referred to in explaining why $C < \mu$). It is easy to guess from this that $q_{XY} \lesssim \frac{3}{4}C/\mu$, and hence $X \gtrsim \frac{4}{3}C^{-1}$, $= 67\%$ in the present case.

When the parameters approach the shaded regions of Fig. 2, the proportions begin to fluctuate until finally extinction occurs. If r is decreased the infection eventually becomes extinct, while if C is increased the population becomes extinct. However, in this parameter region the proportion of infectives is small, and the few that there are tend to group together. Thus, the fluctuations, and perhaps the ensuing extinction, may be due only to the finite size of the simulation area. Interestingly, the more realistic model [Model (1)] appears stable down to lower values of r.

C. DISCUSSION OF SIMULATIONS

The models we have simulated were chosen to include only the most basic features essential for a study of spatial patterns of an endemic disease of territorial animals. We have omitted many features, and made considerable approximations in the features we have included. Hence, before we interpret the results of our simulations, we must discuss some of the shortcomings of our models.

We have apparently neglected natural mortality. However, this is largely taken into account if we assume that most vacancies occurring through natural mortality are soon filled by the offspring of nearby sites, thus keeping the population at the carrying capacity, at least in rabies free areas.

We have only been able to simulate with values of r down to about 2 year^{-1}, even for Model (1). As mentioned in the previous section, we find that the level of prevalence fluctuates for small values of r, but we conjecture that this may only be due to the finite size of the simulation area and the consequent small total population of infectives in these cases; to investigate the stability of the equilibrium for smaller values of r would require simulations on a considerably larger lattice. On the face of it, this is a considerable shortcoming of our present simulations, since values of r appropriate to foxes are about 0.5 year^{-1}. However, against this we must note that our present assumption that territories can only be recolonised by their immediate neighbours 'disenfranchises' a large proportion of susceptibles, whose offspring might in reality be prepared to travel considerable distances in search of empty sites. Even at low population densities, the susceptibles tend to group together, and thus in our model the offspring of the individuals at the edges of such a group really represent the offspring of the entire group. Thus the lower values of r in our simulations ($r = 2$–5, say) may in fact

(a)

Fig. 3. (a) Typical state of Model (1), in apparent equilibrium, for parameter values $r = 4.4$, $C = 2$ (marked A in Fig. 2a). Symbols: susceptible (•), incubating (○), infectious (●), vacant ( ). (b) The same, but with $r = 14.6$, $C = 3.2$ (B in Fig. 2a).

reasonably represent fox population regrowth. However, this aspect of model-ling clearly requires further consideration, particularly in respect of how far foxes travel to find new territories and how efficient they are at identifying vacant territories.

We have generally only allowed for one individual at each site, whereas fox territories in reality are occupied by family groups. Some simulations were also done of a model with two individuals per site, and for a relatively high internal contact rate the results were qualitatively similar to those for the basic model. This suggests that our model will approximately apply to sites occupied by family groups; though in interpreting results, we must allow for likely dif-ferences: for instance, the generation gap for family to family infections may be a

(b)

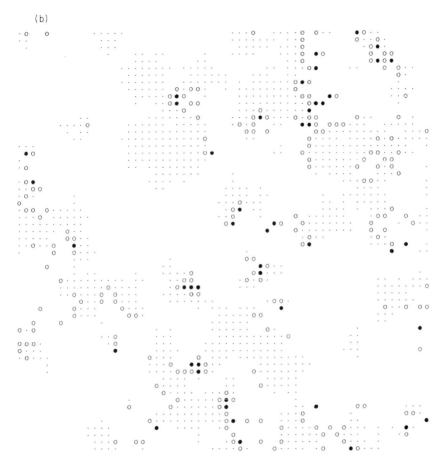

Fig. 3.   (*Continued.*)

compound of several individual generation gaps, and will therefore have a somewhat higher mean (see Chapter 8, this volume). In favour of our basic model, we
may note that its assumption that the directions of contacts made from a site are
independent is rather more reasonable if these represent the contacts made by a
family rather than by a single individual.

We have not allowed for heterogeneity between individuals, and in particular
for the difference between settled and itinerant foxes. In so far as the latter are
important, we clearly need to consider contact distributions allowing longer
range contacts. It would in any case be interesting to examine how threshold
levels (C_0) and endemic patterns depend on the contact distribution. For a start,
we might guess that the scale of endemic patterns, and the velocities with which
they spread, will be roughly proportional to the standard deviation of the contact
distribution.

(a)

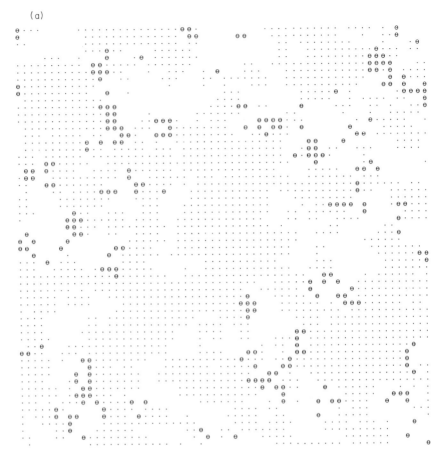

Fig. 4. (a) Typical state of Model (2), in apparent equilibrium, for parameter values $r = 11$, $C = 2$ (marked A in Fig. 2b). (b) The same, but with $r = 176$, $C = 3.2$ (B in Fig. 2b). Symbols: susceptible (•), infectious (⊖), vacant ( ).

Even allowing for all these defects, and other neglected factors such as seasonal variation, we can draw some general conclusions from these simulations. They show how an epidemic which begins by advancing in a regular manner with a fairly well defined velocity can break up into an endemic pattern of quite large wandering 'patches of infection', without any need to invoke geographic or social heterogeneity; that is, we can have heterogeneous behaviour in a homogeneous environment.

The proportions of the various types of individual in endemic equilibrium differ significantly from those expected from non-spatial models; in particular the proportion of vacant sites is much smaller.

The most interesting question raised is whether oscillations in the level of

(b)

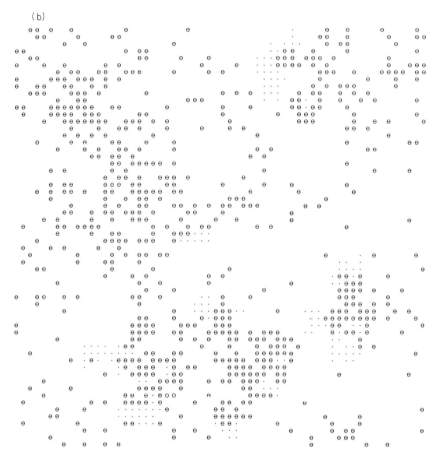

Fig. 4. (*Continued.*)

prevalence can be genuinely cyclical as in the non-spatial case (see Chapters 6 and 9, this volume), or are merely the consequence of considering a large scale random pattern over too small an area; some support for the latter view comes from Macdonald's observation that fluctuations appear more marked in data from small countries (Macdonald, 1980, Table 3.1).

IV. Discussion

The formidable task of developing models for endemic disease may be compared to building a house in a hurry. Practical workers insist on building a complete house, and are not too worried that it may need replacing later. Theoreticians insist on building reliable foundations, and are not too worried if the house is never finished. Both points of view of course have their merits, and ideally we need to combine these.

This chapter lies towards the theoretical end of the spectrum, though it has been framed where possible in terms of parameters with straightforward ecological interpretations, such as the basic reproductive rate and contact distribution. If we are to use complex models to explain rather than just imitate reality, we need to understand which assumptions are crucial for particular results: we need to be able to take a model apart and see what makes it tick. If this chapter assists such understanding, it will have served its purpose as part of the foundations.

References

Atkinson, C., and Reuter, G. E. H. (1976). Deterministic epidemic waves. *Math. Proc. Cambridge Philos. Soc.* **80,** 315–330.

Ball, F. (1983). The threshold behaviour of epidemic models. *J. Appl. Prob.* **20,** 227–241.

Bartlett, M. S. (1957). Measles periodicity and community size (with discussion). *J. R. Statist. Soc. Ser. A* **120,** 48–70.

Bartlett, M. S. (1960). "Stochastic Population Models in Ecology and Epidemiology." Methuen, London.

Bramson, M., and Griffeath, D. (1980). On the Williams-Bjerknes tumour growth model. II. *Math. Proc. Cambridge Philos. Soc.* **88,** 339–357.

Bramson, M., and Griffeath, D. (1981). On the Williams-Bjerknes tumour growth model. I. *Ann. Prob.* **9,** 173–185.

Broadbent, S. R., and Hammersley, J. M. (1957). Percolation processes. I. Crystals and mazes. *Proc. Cambridge Philos. Soc.* **53,** 629–641.

Clifford, P., and Sudbury, A. W. (1979). On the use of bounds in the statistical analysis of spatial processes. *Biometrika* **66,** 495–503.

Downham, D. Y., and Green, D. H. (1976). Inference for a two-dimensional stochastic growth model. *Biometrika* **63,** 551–554.

Durrett, R., and Griffeath, D. (1982). Contact processes in several dimensions. *Z. Wahrscheinlichkeitsth. verw. Gebiete* **59,** 535–552.

Fisher, R. A. (1937). The wave of advance of advantageous genes. *Ann. Eugen.* **7,** 355–369.

Grassberger, P. (1983). Of the critical behaviour of the general epidemic process and dynamical percolation. *Math. Biosci.* **63,** 157–172.

Griffeath, D. (1975). Ergodic theorems for graph interactions. *Adv. Appl. Prob.* **7,** 179–194.

Griffeath, D. (1979). Additive and cancellative interacting particle systems. *In* "Lecture Notes in Mathematics" Vol. 724. Springer-Verlag, Berlin and New York.

Griffeath, D. (1981). The basic contact processes. *Stochastic Processes Applics.* **11,** 151–185.

Harris, T. E. (1974). Contact interactions on a lattice. *Ann. Prob.* **2,** 969–988.

Holley, R., and Liggett, T. M. (1978). The survival of contact processes. *Ann. Prob.* **6,** 198–206.

Kelly, F. (1977). The asymptotic behaviour of an invasion process. *J. Appl. Prob.* **14,** 584–590.

Kendall, D. G. (1965). Mathematical models of the spread of infection. *In* "Mathematics and Computer Science in Biology and Medicine," pp. 213–225. M. R. C., H. M. Stationery Office, London.

Kermack, W. O., and McKendrick, A. G. (1927). Contributions to the mathematical theory of epidemics. *Proc. Roy. Soc. Ser. A* **115,** 700–721.

Kesten, H. (1980). The critical probability of bond percolation on the square lattice equals $\frac{1}{2}$. *Commun. Math. Phys.* **74**, 41–59.

Kolmogoroff, A. N., Petrovsky, I. G., and Piscounoff, N. S. (1937). Étude de l'équation de la diffusion avec croissance de la quantité de matière et son application a un problème biologique. *Bull. Univ. Etat Moscou, Ser. Int., A* **1**(6), 1–25.

Kuulasmaa, K. (1982). The spatial general epidemic and locally dependent random graphs. *J. Appl. Prob.* **19**, 745–758.

Kuulasmaa, K. (1983). Threshold and endemic behaviour of spatial contact models. Ph.D. Thesis, Heriot-Watt University, Edinburgh.

Macdonald, D. W. (1980). "Rabies and Wildlife." Oxford Univ. Press, London and New York.

McKean, H. P. (1975). Application of Brownian motion to the equation of Kolmogorov-Petrovskii-Piscounov. *Commun. Pure Appl. Math.* **28**, 323–331.

Mollison, D. (1972). The rate of spatial propagation of simple epidemics. *Proc. Sixth Berkeley Symp. Math. Stat. Prob.*, Vol. 3, pp. 579–614.

Mollison, D. (1974). Percolation processes and tumour growth. *Adv. Appl. Prob.* **6**, 233–235.

Mollison, D. (1977). Spatial contact models for ecological and epidemic spread (with discussion). *J. R. Statist. Soc. Ser. B* **39**, 283–326.

Mollison, D. (1978). Markovian contact processes. *Adv. Appl. Prob.* **10**, 85–108.

Mollison, D. (1981). The importance of demographic stochasticity in population dynamics. *In* "The Mathematical Theory of the Dynamics of Biological Populations II" (R. W. Hiorns and D. L. Cooke, eds.) pp. 99–107. Academic Press, London.

Richardson, D. (1973). Random growth in a tessellation. *Proc. Cambridge Philos. Soc.* **74**, 515–528.

Schürger, K. (1980). On the asymptotic geometrical behaviour of percolation processes. *J. Appl. Prob.* **17**, 385–402.

Smythe, R. T., and Wierman, J. C. (1978). First-passage percolation on the square lattice. *In* "Lecture Notes in Mathematics" Vol. 671. Springer-Verlag, Berlin and New York.

Whittle, P. (1955). The outcome of a stochastic epidemic—a note on Bailey's paper. *Biometrika* **42**, 116–122.

Williams, T., and Bjerknes, R. (1972). Stochastic model for abnormal clone spread through epithelial basal layer. *Nature* **236**, 19–21.

A Spatial Simulation Model for Rabies Control

13

Dennis R. Voigt
Wildlife Branch,
Ontario Ministry of Natural Resources,
Maple, Ontario, Canada

R. R. Tinline
Department of Geography,
Queen's University,
Kingston, Ontario, Canada

L. H. Broekhoven
Department of Mathematics and Statistics,
Queen's University,
Kingston, Ontario, Canada

I. Introduction

The success and strategy of rabies control in the future will depend on a host of interacting factors. Previous chapters have clearly demonstrated that many vari-

POPULATION DYNAMICS OF RABIES IN WILDLIFE

ables influence rabies epizootiology in a complex fashion. The purpose of this chapter is to describe a spatial simulation model of a fox population with rabies, in an attempt to incorporate many of the variables identified earlier. We describe our model components and operation in detail to illustrate the requirements and assumptions of such models based on current knowledge of fox-rabies epizootiology.

We simulated the spatial and social behaviour of Red Foxes (*Vulpes vulpes*) in southern Ontario, Canada, where wildlife rabies has been enzootic for over 20 years. The key role of the fox in the epizootiology of rabies in Ontario was reviewed by Macdonald and Voigt (see Chapter 4, this volume). The annual cost of rabies in Ontario is estimated at $20 million. A control program directed at the fox could contribute greatly to reducing the human health hazard (2000 people treated after rabies exposure in 1982), the domestic animal loss (400 head in 1981) and the annual loss of foxes.

Ontario has opted for an oral vaccine control strategy based on delivery of a bait to wildlife vectors (Johnston and Voigt, 1982; see also Steck *et al.*, 1982a,b), principally Red Foxes and Striped Skunks (*Mephitis mephitis*). Alternatives to that strategy were either to ignore rabies in wildlife and concentrate on the vaccination of pets and livestock or to kill foxes and skunks by trapping, hunting, and gassing dens. Both alternatives were estimated to be more expensive, less effective, and temporary in nature compared to mass immunization and vaccinating pets does not control wildlife epizootics. Fox control has not been proven to be successful in eradicating rabies in Red Foxes where it has become enzootic (Parks, 1968; Muller, 1971; Wandeler *et al.*, 1974; Bogel *et al.*, 1974, 1976, 1981). Field trials with baits containing the biomarker tetracycline indicated that over 70% of the fox population in an area of 500 km² ingested at least one bait (Johnston and Voigt, 1982). Thus, free-ranging foxes could be immunized if an effective vaccine was available.

Our simulation studies were designed to model fox-rabies epizootiology in order to assess control strategies and evaluate tactics of oral vaccination. Considerable development of vaccine delivery was still required, and, thus, field data from vaccine control attempts in Ontario were nonexistent. Our model was based on the social organization and spatial behaviour of foxes in Ontario, but it incorporated parameters that we identified as being universally important. The student who understands fox social and spatial behaviour in Germany, England or the United States, for example, should be able to assess and modify our subroutines to more closely simulate conditions in their areas. Since we did not simulate details of fox behaviour as much as the *effects* of that behaviour on fox-to-fox contact and fox location, such modifications should be minimal. For example, Ball (Chapter 8, this volume) demonstrated the effect of increasing the size of the fox group (as in a fox family) on the rate of spread of rabies. Our model had provision for a variable group size to allow for that effect. However, fox group composition could cause different inter- and intra-family spacing and, thus, contact rules. In such cases, parameters and algorithms may require adjustment.

The version of the model described here was experimental in nature, and the purpose of this chapter is to illustrate model features, operation and behaviour rather than determine management options and test biological hypotheses. From the outset, however, our rabies model was designed to investigate five related problems important in all fox rabies areas. In the future, we will attempt to further research these problems.

The first major problem was that the vaccine was still under development, and the field immunization rate required for the control of rabies was unknown. It was unlikely that all foxes that ate a bait containing the vaccine would be immunized. An acceptance rate of 70% and vaccine conversion rate of 70% would result in an immunity rate of only 49%. Thus, the immunity rate of foxes would be less than the acceptance rate unless repeated applications of vaccine were made or many foxes were previously immunized. Large-scale serological surveys demonstrated that rabies antibody was present in less than 3% of the free-ranging foxes in Ontario (D. R. Voigt, unpublished data). We undertook to simulate the density and behaviour of Ontario foxes to assess the minimum immunity rate which would affect rabies spread.

A second problem was to determine if all areas with rabies in foxes required similar immunity rates in foxes to prevent epizootics. Portions of Ontario had different carrying capacities for foxes (Voigt and Tinline, 1982), and rabies persisted at fox densities (Voigt et al., 1983) that were lower than densities of foxes in Europe where rabies disappeared. Although the density of confirmed rabies cases in Ontario was lower than in Europe, rabies epizootics have persisted throughout southern Ontario in distinct spatial and temporal clusters since the late 1950s (Johnston and Beauregard, 1969; Voigt and Tinline, 1982). During that time, Ontario reported 90% of the rabies in Canada (Tabel et al., 1974; Tinline, 1981). The threshold theory of epidemics described earlier (see Chapters 6 and 9, this volume) explained how densities of foxes at critical levels caused regular epizootics, but not the contribution of other important variables (but see Chapters 7, 8, 9, 11, and 12, this volume). We attempted to simulate the effect of control programs in both those areas undergoing an epizootic and those areas ahead of a rabies front (Tinline and Pond, 1976).

A third problem involved the economics of large-scale vaccination. At a vaccine cost of $1 per dose, it would require $40,000 per 1000 km²; treatment of Ontario's entire rabies enzootic area would cost $3.7 million. The spatial and temporal segregation of rabies epizootics suggested that control programs might be restricted to specific areas in some years, but we did not know whether any areas would require annual treatment. A model was required that could test selective tactics to reduce the expense of a control program.

The fourth problem concerned the interaction of mortality factors affecting fox populations. Voigt and Tinline (1982) demonstrated that an increased harvest of foxes during escalating fur prices, altered the timing and severity of rabies outbreaks. While trapping and other kill tactics might not eliminate rabies, we considered that they could be either complementary to a control program of vaccination (Bacon and Macdonald, 1980, Chapter 7, this volume) or that they might induce further movements (local and ingress) and therefore increase contact among foxes.

The final question was perhaps the most important. If rabies was controlled in enzootic areas where it was a significant fox mortality factor, other mortality factors would eventually limit foxes but would densities, reproduction, movements and social behaviour change and thus cause a renewed problem? Since protection by the vaccine may be short-lived (1–2 years) and since there was a high turnover in fox populations (75% of the population was less than 1-year-old, as also reported by Lloyd *et al.*, 1976, in parts of Europe), we wished to assess the possibility of a major rabies epizootic several years after vaccination. The possibility of epizootics of measles infections, delayed for several years after vaccination in humans, was described by Bartlett (1973) under a system of partial vaccination and that possibility could also exist for rabies.

These questions suggested that in the absence of good information, large field control programs could be an economic or ecological risk. Because of that, our simulation model of a fox population with rabies was designed as an additional tool (Tinline *et al.*, 1982) to evaluate the strategies and tactics of vaccine control and its impact on rabies and fox populations. The model was also designed to identify specific problems that could be tested in smaller field trials.

The design requirements for similar models were discussed in previous chapters. We believe realistic spatial simulation models should include the following:

1. Spatial components to assess accurately the effects of (a) the movement behaviour of the vectors, (b) the social behaviour of the vectors, (c) variation in vector densities, (d) physical factors that influence movements and animal densities, (e) other factors unique to an area.

2. Output statistics that match the biological information from the field.

3. Output statistics that permit sensitivity testing of the model's parameters.

4. Relationships structured to allow assessment of research questions and behaviour of foxes, which cause output variance.

5. Flexibility in specifying relationships and components to eliminate the need for modelling individual fox behaviour where sensitivity testing has shown that mean values would be acceptable.

Long-range targets of such models include reduced running costs and complexity and increased usefulness as a management tool. A summary of the process of developing and using the model is shown in Fig. 1.

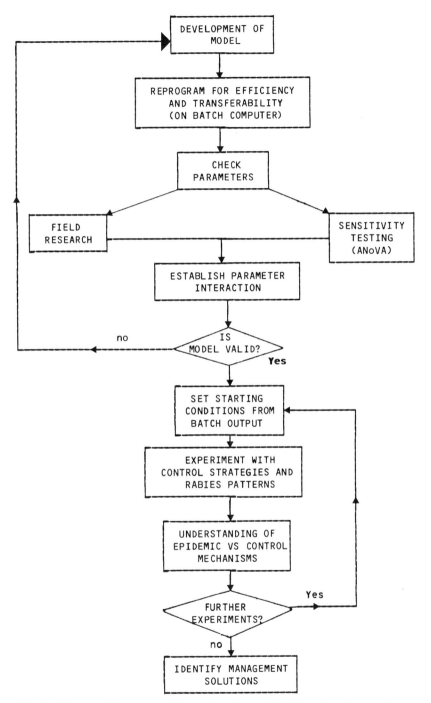

Fig. 1. Diagram of the process of developing and using the Ontario fox rabies model.

II. Model Components

The simulation model was written in FORTRAN and consisted of a series of subroutines, which were linked to describe the activities of foxes important in relation to rabies (Fig. 2). Since fox behaviour changes seasonally, a different series of subroutines were called each season. The four seasons used were winter (January–March), spring (April–June), summer (July–September), and fall (October–December). Those seasons conveniently divided a year into periods equivalent to major events of a fox's year: breeding, denning, pup rearing, and dispersal. We assumed those four seasons effectively summarized a more detailed monthly description. Seasons occurred sequentially and were repeated a specified number of years.

The study area of the model was a grid of rectangular cells with each cell representing a potential fox family range. A family was a group of foxes generally comprising one adult male, one adult female, and their offspring, of either sex. Each cell was described by a variable for identifying its desirability for fox residency. A fixed value lying between 0 and 1 represented the probability that a fox would reside in that cell. The more desirable the cell, the higher the probability of residency by a fox. Study area heterogeneity including habitat suitability, interspecific competitors, and urban areas could be mimicked using the desirability variable since values could be assigned either randomly or in a specified manner. The size of the study area was also varied by specifying the number of rows and columns of cells. In the simulations described here, the study area was 10 cells × 10 cells. Since cells (home ranges) were 10 km², the study area was 1000 km².

There were 20 population variables that described foxes. Foxes were classified as male or female and adult or juvenile. For each of those four groups there were five disease states. Those were as follows:

State 1. Disease free but susceptible.
State 2. Rabid and infective.
State 3. Rabid incubating (late, non-infective incubation).
State 4. Rabid incubating (early, non-infective incubation).
State 5. Disease free and immunized; not rabies susceptible.

There were five groups of subroutines. *Demographic subroutines* dealt with reproduction and non-rabies mortality. *Spatial subroutines* moved foxes either to nearby cells or to any cell in the study area through the mechanism of dispersal. Spatial subroutines did not simulate movements within a cell. *Disease subroutines* determined the incubation of infected foxes but, more importantly, determined the contact between foxes. That contact was important to us only if a rabid fox was present. Thus, the day-to-day activities and contact between healthy foxes within a cell were not simulated. The rules for contact varied

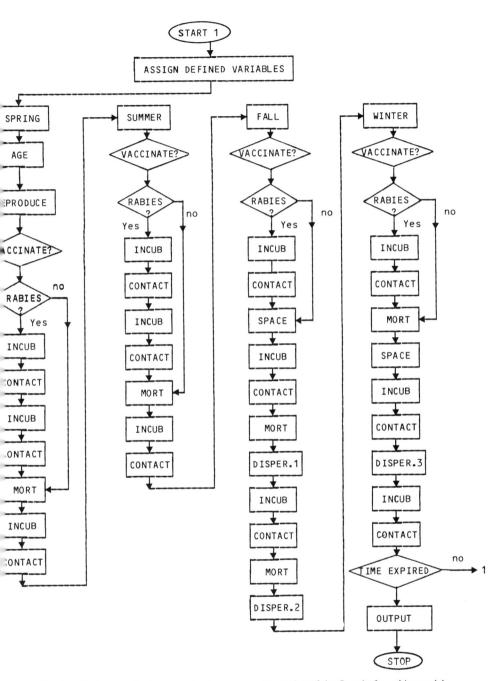

Fig. 2. A diagram of subroutines to show seasonal operation of the Ontario fox rabies model.

seasonally and, as other authors have clearly shown, are extremely important (Macdonald and Bacon, 1982; see Chapter 7, this volume). The *output subroutine* dealt with the content and format of output. A series of *bookkeeping subroutines* were necessary to deal with random number generation, aging animals, parameter value specification, and similar tasks.

In the version described here, representative values for population and disease parameters were used as shown in Table I. They are referred to as P1, P2, . . . , P34 throughout the text. Their values were based on data from Ontario, although in some cases, data were not available and a range of values was tested.

The subroutines were linked together (Fig. 2) to simulate seasonal fox biology and rabies epizootiology as described in MODEL OPERATION (Section III). A brief description of the major subroutines follows.

A. DEMOGRAPHIC SUBROUTINES

Subroutine REPROD controlled the reproduction of model foxes in the spring. Unless classified as barren (P5, P6), each female produced a litter from a specified normal distribution (MU1, MU2), and juveniles were added to her range. Reproduction rates were based on data from Ontario.

MORT controlled all non-rabies mortality. The mortality proportions varied seasonally by sex and age (MORT 1, . . . ,16). Each fox was exposed to the appropriate mortality and withdrawn from the population if killed. Mortality were based on data from Ontario.

A control method was applied to the mortality figures in order to keep the populations of foxes reasonably stable in the absence of rabies. If the population was higher than expected, the mortalities were adjusted upwards and vice versa for lower than expected populations.

The first step in the adjustment was to multiply each of the mortality proportions by the same factor. The factor was determined by equating the expected number of deaths to the expected number of births and solving the resulting equations. That was done because reproduction values were good estimates and it was believed that the mortalities were in the correct seasonal ratios, but their total values were dependent on total population size which was unknown. The procedure to modify the mortalities supplied to the model was done at the beginning of the model operation.

The mortalities were also adjusted yearly since, if they were not, the process would be a random walk. In a random walk the population would vary from its original value with ever increasing variance. Both unreasonably high populations and zero populations would become increasingly likely as time passed. Since that was unrealistic, some control process was required. Our model used a simple process based on mortality. The procedure was to first convert mortalities, which were probabilities, to logits by the equation

TABLE I

Values for Parameters Varied in the Ontario Fox Rabies Model

Parameter	Value	Description
P(1)	0.15(1) = 0.15	Probability juvenile infecting neighbour juvenile summer (weighing = 1)
P(2)	0.15(1) = 0.15	Probability adults infecting neighbour adults all seasons (weighing = 1)
P(3)	0.15(2) = 0.3	Probability of foxes infecting other cell members (except spring) (weighing = 2)
P(4)	0.15(1.5) = 0.225	Probability of males infecting neighbour females winter (weighing = 1.5)
P(5)	0.15	Probability juvenile female barren
P(6)	0.05	Probability adult female barren
P(7)	0.5	Probability offspring male
P(8)	0.6	Constant in formula for probability of contact in time T
P(9)	0.75	Probability of getting rabies given contact
P(10)	0.8	Probability of directed dispersal (DI) by female
P(11)	0.8	Probability of directed dispersal (DI) by male
P(12)	1.0	Probability of drift dispersal (DR)
P(13)	0.8	Probability of female dispersing
P(14)	1.0	Proportion of ingressing foxes (of egressing foxes)
P(15)	7.1	Mean distance female foxes disperse (km)
P(16)	26.6	Mean distance male foxes disperse (km)
P(17)	0.85	Probability ingressing fox is in health state 1
P(18)	0.90	Probability ingressing fox is in health state 1 + P(17)
P(19)	0.90	Probability ingressing fox is in health state 2 + P(18)
P(20)	1.0	Probability ingressing fox is in health state 3 + P(19)
P(21)	1.0	Probability ingressing fox is in health state 4 + P(20)
P(22)	0.4	Probability ingressing fox is female
P(23)	0.4	Probability of dispersing if $K = 1$
P(24)	0.666	Probability of dispersing if $K = 2$ + P(23)
P(25)	1.0	Probability of dispersing if $K = 3$ + P(24) = 1.0
P(26)	1.0	Probability state 2 to death in INCUB
P(27)	1.0	Probability state 3 to state 2 in INCUB
P(28)	0.0	Probability state 4 to state 3 in INCUB
P(29)	0.42	Probability state 4 to state 2 in INCUB
P(30)	0.2	Mortality adjuster
P(31)	10.0	Control point for fox density (foxes per cell after reproduction)
P(32)	1.00	Parameter for directed dispersal times for females
P(33)	0.25	Parameter for directed dispersal times for males
P(34)	20.0	Parameter for drift dispersal time
V(1–8)		Number of vaccinations (1), Year (5), Season (4), Rate (0.00), LLR (1), LLC (1), URR (10), NRC (10)
ROW	10.0	Number of rows in simulation area

(*continued*)

TABLE I (*Continued*)

COL	10.0	Number of columns in simulation area
MU(1)	7.9	Mean litter size for juvenile females
MU(2)	8.2	Mean litter size for adult females
		Mortality rate proportion
		Winter
MORT(1)	0.20	Juvenile female
MORT(2)	0.14	Adult female
MORT(3)	0.20	Juvenile male
MORT(4)	0.12	Adult male
		Spring
MORT(5)	0.10	Juvenile female
MORT(6)	0.05	Adult female
MORT(7)	0.10	Juvenile male
MORT(8)	0.05	Adult male
		Summer
MORT(9)	0.14	Juvenile female
MORT(10)	0.05	Adult female
MORT(11)	0.16	Juvenile male
MORT(12)	0.05	Adult male
		Fall
MORT(13)	0.26	Juvenile female
MORT(14)	0.16	Adult female
MORT(15)	0.34	Juvenile male
MORT(16)	0.18	Adult male
ROWSIZ	3.16	Horizontal size of cell (km)
COLSIZ	3.16	Vertical size of cell (km)

$$L_i = \text{Log} \left(\frac{P_i}{1 - P_i} \right) \tag{1}$$

That was done because the L_i has a range of $-\infty$ to ∞, which was more suitable for arithmetic than P_i, which ranges from 0 to 1. The second step was to choose a control point density of foxes D_0, which was a parameter of model (P31). That control point acted as a carrying capacity density. The density at the beginning of the year was calculated (D), and the logits, corresponding to mortalities actually used, were estimated by the following equation:

$$L_{i'} = L_i + K(D - D_0) \tag{2}$$

In Equation (2), K was also a parameter of the model (P30). It affected the rate of adjustment. The mortalities to be used were given by

$$P_{i'} = \frac{e^{L_{i'}}}{1 + e^{L_{i'}}} \tag{3}$$

B. SPATIAL SUBROUTINES

SPACE moved foxes among ranges according to rules based on field observations in Ontario. Simulation of the social organization of foxes differing from that in Ontario (e.g. more groups of adult females) might require changes in the SPACE rules, although most of the variation currently recognized (Voigt and Macdonald, 1985; see Chapter 4, this volume) in fox behaviour could be mimicked. SPACE operated only in the fall and winter seasons and allowed the movement of foxes from locally high density areas to low density areas. It also allowed pairing of male and female foxes in the same cell.

DISPER caused juvenile foxes to disperse during the fall and winter. Dispersal distributed both the disease and the foxes. The rules for dispersal were based on data from Ontario. Rabid, dispersing foxes spread the disease, and healthy foxes that passed through cells with rabid animals could be infected. Dispersal occurred in three stages—twice in the fall and once in the winter. The model study area was *not* closed; foxes could enter from, or depart to, the 'outside'.

C. DISEASE SUBROUTINES

The subroutine CONTAC was used to simulate transmission of rabies. If a fox was infective, then foxes in the same cell or neighboring cells could be infected. The rules and probabilities varied depending on the season, age, and sex of the fox. Those rules and probabilities were a synthesis of the effects of fox behaviour and movements, and they are described in Section III,D.

INCUB advanced foxes through rabies incubation. When a fox was infected, it was put into state 4 and later progressed either to state 3 or 2. State 2 was the infective state reached by all rabid foxes, if not killed by other means. Shortly after reaching state 2, foxes died and were withdrawn from the population. Only foxes in state 2 were infective. Although most foxes incubated rabies for 19–20 days, the mean incubation period was longer. In the simulation described here, foxes advanced directly from state 4 to state 2 by probabilities calculated from Sikes (1962) and K. F. Lawson (unpublished data).

D. BOOKKEEPING SUBROUTINES

NEIGH was used by SPACE to determine the subscripts of neighboring cells. RAN generated random numbers.

DEAL generated a random order for the cells. To minimize possible bias, subroutines such as SPACE and CONTAC accessed DEAL for a new operating order each time those routines were called.

INIT generated various constants required by the program. For example, the number of rows and columns of the study area and cell size were variable. It was necessary to generate coordinate positions for the cells for each set of initial conditions.

CONST contained various constants and parameters required by the program, such as the probability of being infected if a contact was made. Values for mortality and reproduction rates were stored here. Some of those values were established from field observations, and others were estimated from laboratory observations. All the parameters that required sensitivity testing were stored as variables in CONST.

AGE was used each spring after REPROD and changed all juvenile foxes who were born in the previous spring into adults.

OUTPUT generated reports and statistics after each model operation.

III. Model Operation

Operation of the model occurred in three modes: RABIES-FREE, RABIES, and VACCINE. We will describe operation for a typical year, in RABIES-FREE mode, and then introduce rabies and vaccination. Three of the subroutines (SPACE, CONTAC, DISPER) summarized in Model Components (Section II) made this model different from other rabies models. They will be explained in detail in this section.

A. SPRING

The starting conditions were user determined in the INIT subroutine. Typically, cells were assigned a pair of foxes (one male, one female), according to cell suitability and a specified fox density. The density values used were similar to averages for large areas (> 500 km^2) that included areas vacant of foxes because of water, cities, unsuitable habitat, and interspecific competitors such as Coyotes (*Canis latrans*) (Voigt and Earle, 1983).

In southern Ontario, a density of 0.10 foxes per km^2 before parturition was observed over large areas. Densities were 3 to 4 times higher in local areas of several 100 km^2 (D. R. Voigt, unpublished data). Densities after parturition varied from 0.5 to 2.0 foxes per km^2 because of high reproduction. Ontario fox densities were lower than those reported for Europe (Lloyd, 1980). They were, in fact, lower than densities believed to be necessary to support rabies in Europe (Bogel *et al.*, 1974, 1976), and yet they have, in the past, supported North America's highest incidence of rabies in wildlife! Since some previous models showed that rabies in Europe would disappear at low densities with implied low contact rates (Anderson *et al.*, 1981; David *et al.*, 1982; David and Andral, 1982; Bacon and Macdonald, 1982, but see Mollison, Chapter 9, this volume), we hypothesized that the maintenance of rabies at the low Ontario densities would require either the spacing and dispersal effects (as in this model), some reintroduction mechanism for rabies or a higher contact rate.

Routine REPROD randomly selected all vixens to breed or not, according to proportions observed in Ontario. The proportions differed for yearlings (last year's juveniles) and older vixens. Vixens were also randomly selected for a litter size and sex ratio of pups based on a normal distribution derived from data from Ontario. In our model, we have not made reproductivity density dependent, although we recognized that it could be assessed as a density-dependent parameter (Englund, 1970; Macdonald, 1980). We chose instead to prevent unrealistic population explosion or extinction by relating non-rabies mortality (MORT) to density, such that when densities were high, mortalities were biased to be slightly higher. Without this provision, the high mortalities of foxes (even if 'balanced' with high reproductive rates) could result in extinction in a stochastic model by random chance alone. Therefore, mortalities varied according to density, but the relative proportions of mortality among sex and age classes by season did not vary from year to year. The year-end result was similar to varying both mortality and reproduction in a density-dependent fashion. In SPRING, all foxes were thus subjected to a chance of dying (MORT 5, 6, 7, 8) due to a non-rabies cause.

There was no provision to move foxes among cells during SPRING. The model allowed contact among foxes (CONTAC), such as within the family and between neighbours, but since that contact was only important in the model if it presented a chance for rabies transmission, we did not 'CONTAC' foxes during the RABIES-FREE mode.

B. SUMMER

During the SUMMER season, the major subroutine used in the RABIES-FREE mode was MORT. It operated as in SPRING, but according to different probabilities (MORT 9, 10, 11, 12). We did not allow intercell movement although radio-tracking studies clearly demonstrated that juvenile foxes contacted their siblings, as well as neighbours, during July, August, and September. That movement was simulated by CONTAC rules only if in RABIES mode. Our model did not allow foxes to leave their ranges permanently until FALL.

C. FALL AND WINTER

During the FALL season, operation of our model was more complex. The subroutine SPACE distributed the population of model foxes as would occur in the real world during October, November, and December. It allowed foxes to move into nearby cells according to rules established during radio-tracking studies. SPACE did not simulate long-range movement (see DISPER) or contact among foxes. However, by redistributing foxes, SPACE allowed new contacts to occur when CONTAC was operated with rabies present. Other authors (Preston, 1973; Montgomery, 1974; Grant, 1977) simulated movement behaviour using a random walk or related algorithms for individual foxes. That strategy can greatly increase the running costs of models, which may reduce their usefulness as management tools. SPACE and DISPER are alternate strategies in that they mimic only the end results of a random walk (contact probabilities) rather than the intermediate steps.

Cells (home ranges) in the study area were arranged in a random order by subroutine DEAL and examined in that order during SPACE. For each range the eight adjacent ranges were called A ranges and recorded in NEIGH. The next 16 most adjacent ranges were called N ranges. SPACE (Fig. 3) assessed the number of adults and juveniles in range C_{ij} and then attempted to move juveniles to adjacent ranges (A cells) or next to adjacent ranges (N cells). If there were no adults, it moved the juveniles until only one was left. If there were adults, it would try to move all juveniles. $A_{C_{ij}}$ ranges were searched first and then $N_{C_{ij}}$ ranges were searched. If an empty range was found, a juvenile was randomly chosen to move. That process continued until either all the scheduled juveniles were moved, or there were no more empty ranges nearby. In effect, we gave all juveniles a chance to move.

SPACE then determined if more than one adult male was in the range. If true, then A and N ranges were searched for male-free status. If such a range was found, an adult male was randomly chosen and moved to that range. SPACE next determined if males were present in ranges without females. If so, then A and N ranges were searched for females without males. If such a range was found, a lone adult male was randomly chosen and moved to that range. The process continued until all the remaining ranges were treated in similar fashion.

The subroutine MORT, which determined non-rabies mortality, was called several times during the FALL season. The problem of simulating a continuously occurring event in a discrete-time model was considered in relation to some events such as mortality. A simulation model could subject foxes to events such as mortality, or contact, each second of their life. Computer storage requirements, time constraints, and stochastic considerations all suggested using some more reasonable time interval. Many modellers of wildlife populations choose monthly or annual intervals. We chose four seasons as reasonable time intervals and as approximations of the largest time groups of similar fox behaviour and activity during a year. However, some subroutines (MORT, DISPER, INCUB, CONTAC) that were dependent on the results from other subroutines ran several times within a season for realism. MORT was run before and after dispersal. The calculation of appropriate proportions per run would allow the routine to be

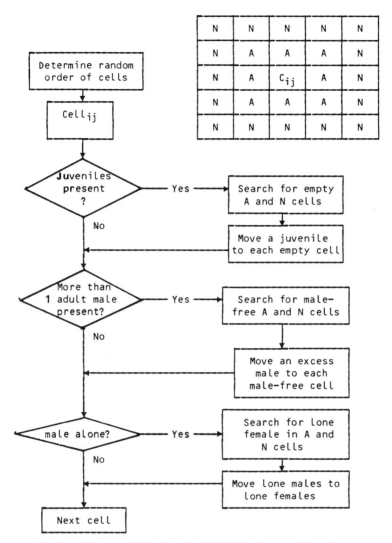

Fig. 3. A diagram of the subroutine SPACE showing operation rules.

called many times in a season until the total mortality for the entire season was obtained.

The next routine called was DISPER (Fig. 4), which simulated the dispersal behaviour of foxes in Ontario. DISPER permitted long-range movements, but also allowed the spread of rabies during movement. That was unlike SPACE, which did not allow disease spread until the subroutine CONTAC was run.

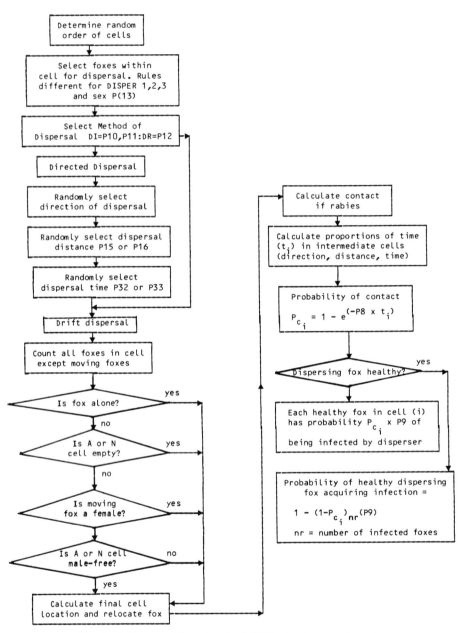

Fig. 4. A diagram of the subroutine DISPER showing operation rules.

Explanation of the spread of rabies during dispersal is in Section III,D. During field studies in Ontario, three patterns of dispersal by foxes were observed. Patterns of dispersal were named drift, exploratory, or directed (D. R. Voigt, unpublished data).

Drift dispersal (DR) occurred over short (2 days) to long (60 days) time periods. A fox gradually shifted its movements (and thus its territory) to a new location. That new location was one or two home ranges distant.

Exploratory dispersal was exhibited by foxes that oscillated between a new location and their old location. These were distinct trips between two locations 1 to 10 km apart. In some cases, those movements were fore-runners of longer trips on that vector. Longer trips were zigzag in nature and did not always show a favoured direction.

Directed dispersal was generally a longer distance and unidirectional. Straight-line distances ranged from 5 to 150 km. The distinction between exploratory dispersal and directed dispersal was not always clear, since some foxes illustrated components of both. A feature of exploratory movements was their oscillatory nature which, in relation to rabies spread, increased contact potential by increasing the total time spent in other ranges.

In order to simplify the operation of DISPER, we chose to simulate exploratory and directed dispersal by one type of dispersal called DIRECTED (DI). In DI dispersal, a fox moved in a straight line for a predetermined distance. When it arrived at its destination it explored the local available ranges (for mechanism, see DR dispersal) to find the most suitable range and settle there. The direction that a fox took in that mode of dispersal was determined by randomly choosing a number from a uniform distribution in the current version. The distribution used could have been with most of its density in certain preferred directions to simulate a particular area that was influenced by physiography, for example, mountain or lake barriers. The distance a fox travelled under DI was chosen randomly from an exponential distribution, which correlated with a distribution of dispersing foxes observed during radio-tracking studies (mean distance for females: P15; mean distance for males: P16). Although foxes probably decided on where to stop based on population factors (such as sex, age, density of nearby foxes) and habitat requirements, the exponential distribution acted as a fixed average of those dynamic processes. The use of the exponential distribution assumed that at every unit of distance the fox had a constant probability of continuing to disperse. The probabilities of DI were separate for females (P10) and males (P11).

DIRECTED assumed that a fox went directly from its origin to its destination. The travel time was calculated from observed distributions of travel times versus distances.

$$\text{For males} \qquad T = .04D - D(\text{P32}) \ln R \qquad (4)$$

$$\text{For females} \qquad T = .04D - D(\text{P33}) \ln R \qquad (5)$$

where T is the total dispersal time in days, D is total dispersal distance in km, and R is a random number from 0 to 1. The program calculated, from geometrical principles, the length of the path of the fox in each of the ranges it passed through. It then calculated the amount of time the fox was in each range. Time spent in a range was proportional to the length of the path in the range and the total time of dispersal

$$t_i = (d_i/D) \times T \tag{6}$$

where t_i is time in range i, d_i is length of path in range i. Those times were then used to determine the probability of contact between the dispersing fox and other foxes in the range (see Section III,D). Zigzag routes observed by exploratory type dispersing foxes in Ontario were mimicked, partially at least, since the travel distribution included those data. All DI dispersal foxes were subjected to drift dispersal after their relocation to assist in locating them in a suitable cell.

Drift dispersal (DR) was similar to SPACE except that it applied only to juvenile foxes in the fall and winter. The drift dispersal fox did not travel very far since it assessed neighboring range (A and N ranges) to see if any range was more desirable (Fig. 4). The rules were similar to those used in SPACE.

The travel time for drift dispersal was determined from Equation (7), which was developed from the observed distribution of travel times by drift dispersing foxes in Ontario.

$$T = -(P34)\ln R \tag{7}$$

The amount of time spent in each neighboring cell was proportional to the total time and whether the cell was adjacent or next adjacent (A or N). Those times were used to determine the probability of contact.

Although the study area was bounded, it was not closed. We permitted ingress and egress during operation of DISPER. A number of foxes left the simulation area because of the distance of their dispersal. An option allowed the user to specify the number of foxes to enter the study area. The number entering was expressed as a proportion (P14) of the number of directed dispersals leaving and could be smaller, equal, or greater to test effects of ingressing healthy and/or rabid foxes. The direction, length of travel, point of entry, sex, age, and disease states of those foxes could be varied to test different modelling situations. Once the characteristics of the ingressing fox were determined, the dispersal of that fox proceeded as for foxes within the study area. Thus, the model allowed for the provision of rabies entry and the model population could be exposed to 'external' effects. In this version, ingressing foxes were given a disease state based on the average disease state of the model fox population after 10 years. Thus, during operation with rabies, P17 was 0.85, P18 was 0.90, and P19 was 0.90. That was equivalent to ingressing foxes being 85% in a healthy state, 10% in a incubative state, and 5% in a rabies infective state on average.

D. OPERATION WITH RABIES

In RABIES mode, the CONTAC and INCUB subroutines were used to model the effects of rabies in an Ontario fox population. That differed from the RABIES-FREE mode, which was a simple birth–death population model with spatial components effected through SPACE and DISPER. In the RABIES-FREE mode, we were not concerned with fox-to-fox contact or the disease state of foxes.

The subroutine for rabies incubation (INCUB) of infected foxes operated three times each season. That allowed an equivalent to monthly up-dating of the disease state of each fox. Since the incubation period for most foxes is less than 1 month (Sikes, 1962), monthly operation was a solution to a continuous event in a discrete-time model. Each fox that became infected entered disease state 4 (rabid incubating). Each fox was then randomly chosen, according to an exponential distribution (probability = P29), to advance from state 4 to state 2 (rabid infective): That exponential distribution fits data of Sikes (1962) and K. F. Lawson (unpublished data). Thus, in the version of the model described here, we did not implement state 3 in incubation. Other versions with different distributions could use state 3.

CONTAC determined disease spread and was designed on the basis of seasonally variable rules (Fig. 5). Those rules were based on social and spatial behavior of foxes. Ranges were processed in random order and their A and N ranges determined (NEIGH). CONTAC was operated after each INCUB to allow for disease spread after disease state changes. The values for parameters P1, P2, P3, and P4 (Table I) were reduced whenever CONTAC operated more than once per season by calculating new probabilities

$$P' = 1 - (1 - P)^{1/x} \tag{8}$$

where x is the number of operations per season. The seasonal totals remained the same.

Spring rules: Because of the close contact within a family during the spring, rules were simple. If any adult became infective, all foxes in its range were infected.

Summer rules: In summer, some contact between juveniles in neighbouring ranges was allowed. For each juvenile with infective rabies, juveniles in adjacent ranges were exposed to a risk (P1) of infection.

Fall rules: See *All-seasons rules.*

Winter rules: The winter rules simulated the contact effects of mating activities of foxes. If there was a male fox with infective rabies it was liable to spread the disease to all females in neighboring ranges. Thus, for each infective male, all the females in adjacent ranges were exposed to a risk (P4) of infection. P4 was given a value 1.5 times as large as P1 and P2.

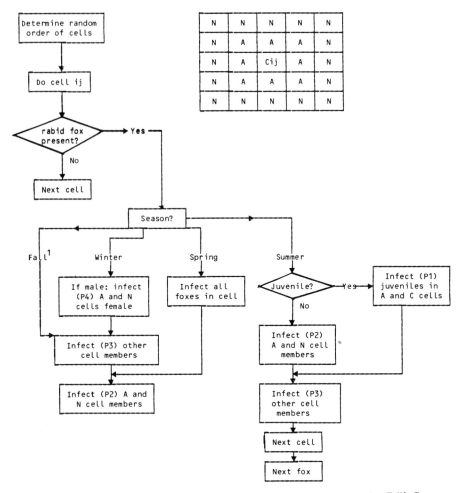

Fig. 5. A diagram of the subroutine CONTAC, showing seasonal operation rules. Fall[1]: Contact by juveniles also occurs during DISPER.

All-seasons rules: In all seasons adults were allowed to contact neighboring adults. The rules were therefore the same as for neighbouring juveniles in the summer except that the probability of passing the infection was P2.

All-seasons except spring: In all seasons, foxes could infect other foxes within a range at some probability. In spring, this probability was 1. For the other seasons, all foxes within the range were exposed to a risk of infection (P3) if an infective fox was present. P3 was given a value twice as large as P1 and P2.

Contact during Dispersal: Two types of contact by foxes occurred during DISPER: (1) a *healthy* fox that travelled through a range during DISPER could contract rabies if it travelled through a range with a rabid fox, that is, a fox in the infective stage; (2) a *rabid* infective fox that travelled through a range during DISPER could transmit rabies if it 'met' a healthy fox.

If the dispersing fox was healthy, then the program calculated the probability of it acquiring infection in each of the ranges it passed through. For each range, the number of infective foxes was counted (nr). The probability of meeting any fox was based on the assumption that foxes were moving randomly within the range, and the probability of contact was constant for any time t_i. That probability was

$$P_{c_i} = 1 - e^{(-P8 \times t_i)} \tag{9}$$

which goes from zero probability for very short times to almost certainty for very long times. The constant P8 was a parameter of the model. The probability of the fox being infected was

$$\left[1 - (1 - P_{c_i})^{nr} \right] \times P9 \tag{10}$$

where P9 was the probability of infection given a single contact. P9 was a parameter of the model, but Equation (10) was derived from probability theory.

If the dispersing was infective, then it could transmit the disease to healthy, non-vaccinated foxes. The probability of contact P_{c_i} was calculated as in Equation (9). The probability of transmittal was $P_{c_i} \times P9$ per fox, but that was applied to each healthy fox separately in order to determine which were infected.

E. OPERATION WITH VACCINATION

During VACCINE mode the model operated as during rabies mode except for the seasonal option of vaccination. V(1–8) in CONSTANT (Table I) specified the characteristics of vaccination. Although delivery of oral vaccines is most likely during FALL (Johnston and Voigt, 1982), we allowed any season to be specified. The vaccination rate was defined as the immunization rate of the vaccine times the rate of bait acceptance by foxes. In order to simulate control sub-areas and barrier effects, vaccination could be applied to any range or group of ranges. Ranges were specified according to their row and column designation. In the results described here, the entire study area was vaccinated. Foxes were subjected to a chance of vaccination based on desired vaccination rate. Juveniles were born rabies susceptible, even if their mother was vaccinated.

IV. Sensitivity Testing Process

The Ontario rabies simulation model had a large number of parameters, but the accuracy and precision of their values varied considerably. For example, the distribution of litter sizes of Ontario foxes in the enzootic area was known quite accurately, but the probability that a dispersing fox transmitted rabies to other foxes as it passed through territories was very difficult to estimate. Similarly, estimates of mortalities by age and sex were accurate for only some seasons. In designing the model, considerable attention was paid to the social and spatial behaviours of foxes. We could only hypothesize which behaviours were most important and how sensitive they were to particular parameter values. Those uncertainties are common to many models, and an important goal of building any model is gaining experience with its sensitivity to parameters. That is done by deliberately varying parameters in different runs of the model to determine their effects on output. The general procedure, called *sensitivity testing*, determines which parameters may be most important to know accurately. If there are good estimates available for those parameters, then confidence in the model increases if model output matches reality. If there are not good estimates for those parameters, then it focusses attention on the need for better biological information in order to understand better the inherent biological mechanisms. It is important to note that even simple models have as many parameters as those listed in Table I, but values or effects are either assumed or considered to be negligible (see Chapter 5, this volume).

A large number of parameters and the possibility of interactions between those parameters requires simulation experiments to be designed carefully. A factorial experiment is one in which all the different combinations of variable values are used. Factorial experiments are ideal since they give high precision for the estimates and allow for estimates of interactions among variables. An interaction between variables has a precise technical meaning. Consider two variables A and B. The AB interaction is the change in the effect of A for the different levels of B. Thus, if A has a large effect at one level of B and a small effect at another level of B, there is said to be an AB interaction. The idea of interaction can be extended to many factors. Consider three variables A, B, and C. If the AB interaction is large at one level of C and small at another, then there is an ABC interaction. It is easy to show that these definitions (interactions) are symmetrical in the variables. That is, if A interacts with B, then B interacts with A, and both interactions have the same value. Similarly, if AB interacts with C, then AC interacts with B, and BC interacts with A. Consequently, all have the same interaction value.

Two-level factorial experiments are desirable in screening experiments because of their high precision and ability to detect interaction. A two-level factorial experiment in n variables comprises all possible combinations of the two levels of each variable and requires 2^n runs (as in Chapter 7, this volume). If n is a number such as 30 then the number of runs is astronomical and clearly impractical. (The current version of the model has 34 parameters and would require 17,179,869,000 runs!). The full factorial experiment allows for the estimation of all possible interactions, that is all the 2-way, 3-way, . . . , up to n-way interactions. Information on all those interactions is not necessary. It is extremely difficult to interpret high order interactions and in mathematical terms they tend to be unimportant. Also, if there were 30 variables, it is extremely unlikely that all 30 will have effects. It is probable that only a very few will have major effects and those variables which do not have effects will also not have interactions. It is possible to construct fractionated versions of the full factorial designs, which have the following desirable properties. If only a small subset of the variables have effects and the variables which do not have effects are ignored then the resulting design is a complete factorial in the small subset of variables. That would be true for any small subset. Thus, it would be possible to study 30 variables in 16 runs (in 2^4 runs) if four variables had effects. If more than four variables had effects, the experiment might be difficult to interpret, since some main effects might be confounded with some interactions. In that case, the design could be augmented by a further 16 runs, which could be set up so as to clear all main effects from contamination with two-way interactions.

The sensitivity testing of our simulation model used fractional factorial designs (Box *et al.*, 1978). Sensitivity testing is an ongoing procedure in a model of this kind and proceeds in stages. As a first stage, it was decided to test some of the parameters which were in greatest doubt. Initially, the model was tested in all three modes (RABIES-FREE, RABIES, VACCINE) to determine the effects of selected parameters.

Those selected parameters were the probability of a rabid fox infecting other foxes if contacted (P1, P2, P3, and P4), the probability of getting or giving infection if contact is made in DISPER (P9), and the control point for fox density (P31). However, the total number of parameters tested was only four since the first three parameters (P1, P2, P3) were varied as a group in the proportions 1 : 1 : 2, respectively. They represented similar phenomenon, and it was believed that the relative magnitudes were understood although the actual levels were in doubt. P4 was specifically related to mating activities of male foxes. P9 was a poorly understood parameter that included various aspects of fox behaviour, and since it was related to other parameters, (P8, P32 and P33), it was varied over a wide range. The control point for fox density (P31) was varied because it was believed to be of fundamental importance as a carrying capacity determinant and it would interact with many other variables.

The six dependent or test variables (responses) that were measured were the total population just after REPROD in spring, total non-rabies mortality per year, the total rabies mortality per year, the total number of infections transmitted in CONTAC, the total number of infections transmitted in DISPER, and the total number of infections transmitted by INGRES. A simulation of 25 years in RABIES mode was made, but the first 5 years were excluded from analysis to avoid transient and start up effects. The averages, standard deviations, and correlations between test variables were recorded. The design was a 2^4 factorial expression, that is, each factor (parameter) had two levels and all 16 combinations of the factors were run. In a 2^4 level experiment, it is possible to estimate four main effects, 6 two-factor interactions, 4 three-factor interactions, and 1 three-factor interaction. These interactions were recorded for each response and examined. The high and low values for each factor are shown in Table II.

In addition, four simulations of 25 years each were made in RABIES-FREE mode. The parameter for control density (P31) was given the values 5, 10, 20, and 30 (equivalent to 0.5, 1, 2, and 3 foxes per km²). Four further simulations of 55 years each were made for an initial investigation of model behaviour in VACCINE mode. Those simulations were for a 1000 km² area and comprised 25 years of RABIES mode, followed by 25 years of VACCINE mode, followed by 5 years of RABIES mode. Two levels of vaccination (50 and 70%) and two levels of P31 (10 and 20) were tested at low level P1, P2, P3 and P4, and high level P9. Foxes throughout the entire study area were subjected to a chance of vaccination.

A standard analysis of variance using the SAS package (Statistical Analysis System) was used.

V. Results

A. FOX POPULATIONS AND RABIES

The results from the initial 25-year simulations in the RABIES-FREE mode demonstrated the effect of the control point density (P31) and the mortality adjuster (P30). Control point densities should not be misconstrued with any gassing, hunting, or trapping control figures (HIPD) but they are the densities at which the environment strongly affects populations. A control point density of 5 foxes was equivalent to a carrying capacity of 0.5 foxes per km² or a population of 500 foxes in the 1000-km² study area. At that control point, the total population from year 6 to 25 averaged 393 ± 51 (1 SD) and mortality averaged 79% (Table III). The total population ranged from 71 to 99% of the carrying capacity

TABLE II

Values of the Response Parameters Assessed in the First Sensitivity Analysis of the Ontario Rabies Simulation Model

Level	Factor (parameter)					
	P1	P2	P3	P4	P9	P31
Low	0.05	0.05	0.10	0.225	0.25	10
High	0.15	0.15	0.3	0.75	0.75	20

TABLE III

Annual Population and Deaths of Foxes in a 20-Year RABIES-FREE Simulation at Control Point Densities of 5, 10 and 20, and 1000 km² Study Area[a]

Control point density	Annual population maximum	Annual number of deaths
5	393 ± 51 (284–493)	311 ± 53 (205–418)
10	816 ± 97 (663–987)	614 ± 107 (476–806)
20	1149 ± 1220 (1–3243)	908 ± 1276

[a] Values are the mean ± 1 SD, and the range is in parentheses

population level with an average of 79%. Results from the simulation with a control point density of 10 were similar in that the annual population ranged from 69 to 99% of the carrying capacity population level with an average of 82%. In that simulation the annual mortality of foxes averaged 75% and fluctuations were moderate ($\bar{x} = 816 \pm 97$), with irregular oscillations (Fig. 6).

A control point density of 20, equivalent to a carrying capacity population

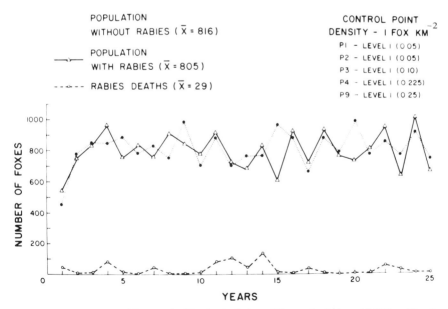

Fig. 6. The number of foxes and rabies deaths during a 25-year simulation with P31 = 10 and contact parameters P1, P2, P3, P4, and P9 at a low level.

level of 2000 or 20 foxes per territory, demonstrated large fluctuations. The total population varied from one (in year 20) to 3243 ($\bar{x}$ = 1149 ± 1220). The extremes in density caused variable mortality that averaged 79% but ranged from 0 to over 99%. Furthermore, fluctuations became more extreme with time. The population only reached 57% of the carrying capacity population level on average but in individual years it ranged from 0 to 162%. Thus, in the absence of rabies, but with high reproductive parameters and a high carrying capacity, the mortality adjustment needs to be limited.

The results from a 25-year simulation in RABIES mode were designed to show interactions between the control point density and rabies contact parameters. A simulation with a control point density of 10 (one fox km^{-2}) and low level contact parameters (P1, P2, P3, P4, and P9) showed little difference from the RABIES-FREE mode results at the same control-point density. Fluctuations were irregular and population levels (Fig. 6) were similar (805 ± 112). Rabies incidence was low (annual $\bar{x}$ = 29 deaths), and in several years, extinction of rabies would have occurred if it had not been reintroduced by ingressing foxes. Annual non-rabies mortality averaged 73% and the maximum annual number of foxes ranged from 60 to 100% of the carrying capacity population level.

A simulation with an increase in the value of contact parameters with no change in the control point density showed 3- to 4-year cycles in rabies incidence and total fox population (Fig. 7). The mean population level ($\bar{x}$ = 461 ± 151) was less than one-half of the carrying capacity level (1000), and the non-rabies

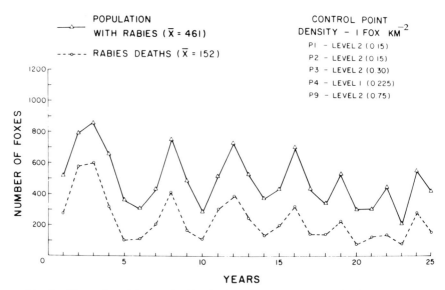

Fig. 7. The number of foxes and rabies deaths during a 25-year simulation in RABIES mode with P31 = 10 and contact parameters P1, P2, P3, and P9 at a high level.

mortality rate was only 43%, although it ranged from 25 to 54%. The rabies mortality averaged 33% and ranged from 12 to 55%. The number of cases of rabies per year ranged from 31 to 267.

A simulation with an increase in the control point density (two foxes km^{-2}) but lower value contact parameters also showed 3- to 4-year cycles in rabies incidence and total fox population (Fig. 8). However, as an earlier simulation with a control point density of 20 had shown, fluctuations were extreme. The total population averaged 1013 ± 594 but ranged from 201 to 2227. Those values are 10 and 111%, respectively, of carrying capacity levels. Unlike the RABIES-FREE mode simulation with P31 = 20, this RABIES mode simulation showed less violent oscillation and 3- to 4-year periodicity in the fox population and rabies incidence. Rabies deaths averaged 470 ± 381, and non-rabies deaths averaged 291 ± 338. The interaction between rabies and non-rabies mortality smoothed the response by the fox population in comparison to the RABIES-FREE mode simulation. Thus, rabies mortalities varied from 2 to 65% ($\bar{x} = 46$)

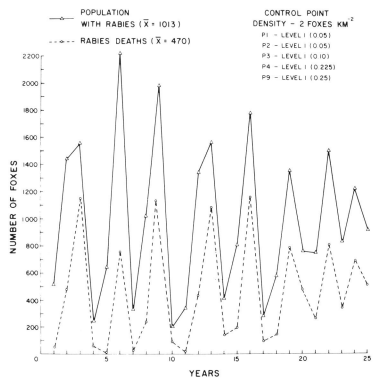

Fig. 8. The number of foxes and rabies deaths during a 25-year simulation in RABIES mode with P31 = 20 and contact parameters P1, P2, P3, P4, and P9 at a low level.

and non-rabies mortality from 5 to 62% ($\bar{x} = 29$). Annual mortalities due to both causes varied from 9 to 96%, which is more realistic than 0 to 99% shown in RABIES-FREE mode. Both simulations do suggest, however, that minimum and maximum non-rabies mortalities should have minimum and maximum values, and adjustments should be made during each season of the year when carrying capacity values are high.

The 55-year simulations with a control density of 1 fox per km² produced equal populations and rabies deaths during the first 25 years since starting conditions were the same (Fig. 9). An annual vaccination rate of 50% during the next

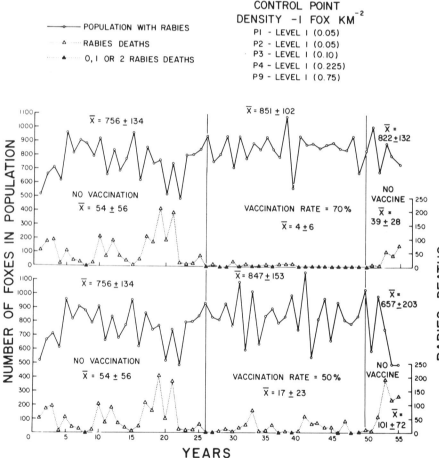

Fig. 9. The number of foxes and rabies deaths during a 55-year simulation with 25 years of RABIES mode, 25 years of VACCINE mode, and 5 years of RABIES mode. Results with vaccination rates of 50 and 70% are shown. P31, P1, P3, and P4 were at a low level. The ▲ indicates 0, 1, or 2 rabies deaths.

25 years increased that population from a mean of 756 ± 134 to 847 ± 102. The average densities during VACCINE mode were almost the same, but the variance was less at the high vaccination rate. The lower vaccination rate population exceeded the carrying capacity in 4 years, however. A more dramatic response was seen in the annual number of rabies deaths after vaccination. At the 50% rate, those deaths dropped in number from an average of 54 ± 56 to only 17 ± 23. In 7 years during vaccination, rabies deaths dropped to 0, 1, or 2 cases, but the ingress of rabid or incubating foxes in many years initiated further epizootics. Prior to vaccination, rabies deaths had dropped to 1 case in only 1 year. The 70% vaccination rate was even more effective in controlling rabies. Annual rabies deaths dropped to 4 ± 6 foxes and in 18 of the 25 years there were only 0, 1, or 2 cases of rabies (Fig. 9). However, the persistent ingress of rabid foxes meant that rabies outbreaks were always possible, and in both simulations, an epizootic started within 2–3 years of ceasing vaccination.

Simulation for 55 years with a control point of two foxes per km^2 showed comparable results in that a 70% vaccination rate was far more effective (rabies deaths $\bar{x}$ = 95) in controlling rabies than a 50% vaccination (rabies deaths $\bar{x}$ = 287). Before vaccination, the rabies deaths averaged 448 foxes annually. However, at the much higher densities and more cyclic conditions, control was much less effective than that shown in Fig. 9. Populations increased before vaccination from a mean of 866 foxes to a mean of 1321 and 1446 foxes after vaccination rates of 70 and 50%, respectively. Since populations built up quickly after rabies deaths declined, the ingress of rabid foxes initiated severe epizootics. Epizootics were also more severe within 2 years after vaccination ceased. The peak populations in vaccine mode were frequently over carrying capacity levels and before non-rabies mortality increased in response, rabies outbreaks ensued. These findings are similar to the compensatory relationships observed between rabies deaths and fur harvest deaths observed in parts of Ontario by Voigt and Tinline (1982).

In the simulations described above, clusters of rabies cases were usually localized during the initial rabies epizootic. Those outbreaks spread in subsequent seasons in a pattern similar to that shown in Fig. 10. Rabies incidence varied seasonally with lows in the summer and peaks from the fall through spring as observed in Ontario.

B. ANALYSIS OF VARIANCE

The analysis of variance of the RABIES mode simulation results showed that, in general, the interactions terms were smaller than the main effects. Thus, data were re-analyzed by extracting only main effects and putting all interactions into the error term. This procedure was followed in order to simplify the presentations of results despite the fact that there were significant interactions for some variables. Those significant interactions are discussed later.

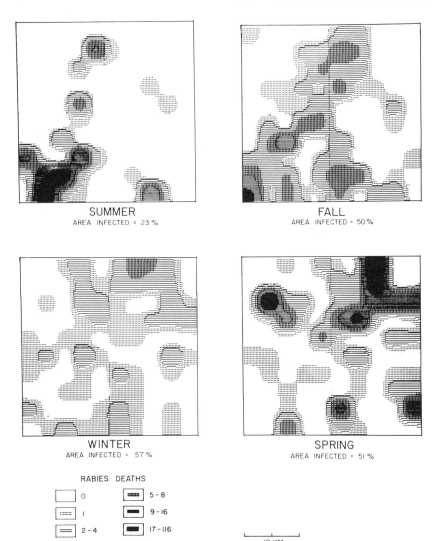

Fig. 10.   The spatial distribution of rabid foxes during four seasons of a year from a simulation of 1000 km².

The significance probabilities of each of the four main effects for each response are summarized in Table IV. The results appear surprising initially. The effect of P31, which supposedly directly controls the population level by simulating carrying capacity had no significant effect on the population level. However it did have a highly significant effect on the other test variables. The effects of P1 and P4, which relate to the probabilities of transmitting infection, had few effects

TABLE IV

Significance Probabilities of the Main Effects on the Response Variables Based on the Yearly Averages from the First Sensitivity Analysis[a]

Factor	Test variable					
Main effect parameter	Total population	Non-rabies deaths	Rabies deaths	CONTAC infections	DISPER infections	INGRES infections
P1	<0.000	0.002	0.264	0.498	0.041	0.005
P4	0.003	0.43	0.845	0.576	0.466	0.478
P9	<0.000	0.01	0.839	0.477	0.005	<0.000
P31	0.110	<0.000	<0.000	<0.000	0.001	0.001

[a] Values for P1 include P1, P2, and P3

on the number of infections or rabies deaths but had very significant effects on the total population (recall that P1, P2, and P3 are combined under P1 since all were varied as a group). P9 had an effect on DISPER infections and INGRES infections as expected, but no direct effect on rabies deaths.

The factor P4 had the least number of significant effects. The effect on P4 on total population was consistent at all levels of the other factors, and its effect was to reduce the total population by 105 foxes on average. Similarly, for non-rabies deaths, the effect was to decrease the number of deaths by 81 on average. The effect on the other response variables was not significant though in each case the measured effect, though small, was opposite to what one might expect. Thus, the number of rabies deaths, CONTAC infections and DISPER infections were reduced. This illustrates the counter-intuitive nature of the results which showed that the number of non-rabies deaths and total population were reduced at the same time. Presumably, P4 did increase the rate of infection though the effect was not measurably significant. That put increased pressure on the population and reduced it, possibly because more females at the reproductive stage were infected. The reduced population then had lower mortality, partly because there were fewer foxes to die and partly because lower densities resulted in lower mortalities.

The values of test variables at each level and each combination of factors is depicted by the vertices of cubes in Fig. 11. The factor P4 is left out of this diagram for simplification and consequently values for test variables are average values from simulations of both levels of P4. The effect of each factor, with the others constant, can be determined by moving from one vertex to another along the edge of the cube. Viewing a set of four edges gives four estimates of the effect of the factor at the different levels of the other factors. Thus for example in the total population cube, the effect of P31 at the low level of the other factors is to increase the population from 797 to 913 or by 116. At the other levels of the

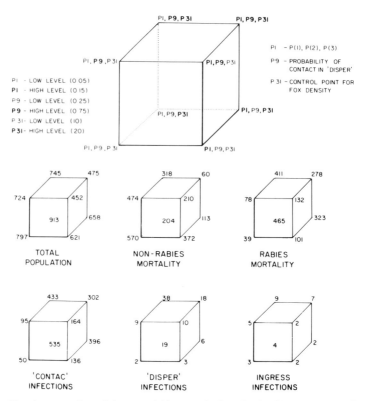

Fig. 11. Average values of six test variables at each of two levels of three parameters from a 20-year simulation run.

factors, the increases are 21, 37, and 23 for an average increase of 49. The analysis of variance indicates that an increase of that magnitude could have occurred by chance. The rabies deaths and CONTAC infections responses showed a strong interaction between P31 and P1 and P9. Thus, at the low level of P31, P1 caused an increase in the number of deaths and infections whereas at the high level of P31 those were reduced. The same was true to a lesser extent for P9. As a consequence, no further reductions of the data by averaging were justified as they were best described as in Fig. 9. The same was true for DISPER infections where P9 had a strong effect each time, but the combinations of low P1 and high P31 caused a larger response.

The average effect of the three factors on the test variables is shown in Table V. The use of averages was reasonable for those cases where the interactions between the factors were small such as the responses for total population and non-rabies deaths. A number of interesting features emerged from the data in Table V. The most obvious was that P31 had such a small influence on total

TABLE V

The Average Effects of Three Factors (Response Parameters: P1, P9, P31) on the Test Variables

Factor and level	Average value of test variables					
	Total population	Non-rabies deaths	Rabies deaths	CONTAC infections	DISPER infections	INGRES infections
P1 Low	795	345	248	278	17	5
P1 High	552	204	208	249	9	3
Difference	−243	−141	−40	−29	−8	−2
P9 Low	747	330	232	279	8	3
P9 High	590	219	225	249	19	0
Difference	−148	−111	−7	−30	11	3
P31 Low	649	406	87	111	6	3
P31 High	698	143	369	417	20	6
Difference	49	−263	282	306	14	3

population. Even more dramatic was how mortality shifted from non-rabies deaths to rabies deaths while the total population was relatively unchanged. P1 had a large effect which reduced both population and total mortality (similiar to P4, discussed previously). P9 had a large effect on populations, reducing it on average by 148, but a small effect on DISPER infections, increasing those on average by 11. It was interesting that the total number of infections transmitted by DISPER was small, on average only 19 at the high level of P9 and yet the effect on the population was large. Infections that occurred in the fall and winter may have had a disproportionate effect on breeding.

VI. Discussion and Conclusions

A. VALIDATING THE MODEL

It is always difficult to prove that a model is a valid approximation of reality. The usual strategy is to identify factors that are believed to be important characteristics of the real situation and to check that the model can reproduce them. In our fox rabies model, the temporal and spatial characteristics of rabies in foxes were of major interest, e.g. did the model reproduce the cyclical variations in rabies incidence and the rates of spread that were observed in the field? One difficulty was that the real world has stochastic elements, evolutionary strategies, genetic variation, and a changing environment. The characteristics of any given situation represent only a single realization of a large number of possible situations. Given a one-sample estimate of reality, it is impossible to estimate the variance to be used to test whether model output is a member of the real world populations. However, the situation can usefully be viewed in reverse. Since a stochastic model is a closed (completely defined) system, the distribution (variance) of any of its output characteristics can be established. Thus, tests can be conducted to see if the real world sample can be considered to be a member of the population distributions produced by the model. The difficulty with that strategy is that several models with very different structures and assumptions may produce similiar results. The problem of an 'under-identified model' (Harvey, 1969) has no easy solution. Our goals were (1) to ensure that each component of the model had biological significance based on available field evidence, (2) to compare as many real world situations as possible with model results, and (3) to concentrate on validating the output characteristics of the model that could be directly related to field evidence.

Validating a model is an ongoing procedure. Final validation can only be shown after prediction of all events in advance. Some events may, however, be accurately predicted when others are not. After the initial simulations described in this paper, we assessed the validity of the model by using three methods.

First, we used birth and death rates derived from Ontario studies of foxes to observe whether our model produced a 'steady state' fox population (Murray, 1979) with a realistic juvenile:adult ratio, in the absence of rabies. That was shown in the rabies-free simulation (Fig. 6) and in the high mortality biased to juveniles.

Secondly, we observed whether the model with rabies showed the 3- to 4-year cycling in rabies incidence and long-term maintenance in areas of several townships (600–1000 km²). The 3- to 4-year cycling (Figs. 7 and 8) occurred frequently in our simulations. Autocorrelations showed significant probabilities at 3 and 4 years consistently when control densities were high (two foxes per km²). However, maintenance of rabies in our study area usually required at least a small proportion of ingressing foxes to be rabid.

Finally, we observed whether the distribution of rabies deaths demonstrated the spatial clustering of epizootics and rate of advance across areas typical of the situation in Ontario. Figure 10 demonstrates that the model produced such patterns and that rabies moved through the study area in 1 year.

The temporal and spatial patterns of rabies incidence produced by the model were complex and require further investigation. However, they do compare favourably with the variation in patterns observed under various levels of mortality pressure from trapping and hunting (Voigt and Tinline, 1982).

B. FUTURE DEVELOPMENT

It is impossible to claim yet that the Ontario model accurately mirrors a reality, and care must be taken in interpreting results from the model. Nonetheless, it is true that a number of plausible procedures have been put together, and at the very best, the true state of reality must be more complex than the model. The procedures that have been put together produce often surprising results showing the complex interactions taking place. Those results stimulate our imagination and hopefully further our knowledge of what is happening in nature. A further evident feature is that a model of this type will never be completed and will continue to be developed as it continues to be used. Our results illustrate the nature of model building and although conclusions are tentative they do point to the importance of the factors such as contact probabilities (P1, P9) and density control (P31). It is clear that efforts should be made to obtain figures as realistic as possible. The results also show that a variety of responses are possible with the same model structure but with changes in selected parameters.

Our experience to date with the model suggests several changes that would be desirable for greater accuracy or for extreme situations. For example, it would appear that at some levels the effect of P31 (control point density parameter) on non-rabies deaths was too strong. The results indicate that the controller does indeed work but further tuning would be beneficial for extreme cases. The value of P31 is in a sense the carrying capacity of the area, but populations rarely reached it. The mortalities of foxes fluctuated too widely to be considered reasonable. We therefore propose to put a lower limit on mortalities such that the expectation of survival of a fox in a low density area with a high carrying capacity would not exceed 4 years. The average age of a fox in a rabies-free population in Ontario was estimated by assuming the maximum age of a fox would be 10 years, the mortality of juveniles was 65%, and the shape of the survivorship curve was exponential. Since high levels of mortality can cause extinction of populations, we propose to effect the controller several times during the year rather than applying high mortalities throughout the whole year (based on initial figures) even when populations have already been considerably reduced. Similarly, there should be an upper limit on mortality at some rate less than 100%. Such limitations and adjustments that assist in the fine tuning of a model are legitimate 'a posteriori' changes if they have credible basis. They are, perhaps, more important in stochastic models where random chance could produce unrealistic extremes.

It was obvious from our simulations that in a 1000-km^2 area, ingressing rabid foxes were necessary to maintain rabies. Because fox dispersal distances are finite, it is reasonable to assume that the effects of ingressing foxes are negligible at some larger size of area. We believe it will be important in future research to identify the relationship between the 'size of the control area' and the threat of the reintroduction of rabies. In Ontario, that area will probably not exceed 10,000 km^2 because of water barriers unless reintroduction occurs by bats or some similar long-range carrier.

The influence of fox density on a variety of parameters should be investigated in future versions of our model. We believe that density dependent relationships with dispersal, egress, territory size, and reproduction may prove to be important effects and necessary for greater accuracy in the case of extreme situations.

In general, the population levels and temporal patterns from our simulations are very similar to levels and patterns observed in Ontario. Those values and the results of other simulations raise some intriguing possibilities about rabies spread and maintenance. In several years rabies incidence was very low or zero, but the provision for ingressing foxes of which only 5% were rabid and 10% were incubating rabies insured a subsequent epizootic. Earlier simulations with our model had shown the disappearance of rabies without some reintroduction. Although our model used ingressing, dispersing foxes to maintain rabies, the mechanism in the wild could be long-term incubation of rabies in skunks or another ingressing vector such as bats. The role of skunks in maintaining or initiating rabies outbreaks in Ontario is unknown, but in several urban areas, skunks are the major wildlife species diagnosed rabid and in the provinces, they account for over 20% of all cases annually. In the prairie provinces and states of North America, skunks maintain an enzootic in the absence of any obvious role of Red Foxes. In Europe, however, Red Foxes maintain rabies in the absence of skunks (see Macdonald and Voigt, Chapter 4, this volume). The simulation of Ontario rabies excluding skunks may be criticized if it is demonstrated that skunks are essential in the maintenance of rabies. While ingressing foxes in our model may well mimic the long-term incubation of skunks (and thus 'reintroduction' into foxes), we recognize that social behaviour, and thus contact rate between skunks, differ from foxes. Our fox model could be valid, however, if control of rabies in foxes eradicated all rabies. The matching of model output with field data may also mitigate against the need to model skunks directly, since field data on rabies incidence in foxes and population dynamics of foxes are from an environment that includes effects of both foxes and skunks.

Our model suggests the number of infections caused by 'introduced' or 'ingress' rabies is small but critical for an epizootic. Our study area of 1000 km^2 approximates units in Ontario that predictably produce 3- to 4-year peaks in rabies incidence. Those areas are adjacent to similarly sized units that may be out-of-phase but important in seeding an adjacent unit. That situation should be the topic of future simulation research.

Our results also suggest that epizootics require either a threshold population or a threshold contact level. For long-term maintenance of rabies, simple theory dictates that contact rate must be 1.0 or greater on average (May, 1983; but see Chapter 12, this volume, for discussion of spatial aspects). However, our model produced peaks of rabies outbreaks when either control densities or contact rates were high, but low levels of rabies when contact and control densities were low. That behaviour of the model and the role of dispersal suggest that the factors may be fundamental to the long-term maintenance of rabies. First, the border of the enzootic area must be large enough to allow reintroduction from outside sources.

Second, the contact rate among vectors must be high enough to perpetuate the disease on a short-term basis. The latter factor in fox epizootic areas probably would require both a high population (and carrying capacity) and an initial amount of virus sufficient to cause an epizootic. Those conditions could explain the enzootic nature of rabies in Ontario and parts of Europe as well as the anomalous lack of rabies elsewhere in regions that appear ecologically similar. Indeed, even within Ontario, peninsular areas with lower reintroduction potential have lower rabies incidence. Some recent virological studies also suggest that viral strain differences may add another level of complexity (Schneider, 1982).

Our model has produced some results similar to those from much simpler models. However, the complex and stochastic nature of our model will permit future research into the effects and interactions of many fox–rabies parameters. The actual values for parameters in different areas will depend directly on the social and spatial behaviour of the foxes and the environmental carrying capacity. We hope that investigations of those parameters, through models such as ours, will be useful in better explaining the epizootiology of fox rabies around the world.

Acknowledgements

If this model proves to be a useful simulation, it will be largely due not to our efforts as modellers, but to the team of rabies researchers with which we have worked. The Rabies Research Unit of the Ontario Ministry of Natural Resources played a key role by collecting the basic ecological data and providing the ecological basis of the model. Staff included D. H. Johnston, I. D. Watt, F. O. Matejka, P. Bachmann, B. D. Earle, R. N. Bramwell, J. B. Broadfoot, W. M. Lintack, R. Rosatte, O. C. McNeil, M. Collins, and E. Brolly (who also retyped many drafts of the manuscript). C. M. MacInnes, Wildlife Research Supervisor, provided constant encouragement as well as a great many ideas from inception onwards. Continual support for this project was provided by the Rabies Advisory Committee under the Chairmanship of Dr. A. J. Rhodes. A committee member, K. Charlton, of Agriculture Canada, also arranged for initial access to rabies incidence records which provided the epizootiological basis for much of the model. K. F. Lawson, of Connaught Laboratories, provided data on incubation periods of red foxes infected with rabies. In the latter stages of development, B. Pond, of Queen's University, provided the programming expertise and stimulation to get the job done—a special thanks. Finally, many fox and rabies biologists around the world played a perhaps unknown, but nonetheless essential, role in providing data, ideas, and synthesis. We thank all the above for their contribution but at the same time we, as authors, take full responsibility for shortcomings of the model.

References

Anderson, R. M., Jackson, H. C., May, R. M., and Smith, A. D. M. (1981). Population dynamics of fox rabies in Europe. *Nature (London)* **289,** 765–770.
Bacon, P. J., and Macdonald, D. W. (1980). To control rabies; Vaccinate foxes. *New Sci.* **87,** 640–645.

Bartlett, M. S. (1973). Equations and models of population change. "The Mathematical Theory of the Dynamics of Biological Populations" (M. S. Bartlett and R. W. Hiorns, eds.), pp. 5–21. Academic Press, London.

Bogel, K., Arata, A. A., Moggle, H., and Knorpp, F. (1974). Recovery of reduced fox populations in rabies control. *Zentralbl. Veterinaer med., Reihe B* pp. 401–412.

Bogel, K., Moegle, H., Knorpp, F., Arata, A., Dietz, K., and Diethelm, P. (1976). Characteristics of the spread of a wildlife rabies epidemic in Europe. *Bull. W.H.O.* **54**, 433–447.

Bogel, K., Steck, F., Krocza, W., and Andral, L. (1981). Assessment of fox control in areas of wildlife rabies. Bull. W.H.O. **59**, 269–279.

Box, G., Hunter, W., and Hunter, J. (1978). "Statistics for Experimenters: An Introduction to Design, Data Analysis and Model Building." Wiley, New York.

David, M. M., and Andral, L. (1982). Modelling of spatial evolution and dynamics of a population of healthy and rabies infected foxes. *Comp. Immunol. Microbiol. Infect. Dis.* **5**(1–3), 351–358.

David, M. M., Andral, L., and Artois, M. (1982). Computer simulation model of the epi-enzootic disease of vulpine rabies. *Ecol. Model.* **15**, 107–125.

Englund, J. (1970). Some aspects of reproduction and mortality rates in Swedish foxes (*Vulpes vulpes*), 1961–63 and 1966–1969. *Viltrevy* **8**, 1–82.

Grant, G. C. (1977). A simulation study of a red fox population with rabies. M.A. Thesis, Queen's University, Kingston, Ontario.

Harvey, D. (1969). "Explanation in Geography." Arnold, London.

Johnston, D. H., and Beauregard, M. (1969). Rabies epidemiology in Ontario. *Bull. Wildl. Dis. Assoc.* **15**, 357–370.

Johnston, D. H., and Voigt, D. R. (1982). A baiting system for the oral rabies vaccination of wild foxes and skunks. *Comp. Immunol. Microbiol. Infect. Dis.* **5**(1–3), 185–186.

Lloyd, H. G. (1980). "The Red Fox." Batsford, London.

Lloyd, H. G., Jenson, B., Van Haaften, J. L., Niewold, F. J., Wandeler, A., Bogel, K., and Arata, A. A. (1976). Annual turnover of fox populations in Europe. *Zentralbl. Veterinaer med., Reihe B* **23**, 580–589.

Macdonald, D. W. (1980). Social factors affecting reproduction amongst red foxes (*Vulpes vulpes* L., 1758). *In* "The Red Fox" (E. Zimen, ed.), Biogeogr. No. 18, pp. 123–175. Junk, The Hague.

Macdonald, D. W., and Bacon, P. J. (1982). Fox society, contact rate and rabies epizootiology. *Comp. Immunol. Microbiol. Infect. Dis.* **5**, 247–256.

May, R. M. (1983). Parasitic infections as regulators of animal populations. *Am. Sci.* **71**, 36–45.

Montgomery, G. G. (1974). Communication in red fox dyads: A computer simulation study. *Smithson. Contrib. Zool.* **187**, 1–30.

Muller, J. (1971). The effect of fox reduction on the occurrence of rabies. *Bull. Off. Int. Epizoot.* **75**, 763–776.

Murray, B. G., Jr. (1979). "Population Dynamics: Alternative Models." Academic Press, New York.

Parks, E. (1968). Control of rabies in wildlife in New York. *N.Y. Fish Game J.* **15**, 98–111.

Preston, E. M. (1973). Computer simulated dynamics of a rabies-controlled fox population. *J. Wildl. Manage.* **37**, 501–12.

Schneider, L. G. (1982). Antigenic variants of rabies virus. *Comp. Immunol. Microbiol. Infect. Dis.* **5**(1–3), 101–107.

Sikes, R. K. (1962). Pathogenesis of rabies in wildlife. 1. Comparative effect of varying doses of rabies virus inoculated into foxes and skunks. *Am. J. Vet. Res.* **23**, 1041–1047.

Steck, F., Wandeler, A., Bichsel, P., Capt. S., and Schneider, L. (1982a). Oral immunisation of foxes against rabies. A field study. *Zentralbl. Veterinaer med., Reihe B* **29**, 372–396.

Steck, F., Wandler, A., Bischel, P., Capt, S., Hafliger, U., and Schneider, L. (1982b). Oral immunization of foxes against rabies. *Comp. Immunol. Microbiol. Infect. Dis.* **5**(1–3), 165–171.

Tabel, H., Corner, A. H., Webster, W. A., and Casey, C. A. (1974). History and epizootiology of rabies in Canada. *Can. Vet. J.* **15**, 271–281.

Tinline, R. L. (1981). The geography of rabies in Canada. Presented at the annual meeting of the Canadian Geographical Association, Corner Brook, Newfoundland.

Tinline, R. L., and Pond, B. (1976). Rabies incidence in Ontario: A Grey County example. *"Queen's" Geogr.* **3**(2), 1–18.

Tinline, R. L., Voigt, D. R., and Broekhoven, L. H. (1982). Evaluating tactics for the control of wildlife rabies in Ontario. *Proc. Int. Symp. Vet. Epidemiol. and Economics 3rd, 1982,* 581–589.

Voigt, D. R., and Earle, B. D. (1983). Avoidance of coyotes by fox families. *J. Wildl. Manage.* **47,** 852–857.

Voigt, D. R., and Macdonald, D. W. (1985). Variation in the spatial and social behaviour of the red fox, *Vulpes vulpes. Acta Zool. Fenn.* **171:** 261–265.

Voigt, D. R., and Tinline, R. R. (1982). Fox rabies and trapping: A study of disease and fur harvest interaction. *In* "43rd Midwest Wildlife Conference, Furbearer Symposium" (G. C. Sanderson, ed.), pp. 139–156. North Central Sect., Central Mountain and Plains Sect., and Kansas Chapter, Wildl. Soc., Wichita, Kansas.

Wandeler, A., Muller, J., Wachendorfer, G., Schale, W., Forster, U., and Steck, F. (1974). Rabies in wild carnivores in central Europe. III. Ecology and biology of the fox in relation to control operations. *Zentralbl. Veterinaer med., Reihe B* **21,** 765–773.

Index